OXFORD INDIA STUDIES IN CONTEMPORARY SOCIETY

SERIES EDITOR
SUJATA PATEL

OXFORD INDIA STUDIES IN CONTEMPORARY SOCIETY is a new series of interdisciplinary compilations on issues and problems shaping our lives in twenty-first century India. The Series appears at an opportune time, when the boundaries of social science disciplines are being redefined, and theories and perspectives are being critically interrogated. Using the frameworks developed by social science interdisciplinarity, this Series captures, assesses, and situates social trends in contemporary India. It affirms the necessity of analyzing issues and themes that have a direct bearing on our daily lives, and in doing so, brings fresh perspectives into play, integrating knowledge from a variety of unexplored sources in conventional social science practice in India. The Series aims to introduce to a wider audience the central importance of interdisciplinarity in contemporary social sciences. It presents novel themes of investigation and builds a fresh approach towards the longstanding debates on methodologies and methods. With its emphasis on the debates on and about 'society' rather than 'social sciences', this Series should find an audience not only among the students and scholars of conventional social sciences, but also among the students, researchers, and practitioners of fields such as law, media, environment, medicine, policy studies, and business studies.

The series editor would like to acknowledge the help of University of Hyderabad's UPE II (C1.2) grants for the support of this work.

Sujata Patel is Professor, Department of Sociology, University of Hyderabad, India.

OXFORD INDIA STUDIES IN CONTEMPORARY SOCIETY

EQUITY
AND ACCESS
HEALTH CARE STUDIES IN INDIA

edited by
Purendra Prasad
and
Amar Jesani

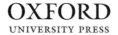

OXFORD
UNIVERSITY PRESS

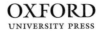
OXFORD
UNIVERSITY PRESS

Oxford University Press is a department of the University of Oxford.
It furthers the University's objective of excellence in research, scholarship,
and education by publishing worldwide. Oxford is a registered trademark of
Oxford University Press in the UK and in certain other countries.

Published in India by
Oxford University Press
2/11 Ground Floor, Ansari Road, Daryaganj, New Delhi 110 002, India

ISBN-13 (print edition): 978-0-19-948216-0
ISBN-10 (print edition): 0-19-948216-0

ISBN-13 (eBook): 978-0-19-909373-1
ISBN-10 (eBook): 0-19-909373-3

Typeset in Adobe Garamond Pro 10.5/12.5
by Tranistics Data Technologies, Kolkata 700 091
Printed in India by Replika Press Pvt. Ltd

Contents

II PHARMACEUTICALS AND EXPERIMENTATION

6. Globalization, Intellectual Property Rights, and Pharmaceuticals 127
Amit Sengupta

7. Access to Pharmaceuticals: Role of State, Industry, and Market 154
S. Srinivasan and Malini Aisola

8. Structure, Organization, and Knowledge Production of Clinical Trial Industry 178
Roger Jeffery, Gerard Porter, Salla Sariola, Amar Jesani, and Deapica Ravindran

9. Body as 'Resource' in Surrogacy and Bio-Medical Research: New Frontiers and Dilemmas 202
Sarojini Nadimpally and Vrinda Marwah

III EQUITY ISSUES IN HEALTH CARE—GENDER, CASTE, DISABILITY, AND VIOLENCE

10. Health, Disability, and Equity: Conversations among Bodies, Discourses, and Law 221
Renu Addlakha

11. Caste, Class, and Gender on the Margins of the State: An Ethnographic Study among Community Health Workers 245
Madhumita Biswal

12. Legitimizing Violence: A Narrative of Sexual Health 263
Asima Jena

13. Violence against Women as a Health Care Issue: Perceptions and Approaches 286
Sangeeta Rege and Padma Bhate-Deosthali

Tables and Figures

TABLES

FIGURES

Acknowledgements

Despite significant advances in medical knowledge and profession in India, the health care scenario continues to present exacerbated inequality, discrimination, and inaccessibility to a large majority of people. In the past few decades, health and health care as a subject has assumed lot of significance and has been much under discussion and debate. While there are numerous research studies on aspects of health care, there is no single volume that captures health equity or inequity across the sectors. Therefore, commissioning fresh set of papers and bringing together scholars from different domains—social sciences, medical profession, policymakers, health activists, legal experts, gender specialists, and others—has been a challenging task. Subsequently, thinking through and creating pathways towards an interdisciplinary field of health care studies in India was both exciting and arduous. This has been possible only because of the commitment, deep reflection, and creative ideas that contributing authors brought to this book that has taken more than three years to complete, from conceptualization to the final document, and we thank all the contributors for their cooperation and patience.

We thank Sujata Patel, the series editor, for her encouragement, discussions, ideas, and critique at different stages of this book. The David and Lucile Packard Foundation, USA, and Indian Council of Social Science Research (ICSSR), New Delhi, India, generously supported the workshop during 6–7 March 2015, upon which this volume is based, and preparation of the manuscript. This workshop provided a unique opportunity for contributors and discussants in debating and generating new ideas for this book. We are grateful to the David Lucile Packard Foundation, California, USA and ICSSR, New Delhi, India.

We express our sincere thanks to the discussants, reviewers, and subject experts at the workshop: Ghanshyam Shah, V.R. Muraleedharan, George Thomas, V. Sujatha, Veena Shatrugna, Padma Prakash, Arima Mishra, Aditi Iyer, Amita Dande, Gopal Dabade, Veena Johari, N. Sarojini, Ravi Duggal, K. Sujata Rao, R. Srivatsan, Sheela Prasad, Kalpana Kannabiran, Narendranath, Chakrapani, Aparna Rayaprol, and V. Janardhan for their insightful comments and meticulous reviews which helped improve the quality of the book immensely.

Starting from the workshop organization to the post-workshop manuscript preparation work, several research scholars from the Department of Sociology helped: Shilpa Krishna, Ch. Satish Kumar, Chandrashekar Reddy, Lalhmangaihi Chhakchhuak, Priyam Sharma, Debapriya Ganguly, Bhupati Reddy, Lalatendu Keshari Das, Abhijit Dasgupta, and Anu Gupta. We particularly thank Shilpa who took on much of the grunge work involved in producing an edited volume and handled the nitty-gritties in transitioning from a bunch of papers to a single volume.

We want to place on record the special contribution by Padma Prakash whose ideas and critique helped in substantially reshaping and enhancing the quality of the manuscript. We remain indebted to her for all the time, energy, and enthusiasm that she brought to this book. We also thank IKF Knowledge Foundation, Mumbai, India, for copyediting the manuscript.

We also would like to place on record our sincere appreciation for the work by the administrative staff of the Department of Sociology, University of Hyderabad, India—Geetha Patil, Sreedharan, Chandra Kumar, and Srinivas.

We are grateful to the team at Oxford University Press, India, for their support and cooperation.

Purendra Prasad
Amar Jesani

Abbreviations

AABY	Aam Admi Bima Yojana
ADRs	American Depository Receipts
AIDAN	All-India Drug Action Network
AIIMS	All India Institute of Medical Sciences
ANM	Auxiliary Nurse-Midwife
APL	above poverty line
ASHA	Accredited Social Health Activists
BA/BE	bio-availability and bio-equivalent
BPL	below poverty line
CEDAW	Convention on the Elimination of All Forms of Discrimination Against Women
CEHAT	Centre for Enquiry into Health and Allied Themes
CGHS	Central Government Health Scheme
CRC	Convention on the Rights of the Child
CRO	contract research organization
CrPC	Code of Criminal Procedure
CSDH	Commission on Social Determinants of Health
ESI	Employee State Insurance
ESIC	Employees State Insurance Corporation
FDI	Foreign Direct Investment
FMP	Family Medical Practitioner
FSW	female sex workers
GDP	Gross Domestic Product
GDRs	Global Depository Receipts
GNP	Gross National Product

HLEG	High-Level Expert Group
ICDS	Integrated Child Development Services
ICESCR	International Covenant on Economic, Social and Cultural Rights
IJME	Indian Journal of Medical Ethics
IRDA	Insurance Regulatory Development Authority
IRDAI	Insurance Regulatory and Development Authority of India
ITPA	Immoral Trafficking Prevention Act
LOCOST	Low Cost Standard Therapeutics
MFC	Medico Friend Circle
NACO	National AIDS Control Organisation
NAPCP	National AIDS Prevention and Control Policy
NCEUS	National Commission for Enterprises in the Unorganized Sector
NDPS Act	Narcotics Drugs and Psychotropic Substances Act
NEN	North East Network
NHS	National Health Service
NLEM	National List of Essential Medicines
NRUHM	National Rural Health and Urban Health Missions
NSDP	Net State Domestic Product
NSSO	National Sample Survey Organisation
OOP	out-of-pocket
PFHI	publicly funded health insurance
PFHI	Public Health Foundation of India
PPP	public–private partnership
PWDVA	protection of women from domestic violence law
RSBY	Rashtriya Swasthya Bima Yojana
SDGs	Sustainable Development Goals
SDP	State Domestic Product
STI	sexually transmitted infection
TRIPS	Trade-Related Aspects of Intellectual Property Rights
UAHC	universal access to health care
UDHR	Universal Declaration of Human Rights
UHC	Universal Health Care
UNCRPD	UN Convention on Rights of persons with dis-abilities
UPA	United Progressive Alliance
VAW	violence against women
WTO	World Trade Organization

Introduction: Health Inequities in India—The Larger Dimensions

Purendra Prasad

The complex relationship of the economy, society, state, and health[1] has given rise to wide-ranging enquiry, analyses, and discourses. This slew of literature has repeatedly drawn attention to enormous inequities in the health sector across caste, class, gender, and spatial locations (Balarajan, Selvaraj, and Subramanian 2011; Hammer, Aiyar, and Samji 2007). There is no denying today that a large proportion of India's population has poor or no access to basic health care. For vulnerable groups, escalating costs, against which there is no social protection, have rendered basic health care rapidly out of reach. In fact, tracking universal health coverage, Global Monitoring Report 2017 by the World Bank and the World Health Organization (WHO), revealed that at least half of the world's population cannot obtain essential health services and each year about 100 million people, including in India are being pushed into poverty because they have to pay for health care out of their own pockets. The report further states that about ten million households or a population of nearly 50 million in India are being impoverished due to health care costs (Jadhav 2017). This scenario has produced a vicious spiral: in complex, multidimensional ways the paucity of basic care is prompting a proliferation of high cost medicare in the form of super-specialty, hospital-based medical care, which pushes affordable basic care even further out of reach, contributing to a sharpening of health inequalities.[2]

This volume attempts to unravel the complex and tense narrative of why inequities in the health sector are growing and access to basic health care is worsening. What are the underlying forces that contribute to this situation? How do we analyse the yawning gap between people's desperate needs and a disoriented health care system? It also provides a narrative that explains the politics of access (distribution, utilization, outcomes) as well as the context in which health inequalities are produced. This is critical not only to our scholastic understanding of health care but to informing the development of health care policy in India at a critical time. In exploring the various elements contributing to the current status of health care, the volume opens up the possibility of constructing a new paradigm for understanding health sector as well as signalling a new field 'health care studies', drawing upon several interdisciplinary insights.

HEALTH CARE STUDIES IN INDIA

We have prominently brought into discussion the sharpening health inequalities in the last two decades to draw attention to the way globalization has influenced India's development trajectory. Health inequalities did exist in India even in 1950s and 1960s, at that time, however, there was a concerted attempt to address the issue with public investments and state interventions directed at reducing such inequalities. The state's commitment to intervene in health care was grounded in the Nehruvian development discourse which posited a government health care system in the long run leading to a progressive reduction in health inequities and ill-health. The 1970s and 1980s, however, witnessed waves of privatization resulting in rising costs, making health care increasingly inaccessible to large numbers of people (Baru 2000). This is quite evident with the recent *World Inequality Report* which states that Indian economic inequality has increased rapidly since the 1980s. This is due to profound transformations in an economy that centred on the implementation of deregulation and opening up reforms. The top 0.1 per cent of earners continued to capture more growth than all those in the bottom 50 per cent combined. This rising inequality contrasts to the 30 years following the country's Independence in 1947, when income inequality was widely reduced and the incomes of the bottom 50 per cent grew as a faster rate than the national average (Chancel and Piketty 2017). In the 1990s the liberalization of the economy unleashed large-scale changes in social, cultural, political, and economic realms. What makes globalization different at the turn of the twenty-first century is that these dimensions are affected with unprecedented intensity (Lee 1998). Therefore, it is important to analyse how these changes impacted health care. Three major trends are discernible.

First, the role of state has significantly changed in the way the state has allowed private capital to enter the health care industry. Several studies point out that India's recent history of health care is not simple state policy intervention but one of state policy governing private enterprise (Baru et al. 2010; Duggal 2000; Hodges and Rao 2016; Prasad 2015). Significantly, the guiding philosophy of state action is grounded in the commitment to make 'public–private partnership' (PPP) the cornerstone of health policy, which, no matter how it is couched, has meant that public investments are increasingly geared to securing private rather than social interests. In so doing the state ends up often being only a market activist in relation to capital accumulation (Harvey 2014).

Second, the market has had increasing influence in the development of health care, such that health care is no longer protected from its vagaries in any sector—pharmaceutical, medical device, medical education, and provisioning aspects. The most evident result of this trend has been the corporatization of health care which is rooted in capital's logic of accumulation and profit maximization. The influence of the market is also evident in the public sector, in its driving principle of profit maximization over people's benefit.

Third, individual patients have been transformed into consumers under medical neo-liberalism. Unlike patients, consumers seeking health care are made to bear the responsibility for the choices they make or fail to make regarding health. Fisher (2007) points out that patients as consumers have embraced the neo-liberal logic of health care so that they too see illness in reductionist terms and seek pharmaceuticals as targeted magic bullets.

Given the above trends, in which health care is fragmented and broken up into different areas of experimentation and intervention under the influence of market forces, institutions have undergone significant change with the active support of neo-liberal state. Indeed several research questions arise here. Is globalization creating new opportunities or obstacles in democratizing the health care system? How do we assess the imperative for the state in its obligations to ensure universal access to health care in terms of caste, class, and gender? What are the implications of rising clinical trials and pharmaceuticals in terms of cost, exclusions, and ethical questions? What is the critical role for communities in the health care system today? The chapters in the present volume attempt to address these questions in depth and provide a direction towards inter-disciplinary health care studies.

While disciplinary sub-fields such as medical sociology, medical anthropology, health economics, community health, social medicine, epidemiology, public health, and others with their own theories, methods, and approaches are able to contribute distinctive dimensions, it becomes essential to engage across the boundaries in a collective manner to understand the complexity of health care that is increasingly shaped by the global market forces and ideologies. Secondly, since it was civil society activism[3] that first posed serious questions about the changing trajectory of health care that was moving away from a state-directed path of welfare, we need to take these on board in coming to a nuanced understanding of dynamics of health care. It is, after all, these developments that have highlighted how sociopolitical factors have shaped health care in India.

Embedded in the study of the social, economic, and political factors impacting health care, is a particular understanding of the concepts of equity,[4] equality,[5] and social justice. It is this understanding that impacts the way we comprehend the complexity of socio-economic and political underpinnings of health and health care. Equity and equality, for instance, may not be viewed as equivalent, nor can they be reduced to simple variables or risk factors (Botero et al. 2012). Breilh points out that equity is the process, while equality is the outcome. Equity/inequity are characteristics of the way social formations distribute the conditions for equality or inequality (cited in Botero et al. 2012).[6] Equality, on the other hand, results from equity just as inequality results from inequity. Inequality is linked to considerable poverty, ill-health and suffering, yet is entrenched in many countries. According to Piketty (2014), it took the combination of the devastation of two world wars, high post-war population growth and the active labour movement to achieve the significant reductions in inequality that occurred between the start of the twentieth century and 1960s. Amartya Sen (1999) points out that in any discussion of equity and social justice, illness and health must necessarily figure as a major concern.

CONCEPTUAL UNDERSTANDING OF HEALTH EQUITY

How is the idea of health equity conceptualized in global debates? How have these debates influenced the understanding of health equity in

India? These two issues are crucial to a nuanced understanding of health equity in India.

The World Health Organization (WHO 2008) that has an overarching influence on health policies indicate that health equity means everyone has a fair opportunity to live a long healthy life. It implies that health should not be compromised or disadvantaged because of an individual or population groups' race, caste, ethnicity, gender, income, sexual orientation, region, or other social condition. An equity framework systematically focuses attention on the socially disadvantaged, the marginalized, and the disenfranchised groups within and between countries, including but not limited to the poor (Braveman 2006; Braveman and Gruskin 2003).

Two policy documents published by WHO, one by Margaret Whitehead in the early 1990s and the second by the WHO Commission on Social Determinants of Health (CSDH) in 2008 have defined the concept health equity/inequity decisively and generated the global debate.[7] Whitehead defines health equity 'as equal access to available care for equal need, equal utilization for equal need, equal quality of care for all' (Whitehead 1990). Variations in health, she points out 'are not only unnecessary and avoidable but are considered unfair and unjust'. Further, 'Equity in health implies that ideally everyone should have a fair opportunity to attain their full health potential and, more pragmatically, that no one should be disadvantaged from achieving this potential, if it can be avoided' (Whitehead et al. 2000).

Commission on Social Determinants of Health has defined social inequity as the existence of unjust and avoidable differences in access to goods, services, and opportunities. Social inequity is defined as a situation in which not all individuals and citizens of a society, community, or country have the same rights, responsibilities, goods, benefits, or access. These two definitions of equity and inequity have been influential in health care research. The World Health Organization policy documents talk about the acceptance of the idea that there are just and unavoidable differences in access to health care thus justifying structural inequalities. Intervening in this debate, Amartya Sen (1999) associates equity with equality of opportunity and the flourishing of human capabilities and human achievement. He makes a distinction between the human capital and capability approach. In the former, everything is ultimately measured against the yardstick of economic activity, whereas the capability approach places the individuals and their capacity to achieve their own goals at the centre. If human capabilities increase, true freedom grows and hence governments should be measured against the citizenry's real capabilities.

However, critics point out that the WHO policy documents restrict their analyses to mere effects and miss the causes of those particular effects. They do not tackle the basic issue that of inequity, while Sen, does not analyse the sources of power in a society and how that power is reproduced (David and Walt 2001; Navarro 2000, 2009). The critical insights from these debates are summarized as follows.

First, inequity generates inequality, which is the obvious, visible, and measurable characteristic; but to understand the inequality we have to know what kind of inequity is producing this inequality. Inequity arises from the appropriation of power and wealth, which leads to social classes and discrimination. Critiquing the CSDH, several scholars argue that 'inequity refers not only to injustice in distribution and access, but to processes which generate this injustice. Inequity is about how the social structure determines social inequalities; they are its consequence' (Gonzalez cited in Botero et al. 2012). Commission on Social Determinants of Health and capability approach in fact avoided the social class construct altogether. The result of this omission is that the WHO report tells us little about the origins of economic and power inequalities and that everyone seems to be equally responsible for health inequities (Navarro 2009, 1999). However, the debates around the Black Report, for instance, had clearly depicted the class inequalities inherent in a society and how this not only contoured health inequalities, indeed generated them (cited in Mukhopadhyay 2008).

Second, it is argued that social inequalities and the inequity that generates them are manifested in living conditions determined by 'political, social and economic forces'. A social group or class does not create or control its living conditions; rather, these derive from the general social structure, from the forms of economic production and social organization. Given inequalities in both health and access to health care services, Breilh says people do not become ill at random; illness occurs in the context of their lives: their work, environment, and the larger political and social context (cited in Botero et al. 2012). Smith (2010) points out that the causes of health inequalities rest with material and social factors such as poverty, poor housing, and social exclusion. Health inequalities are increasingly viewed as an outcome of material, social, and cultural inequalities across societies, which are in turn, the product of inequalities in power, income and wealth, knowledge, and social status and social connections.

Third, at the micro level—within a social class—gender relationships create different patterns of inequity, both in terms of formal employment and within the home. Drawing on feminist work on intersectionality, Kapilashrami, Hill, and Meer (2015) point to the need for incorporating 'multiple layers of advantage and disadvantage (that are) relevant for health inequalities' in explaining health inequalities.

In brief, the global debate on health equity has highlighted the importance of understanding how health inequalities are produced and the underlying politics of distribution and access. Significantly, how does this inequality and asymmetry in power get represented and reinforced in health care? Effacing the inequality of outcomes is not, as Paul Farmer (2001) for instance points out, the same as eliminating the underlying forces of inequality.

This volume consciously adopts a political economy approach positing that inequity and inequality change historically within and across social structures. The chapters analyse the politics of social relations, technological choices, organizational politics, perceptions of different social groups, as well as dynamics of gender, disability, and their implications for inequity in health and health care. The authors in the volume use an interdisciplinary approach within a broader political economy framework, bringing in feminist and Foucauldian critical discourses along with epidemiological and ethnographic analyses to enrich their approach. This theoretical frame is useful to understand power relations within social groups and complex organizational systems. The importance of this volume also lies more in its timeliness as it engages with the issues of health inequities as part of a global conversation.

HEALTH EQUITY POLICIES AND PRACTICES

Health policy documents in India have always integrated the guiding principles of equity in health and health care with a promise to serve the needs of the poor and the underprivileged. The *Health Survey and Development Committee Report* of 1946 drafted under Sir Joseph Bhore set out a detailed vision and plan for providing universal coverage to the population through a government-led health service. Since then, and until recently, health policies and priorities have been outlined in the Five-Year Plans, developed as part of India's centralized planning and development strategy.[8] In the first two decades, public investment on health care in terms of infrastructure, medical personnel, and equipment was substantial. This was an attempt by the state to provide access to health services for the unreached population in rural areas. Hence this phase is termed as the 'golden two decades of public health' in India (Banerjee 2001: 44). However, 'population control' and 'immunization programmes' took the centre stage from late 1970s and 1980s paving the way for target-oriented (family planning, reproductive health) approaches, thus drifting from the government's stated vision of universal access.

The Indian state influenced by the Alma-Ata Declaration announced the first official National Health Policy (NHP) in 1984, which re-stated the need for universal comprehensive care. The policy emphasized the primary health care (PHC) approach, decentralization of the health system, improved community participation, and expansion of the private sector to reduce the burden of the public sector. However, two developments took place after the first NHP: One, a paradigm shift from comprehensive to selective PHC about which the ruling class was already convinced found its grounding with the financial assistance from the international agencies such as Rockefeller and Ford Foundation in mid-1980s, and second, this health policy in fact heralded the corporatization of hospitals. This was evident from the way the Apollo Group of Hospitals that got listed as a public limited company in 1984 received wide-ranging state support. Thus it paved the way for other corporate hospitals to emerge in the 1990s to take advantage of the concessions and benefits offered by the Indian state in terms of land, import subsidies, trained medical personnel, and so on.

The second NHP of 2002 reiterated its commitment to achieve a more equitable access to health services across the social and geographical expanse of the country through comprehensive PHC services (Government of India 2002). However in practice, the state gradually divested its responsibility even from the curative health care as part of the economic reforms. This led to the unfettered growth of private hospitals that found it lucrative to adopt the tertiary-care model. The private sector grew without adequate regulation and eventually resulted in the corporatization of health care. With good-quality health services becoming unaffordable and inaccessible, curative health care today is left to the initiative of the patient reinforcing the neo-liberal idea of individualizing the health care.

In 2009, the Government of India drafted a National Health Bill proposing the legal framework to recognize the 'right to health' and 'right to health care' with a stated recognition to address the underlying social determinants of health. In 2012, the Government of India constituted a High-Level Expert Group (HLEG), which recommended comprehensive universal health coverage. The report highlighted how the Constitution of India places obligations on the government to ensure protection and fulfilment of Right to Health for all without any discrimination. In fact, a third National Health Policy 2017 admitted that the country's health equity concerns have, moved in the reverse direction. It acknowledges 'catastrophic expenditure due to health care costs is growing and is estimated to be one of the major contributors to poverty'. The policy underlined the urgent and critical need to enact the Right to Health Care legislation soon (Government of India 2017). However, in practice, two trends can be observed in health care in the last decade. One, fragmented health care with different providers taking care of different parts of the health system, such as the private sector providing hospital-based care and the government sector providing part-primary care and part-secondary/tertiary care where patients are free to bypass it, a worst possible choice created for the patients. Second, given the rising tertiary health care cost, government introduced health insurance schemes both at the central and state levels starting from 2007, for the below poverty line (BPL) population. This initiative is supposed to provide social security for the working poor but it in fact contributes to the higher demand for hospitalization as much as the increased out-of-pocket expenditure given the unregulated private health sector.

Starting from Bhore Committee, 1946 to the recent National Health Policy 2017, almost all the policy documents of the Indian state reiterated their commitment to health equity in principle and more specifically to improve the access to quality health care for the labouring poor and disadvantaged groups (Bhore, Amesur, and Banerjee 1946; Government of India 2002, 2017). It is quite pertinent here to explain the state's contradictory discourse of health equity on the one hand and prevailing health inequalities on the other in India. Several research studies indicated that health equity and access have been interpreted and operationalized by the national and state governments as equal distribution and utilization of health care services according to their needs (Balarajan, Selvaraj, and Subramanian 2011; Ghosh 2014; Mondal 2013).

Even to realize this limited goal, it is imperative to make a systematic assessment of prevailing inequity in the distribution and utilization of health care services. Many of these health inequalities result from a broad set of social, economic, and political conditions, which influence the level and distribution of health within a population. This explains how state's[9] health equity discourse is in tune with the dominant functionalist perspective of the global health equity discourse, which justified the just and unavoidable differences in access to health care. The present volume attempts to pose this question: Are the growing health inequalities in India a direct consequence of the conceptual misinterpretation, directly rooted in the capitalist structures of Indian society? A brief analysis is provided below.

First, while health inequalities re-emerged as an official policy concern in the NHP, the approach to strengthen health systems has been through 'Missions'- and 'Insurance'-induced initiatives. Therefore, it is necessary to understand whether National Health Assurance Mission (NHAM), National Rural Health Mission (NRHM),[10] National Urban Health Mission (NUHM),[11] Rashtriya Swasthya Bima Yojana (RSBY),[12] and several other insurance programmes launched during 2005–17, reflect a neo-liberal response[13] to the capitalist globalization.

Second, access is not merely about physical infrastructure and resource availability but it is to do with social and political concerns. In fact, previous research studies argued that inequality in India is primarily to do with social access. Discrimination against women, lower classes, and castes in health care services is a common example of intolerable inequality in social access (Hodges and Rao 2016; Kumar 1994; Qadeer, Sen, and Nayar 2001). Several studies also indicated that the poor use health care services less frequently when they are sick than do the rich. The landless labourers and the self-employed (who constitute a sizeable majority of the rural and urban poor), the displaced population, and the tribal and nomadic communities have limited access to health services (Prasad 2015). This is because access is deeply intertwined with health equity which is conditioned by the sociopolitical and economic forces. As Doyal (1991) rightly pointed out, health care policies and medical systems in capitalist countries represent the outcome of a particular moment of the struggle between all these conflicting forces. They are not the rational policies of a benevolent state ensuring healthy lives and rational medicine for all its citizens.

The seventeen chapters in the volume together provide a narrative that explains the politics of access (distribution, utilization, outcomes) as well as the context in which health inequalities are produced. The four sections analyse how state and market forces have progressively heightened the iniquitous health care system and the process through which substantial burden of meeting health care needs fell on the individuals and households, impacting different classes, castes, gender, and other categories. The present volume has brought together scholars (medical doctors, social scientists, public health specialists and activists, policymakers, gender specialists, and legal experts) whose past work has looked at health care in its historical, political, legal, and sociological dimensions, respectively, and have attempted to redraw the contours of health care studies in India with an interdisciplinary perspective. The issue of access and equity in health care is not a single narrative, but is multilayered with several perspectives. This volume attempts to capture this multidimensionality as an intellectually stimulating enterprise, across a variety of methodologies, styles of research communication and writing. We hope that the discussion in the volume will lead to a new thinking on health care studies, set in the context of the diversity of analyses.

State, Market, and Society

The first section points out how state and market forces have significantly shaped the health care system—public, private, and, medical education. The five chapters indicate that the Indian state's neo-liberal economic reforms over the last 25 years have rapidly transformed an emerging public health system into a private sector-led growth (corporatization of health) thus gradually eroding the public system at all levels, on education, and training, delivery of care, and research. The Indian state has failed to incorporate the essence of the PHC approach. This section asks whether the attempts by the Indian state to address issues of access (economic/physical barriers) through NRHM, PPP, and social protection through health insurance in the last two decades have in any way contributed towards equitable health outcomes? In fact the chapters in the section persuasively demonstrate that health care reforms have enhanced social inequality at different levels. Medical education and knowledge have remained exclusive and disconnected from the health care needs of the population at large. Further, the tremendous rise of medical specializations has in fact fostered the growth of private tertiary hospitals undermining primary and secondary care contributing to the increased inaccessibility of health care services.

Ritu Priya, in Chapter 1, scrutinizes the techno-centric capitalist vision of the current PHC approach, tracing how at every turn well-meaning concepts and principles have been twisted out of shape to suit the needs of welfare capitalism. She suggests that change in the health care system is possible only if a dynamic relationship can be established between the community, the state, expert knowledge, and the technologies available from home to hospital.

Purendra Prasad, in Chapter 2, further argues that, even the attempts by the Indian state towards inclusion and offering a range of choices to the working poor through empanelled hospitals, has only served to boost health insurance markets and consequent commoditization of health services. This chapter analyses how the economic reforms have created inefficiency, increased costs and accelerated the expansion of a largely unregulated health care market. A vivid illustration of the neglected lot, are the workers such as in Bholakpur slum in Hyderabad, who depend on high-risk waste-related work.

Rama Baru, in Chapter 3, presents evidence that the consolidation and transformation of markets in the Indian health service system now resembles a medical industrial complex. The complex architecture of the private sector involves a range of actors and institutions, which produce a complex network of power relations that actively engages with the political processes at all levels drawing Indian and foreign capital into robust alliances firmly entrenched within the health service system.

The following two chapters explore the critical impact of neo-liberal health care policies on education and training in the medical system. Neha Madhiwalla, in Chapter 4, points out that the commercialization of medical education has led to the deterioration of standards and institutionalization of corruption, devaluing the process of medical training and the profession itself. Notwithstanding social inclusion policies in education, a techno-centric approach to training results in the entrenching of unresponsive services geared to capital intensive and commodified metropolitan model of medicine.

Anand Zachariah, in Chapter 5, elaborates how training in narrow super-specializations has developed rapidly in the last few decades at the cost of primary- and secondary-care training. He richly illustrates the mismatch between existing and emerging health and illness patterns and the inappropriate training that physicians receive to deal with these problems. Zachariah makes a comprehensive argument for a radical change in the medical education content and pedagogy, with concrete suggestions.

Pharmaceuticals, Market, and Experimental Research

Globalization has not only affected the structure and content of the health care and education system, it has drastically affected the availability of necessary medicines. Perhaps its most visible influence may be seen in the area of pharmaceuticals—the production and distribution of medicines and biomedical research in the clinical domain. This section shows how vulnerable the Indian state has become to global policies and market dynamics affecting political-structural, regulatory, and ethical concerns. The authors in this section argue for a strong state intervention in pricing, provision of medicines, health care services, given the extraordinary crisis of public health in India. As bodies became resources in new ways, the chapters raise questions about the unequal social context in which research is being conducted and how conditions of inequality is being reproduced pointing also to the weak ethical frameworks in the conduct of research.

Amit Sengupta, in Chapter 6, narrates the impact of globalization on intellectual property rights (IPR) and pharmaceuticals in India. He traces the trajectory of India's fall from grace—from a country that could supply affordable medicines to over a hundred countries to one that panders to the demands of multinational industry. With the capitulation of the country to the new agreements on IPR post the Uruguay Round of negotiations in 1986, a series of changes in the market and production of medicines made for rising costs of essential medicines. By the 1990s India embarked on economic reforms and introduced explicit neo-liberal polices, which gave way to lower standards of IP protection. Sengupta argues that the best method of controlling prices of patented drugs would be by breaking the monopoly of the patent holder, which the Indian Patent Act itself has elaborate provisions.

S. Srinivasan and Malini Aisola, in Chapter 7, point out that the availability of medicines in the public health system is erratic and uncertain except in some states, like Tamil Nadu, Rajasthan, and Kerala, that have taken radical measures. Why exactly has this happened? For one, this is a direct impact of dilution of key flexibilities in India's patent laws and second, the deliberate indecisiveness of India's drug policy and its regulatory conditions. The authors contend that the huge production of irrational and harmful fixed dose combination drugs, affects patients in multiple ways. The single most effective way of making drugs more accessible and affordable is to regulate the market, introduce price control that includes more than the national list of essential medicines. The key factor here is the development of a universal public health care system.

Moving on to the realm of biomedical and clinical research, Jeffery et al. in Chapter 8, point out that although the Indian generics industry, and contract research organizations (CROs) seemed well prepared for joining the World Trade Organization (WTO) in 2005, they underestimated the cultural and regulatory shifts needed for Indian firms to establish their position in the complex global assemblage that is the contemporary clinical trials industry. With little experience of structured medical research and plagued by poverty, inadequate public medical facilities, excessively expensive private medical care options, and stark social inequalities, Indian regulatory institutions struggled to achieve their stated goals in the face of mounting public, legal, and parliamentary criticism. While commercial interests quickly took note of the new opportunities that outsourced clinical trials might offer them in India, the procedures to regulate these activities in the interests of wider societal goals were much slower to become established. Jeffery et al. further say, commercial clinical trials in India produced particular forms of 'research culture', which may not neatly fit familiar conceptual frameworks. The authors analyse the ethical implications of clinical trials for India and its 'public health' impact.

Sarojini and Vrinda, in Chapter 9, talk about coming together of assisted reproductive technology and the new markets in biomedicine which has resulted in an unprecedented traffic in body parts, and their renting and selling. While acknowledging fundamental differences between commercial surrogacy, egg donation, clinical trials, and bio-availability and bio-equivalent (BA/BE) clinical trials, this chapter attempts to draw out ethical and regulatory concerns across these categories. Given the class of women from which surrogates are being drawn, the issues are not just of the rights for surrogates in the arrangement but of reproductive justice, autonomy, or oppression. A neo-liberal paradigm that rolls back social securities like universal health and education, generates scant and insecure employment, and individualizes risk, robs people of robust alternatives and creates the conditions for clinical labour to flourish.

Equity Issues in Health Care: Gender, Caste, Disability, and Violence

While the health system in its structure and functioning reveals the underlying causes of inequality in access to health care, social and cultural factors penetrate the system in multiple ways. Marginalized groups—disabled, community health workers, sex workers, survivors of violence, and other vulnerable women facing violence are affected by the dominant health discourse of the state. The chapters map out multidimensional axis of inequality that gets perpetuated through legal, medico-bureaucratic state apparatuses complemented by the patriarchal, dominant class–caste perspectives. The authors argue that violence or marginalization of identities is inextricably linked to larger sociopolitical and economic processes.

Renu Addlakha, in Chapter 10, examines the critical and nuanced interconnection between law and disability. She discusses the health equity and social justice demand raised in the disability sector with a narrative of the kind of social justice demands that prompted the making of Mental Health Care Act 2013 and the proposed disability legislation. Addlakha tries to show how law is an important site for demonstrating this intersection between medical and social model of disability because it straddles the slippery terrain between configuring the phenomenon of disability as both an individual problem of the body and a historically embedded structural issue with deep roots in the culture, economy, and polity. When principles of the market become the default patterns that drive the social system, law becomes the derigeur tool of social change since it does not drastically challenge the status quo. Indeed, health becomes the bridge connecting disability as a form of social oppression to disability as a form of bodily and personal difference.

The principle of universal rationality espoused by the state comes into question in Madumita Biswal's Chapter 11 of this volume, looking at class, caste, and gender bias and how it gets perpetuated in the delivery of health care. An ethnographic study in Boudh district of Odisha, forms the basis of the chapter that draws out in detail the manner in which the community-level health workers by virtue of occupying the space between state and community, become agents of the state, at one level, located at the margins of the bureaucratic structure, and simultaneously as the representatives of the local community at another rung. In effect, caste and gender hegemonies at the local level continue to play a crucial role in the statist process of governance.

Asima Jena, in Chapter 12, points out that while caste, class, poverty, religion, and gender are the more familiar axes of discrimination, sexuality is clearly another axis along which women face certain kinds of violence. This chapter on violence focuses on sexual policing as a form of violence based on a study among female sex workers (FSWs) in Rajahmundry of Andhra Pradesh. It tries to show how surveillance of the FSWs gets legitimized in the name of protecting the health of general population. Disciplining these sexual marginals by the state is rationalized without any concern for the violence it imposes.

While it is recognized that public health care institutions are often the first points of reference to women survivors of violence, Sangeeta Rege and Padma Bhate-Deosthali, in Chapter 13, point out that violence against women (VAW) has only recently been recognized as a public health issue in India. The Protection of women from domestic violence law (PWDVA) 2005, the criminal amendment to rape (CLA) 2013, and law on protection from child sexual abuse (POCSCO 2012) now make it mandatory for all public and private hospitals to provide free treatment to survivors of sexual violence. Despite these amendments, the health sector response to violence in general and violence against women and children specifically remains suboptimal. Documenting the experience of different civil society organizations such as Dilasa, a hospital-based crisis centre in Mumbai, North East Network (NEN) in Meghlaya, Swati, a feminist organization in rural Gujarat, Sneha in Mumbai, and Masum a community-based women's organization in Pune at different levels within health care system, the chapter points to the critical need to incorporate a systemic response to violence against women taking cues from the many initiatives underway.

Right to Health and Universal Health Strategies

A running thread throughout the tapestry of health care system is the emphatic assertion that health equity issues cannot be addressed satisfactorily without some form of a universal health care structure and system. This last section critically scrutinizes the recent policy intent of the Indian state to achieve universal health coverage by 2022 and the need to enact the right to health care legislation announced in its National Health Policy 2017. The discussion in this section opens a window to explore and explain the possibilities of achieving universal access both at the conceptual and pragmatic levels.

Srinath Reddy and Manu Raj Mathur, in Chapter 14, highlight the High-Level Expert Group (HLEG's) report particularly the possibility of a design and delivery of people-friendly Universal Health Care (UHC). The authors discuss the significance of providing free essential medicines and listing all drugs in the National List of Essential Medicines (NLEM) through a public distribution system. They point out how user fee of any kind militated against the vision of UHC and produces health inequality.

Based on their study on UHC in the two districts of Kerala (Malappuram and Palakkad), Sunil Nandraj and Devaki Nambiar, in

Chapter 15, point out that Kerala was seen as an exemplar of good health at low cost in 1984 but in the post-2000, there is a clear preference for private hospital-based care compared to a public hospital or PHC. If Kerala has to move towards UHC, the government sector has to emerge as a viable model in a highly privatized and tertiarized health-seeking context. This may be achieved by placing emphasis on the burdens citizens face, with a focus on prevention, early detection, and promotion of health, as well as quality provision of care for acute management of disease.

In proposing a viable model drawn from Maharashtra state, Ravi Duggal, in Chapter 16, examines the possibilities and bottlenecks for financing the universal access to health care (UAHC). For realizing UAHC, the growing out-of-pocket financing of the health care system has to be replaced with a combination of public finance and various collective financing options such as social insurance, collectives/common interest groups organizing collective funds, and others. To realize its social or public value it has to be organized and regulated using both public and private resources for social benefit.

Kajal Bharadwaj, Veena Johari, and Vivek Divan, in Chapter 17, point out that the complexity of giving robust meaning to the right to health in all its dimensions is undermined by the health policy and law in India. While 'health' falls within the jurisdiction of States to legislate, various aspects impacting health care fall under the central or concurrent lists of the Indian Constitution resulting in health being legislated at both the central and state levels. The courts have held, in the context of the right of persons to emergency health care that providing adequate medical facilities is an essential part of the obligations undertaken by the government in a welfare state. This chapter argues that the approach of the Supreme Court with regard to the obligations of the private sector in relation to health care should be re-examined rather than leave patients increasingly at the mercy of the market.

NOTES

1. The definition of health has undergone substantial changes in the last few decades and widened in its scope. The determinants such as resource distribution, gender differences, violence, armed conflict are also given as much significance in redefining health. However, health care is the maintenance and improvement of health through the provision of medical services (UN Covenant for the Social, Economic and Cultural rights 2000).

2. The recent 71st round of National Sample Survey based on the data between January and June 2014, revealed that more than 75 per cent of the people opted for paid private health services despite the provision for free public health services (Lakshman 2016).

3. Health research and policy in India was influenced by two kinds of activism: one, the movement framework (Networks and civil society organizations such as centre for enquiry into health and allied topics (CEHAT), foundation for research in community health (FRCH), Medico-Friends Circle, Sama, Jan Swasthya Abhiyan, Anveshi Centre for Women, among others); second, academic-activists from Jawaharlal Nehru University's (JNU) community health and Social Medicine centre and other universities produced a counter point highlighting perspectives of the local communities.

4. Equity refers to the qualities of justness, fairness, and impartiality, while equality means 'the state of being equal', which is one of the ideals of a democratic society.

5. In the context of political, social, and economic rights, equality specifically denotes equal access to basic resources and opportunities for all the classes to grow and prosper with human dignity and happiness (WHO 2008).

6. Inequality is linked to considerable poverty, ill-health, and suffering, yet is entrenched in many countries. According to Piketty (2014), it took the combination of the devastation of two world wars, high post-war population growth, and the active labour movement to achieve significant reductions in inequality that occurred between the start of the twentieth century and 1960s.

7. Prior to 1990s, Alma-Ata Declaration of 'health for all' in 1978 generated the first debate on health equity globally. The other influential proponent of equity in health was Carl E. Taylor (1982), who advocated the concept 'surveillance for equity' based on his research evidence from Kerala and Sri Lanka in 1980s. He argued that this concept will help achieve optimal health outputs at low cost without corresponding social or economic equality.

8. Government of India replaced planning commission with National Institution for Transforming India also called as NITI Aayog, established in the year 2015.

9. It is true that state's discourse itself emerges from its constant interaction with civil society. Indian state successfully co-opted the radical ideas thrown by the people's health movements into its policies and transformed them for its own purposes. The examples are community health workers schemes, community participation, community health monitoring, and others.

10. National Rural Health Mission was intended to improve health services in rural areas in states with poor health indicators, but several studies pointed out that it focused mainly on maternal and child health and did not cover many other health conditions.

11. National Urban Health Mission sought to address the health of the urban poor and other disadvantaged sections, and facilitate their access to the health service system.

12. Rashtriya Swasthya Bima Yojana is the national government's subsidized secondary-/tertiary-care funding scheme for informal workers.

13. The manifest purpose of these initiatives is to strengthen public health care systems and contribute towards inclusive health care however the process has resulted in weakening the existing institutions and practices of exclusion.

REFERENCES

Balarajan, Yarlin, S. Selvaraj, and S.V. Subramanian. 2011. 'Health Care and Equity in India', *The Lancet* 377 (9764): 505–15.

Banerjee, Debabar. 2001. 'Landmarks in the Developmentof Health Services in India'. In *Public Health and the Poverty of Reforms*, Imrana Qadeeer, Kasturi Sen, and K.R. Nayar (eds), pp. 39–50. New Delhi: Sage Publications.

Baru, Rama. 2000. 'Privatisation and Corporatisation', *Seminar* 489. Available at: http://www.india.seminar.com/2000/489. Accessed on 26 April 2016.

Baru R., A. Acharya, S. Acharya, A.K. Shivakumar, and K. Nagaraj. 2010. 'Inequities in Access to Health Services in India: Caste, Class and Region', *Economic and Political Weekly* 45(38): 49–58.

Botero, Adriana, Maria Correa, Maria Mercedes Arias Valencia, Jaime Carmona-Fonseca. 2012, 'Social and Health Equity and Equality: The Need for a Scientific Framework', *Social Medicine* 7(1): 10–17. Available at: www.socialmedicine.info. Accessed on 21 February 2016.

Bhore, J., R. Amesur, and A. Banerjee. 1946. *Report of the Health Survey and Development Committee*. Delhi: Government of India.

Braveman, Paula. 2006. 'Health Disparities and Health Equity: Concepts and Measurement', *Annual Review of Public Health* 27: 167–74.

Braveman, Paula and Sofia Gruskin. 2003. 'Poverty, Equity, Human Rights and Health', *Bulletin of WHO* 81: 539–45.

Chancel, Lucas and Thomas Piketty. 2017. 'Indian Income Inequality 1922–2014: From British Raj to Billionaire Raj', *The World Inequality Report, WID*. World Working Paper Series N 2017/11. Accessed on 21 October 2017.

David, A. Leon and Gill Walt. 2001. *Poverty, Inequality and Health: An International Perspective*. New Delhi: Oxford University Press.

Doyal, Leslie. 1991. *Political Economy of Health*. London: Pluto Press.

Duggal, Ravi. 2000. 'Where Are We Today?' *Seminar* 489. Available at: http://www.india.seminar.com/2000/489. Accessed on 26 April 2016.

Farmer, Paul. 2001. Infections *and Inequalities—The Modern Plagues*. California: University of California Press.

Fisher, A. Jill. 2007. 'Coming Soon to a Physician Near You: Medical Neoliberalism and Phamaceutical Clinical Trials', *Harvard Health Policy Review* 8(1): 61–70.

Jadhav, Radheshyam. 2017. 'Health Care beyond Half of the World's Reach'. *The Times of India*, 15 December.

Ghosh, Soumitra. 2014. 'Equity in the Utilization of Health Care Services in India: Evidence from National Sample Survey', *International Journal of Health Policy Management* 2(1): 29–38.

Government of India. 2002. *Draft National Health Policy 2001*. New Delhi: Ministry of Health and Family Welfare. Available at: http://mohfw.nic.in/np2001.html.

Government of India. 2017. *National Health Policy 2017*. New Delhi: Ministry of Health and Family Welfare.

Hammer, J., Y. Aiyar, and S. Samji. 2007. 'Understanding Government Failure in Public Health Services', *Economic and Political Weekly* 42(40): 4049–57.

Harvey, David. 2014. *Mega Cities*, 4 Lectures. Available at: http://www.kas.de/upload/documente/megacities/MegacitiesLectur4worlds.pdf. Accessed on 21 February 2016.

Hodges, Sarah and Mohan Rao (ed.). 2016. *Public Health and Private Wealth: Stem Cells, Surrogates and Other Strategic Bodies*. Delhi: Oxford University Press.

Kapilashrami A., S. Hill, and N. Meer. 2015. 'What Can Health Inequalities Researchers Learn from an Intersectionality Perspective? Understanding Social Dynamics with an Inter-Categorical Approach', *Social Theory & Health* 13:288, August. Available at: https:doi.org/10.1057/sth.2015.16.

Kumar, Shiva A.K. 1994. 'Some Considerations in the Formulation of India's Health Policy: A Note on Equity', *Social Scientist* 22 (9–12): 79–88.

Lakshman, Narayan. 2016. 'Malady Nation—Remedying India's Health Care Colossus'. *The Hindu*, 8 August.

Lee, K. 1998. 'Globalization and Health Policy—Proposed Research Agenda', Discussion Paper No.1. London School of Hygiene and Tropical Medicine, London: UK.

Mondal, Swadhin. 2013. 'Health Care Services in India: A Few Questions on Equity', *Health* 5(1): 53–61. Available at: http://dx.doi.org/0.4236/health.2013.51008. Accessed on 21 February 2016.

Mukhopadhyay, Indranil. 2008. 'Analyzing Health Inequalities—Social Capital and its Infirmities', *Social Scientist* 36 (11–12): 69–93.

Navarro, V. 1999. 'Health and Equity in the World in the Era of Globalization', *International Journal of Health Services* 29: 215–26.

———. 2000. 'Development and Quality of Life: A Critique of Amartya Sen's Development as Freedom', *International Journal of Health Services* 30(4): 661–74.

———. 2009. 'What We Mean by Social Determinants of Health', *International Journal of Health Services* 39(3): 423–41.

Piketty, T. 2014. *Capital in the Twenty-First Century*. Cambridge, MA: Harvard University Press.

Prasad, N. Purendra. 2015. 'State, Community Health Insurance and Commodification of Health Care: A Case of Arogyasri in Andhra Pradesh'. In *Medical Insurance Schemes for the Poor—Who Benefits*, Rama V. Baru (ed.), pp. 61–87. New Delhi: Academic Foundation.

Qadeer, Imrana, Kasturi Sen, and K.R. Nayar (eds). 2001. *Public Health and the Poverty of Reforms—The South Asian Predicament*. New Delhi: Sage Publications.

Sen, Amartya. 1999. *Development as Freedom*. Oxford: Oxford University Press.

Smith, Katherine. 2010. 'Research Policy and Funding—Academic Treadmills and the Squeeze on Intellectual Spaces', *The British Journal of Sociology* 61(1): 176–95.

Taylor, E. Carl. 1982. 'Surveillance for Equity in Primary Health Care: Policy Implications from International Experience', *International Journal of Epidemiology* 21(8): 1043–9.

UN Covenant for the Social, Economic and Cultural Rights. 2000. *CESCR General Comment No.14: The Right to Highest Attainable Standard of Health (Art 12)*. Available at: http://www.refworld.org/pdfid/4538838d0.pdf. Accessed on 21 February 2016.

Whitehead, Margaret. 1990. *The Concepts and Principles of Equity in Health*. Copenhagen: Regional Office for Europe, World Health Organization.

Whitehead, Margaret, T. Evan, F. Didenchesen, and F. Bhuiya (eds). 2000. *Inequities in Health: A Global Perspective*. Oxford: Oxford University Press.

World Health Organization (WHO). 2008. *Final Report of the Commission on Social Determinants of Health Closing the Gap in a Generation. Health Equity through Action on the Social Determinants of Health*. WHO: Geneva.

I

STATE, MARKET, AND HEALTH CARE

1

State, Community, and Primary Health Care

Empowering or Disempowering Discourses?

Ritu Priya

In modern times, the Indian state has taken on the responsibility of providing for health care to ordinary citizens. Even as it has contributed to the welfare of the people, this has also introduced the biopolitics of modern public health and planned health services development into the health care scenario. This chapter examines the relationship between the state, the community, and the primary health care approach (PHC) in the Indian context as a historical flow.

A primary health care approach requires the design of health systems development (HSD) to incorporate, (*i*) centrality of primary-level care, (*ii*) use of appropriate technology at primary, secondary, and tertiary levels of care, and (*iii*) recognition of the determinants of health other than medical care. The Alma-Ata Declaration and the policy framework of the Indian state that preceded it, espoused the PHC approach. Both posited 'health care for all' as the goal, with 'community participation' as an important component for attaining the set goals. Yet, neither has 'health care for all' been achieved nor has 'community participation' towards attaining it become a reality. Why has the PHC approach failed to be operationalized?

This chapter argues that the failure of the mainstream health service system's design to incorporate all the elements of the PHC approach is linked to the policymakers/planners' particular perception of 'the community' and of 'health care'. Secondly, the faulty design has contributed to the failure to reach 'health care for all'. Thirdly, the failure to provide even primary-level care to all is linked to contradictions in the initial articulation of PHC itself. The chapter urges the reader, with the benefits of hindsight, to undertake a critical analysis of HSD and PHC to create a future agenda in the spirit of PHC. Finally, it points to the need for a more holistic frameworks of analyses instead of the tendency for fragmented ones.

The state of health and the history of health services development are well-documented and is available in the reports of official committees (from the Royal Commission of 1859, Bhore Committee (BC) of 1946, to the present Government of India planning committees), writings of political streams as well as civil society actors contributing to the envisioning of this domain (ICSSR-ICMR 1981; MFC Bulletin 1976–2015; National Planning Committee 1948; Roy 1982; VHAI-ICDHI 1995–2015; JSA 2000–15), and academic health system analyses beginning from the 1960s (Antia 1981; Banerji 1967, 1969, 1985; Bose and Desai 1983; Jeffery 1988; Qadeer 1985a) with a virtual explosion since the 1990s (FRCH 1994). In addition there are the sociological and anthropological studies of health practices of various communities and socio political analyses of medical pluralism (Banerjee 2009; Banerji 1973, 1979; Priya 2001a, 2012; Sujatha and Abraham 2012). We will use these various contemporary sources to reconstruct the role played by the state, the community, and PHC in the development of health care in India.

Three broad strands of analyses can be found in literature to explain the lack of provisioning to cover all citizens by the public service system. They are as follows:

1. The nature of the Indian state and the ruling class has not been adequately democratic and welfarist (Drèze and Sen 2013; Reddy et al. 2011). The ruling class has prioritized economic growth and defence expenditures over social welfare and people's well-being. Consequently, public expenditure on health (and on other welfare sectors) has been low, with public services remaining limited in coverage and content.

2. The capitalist economy, aided by the technocratic public administration, has accorded a low priority to health and has moved health care towards an over-medicalization of health. In the absence of attention to the environmental and social determinants of health, enhancing medical technology-based services was neither

cost-effective nor suited to the health priorities of the majority of India's population. That the medical industry has been allowed to dictate policy, and the private sector has been allowed to flourish unregulated, form part of this strand of critique (Qadeer 2000; Phadke 2004). After the 1990s, the analysis shifted from 'a capitalist mode of development continuing from the colonial period' to 'globalization since the 1990s' being the major reason for the thwarted development of a public service for universal coverage. The analysis broadly sees a break between the developments of the first four decades after Independence to the time when there was a policy move from the public to private sector development, from health care being a 'service' to an 'economic good', and commercialization was accompanied by the corporatization of the economy and the health sector (Baru 2000; Rao 1999; Sengupta 2013).

3. The 'globalization' of the eighteenth and nineteenth centuries through colonial hegemony by capitalist societies of Western Europe and the US introduced the medical service system that was later adopted as a model for India and other developing countries. Besides encouraging reliance on modern medical technology and its commodification, the model also delegitimized the 'native', lay people's perceptions, and the folk practices related to health and illness that were most accessible, as well as potentially cost-effective and empowering (Antia 1981; Banerji 1985, 1986; Nandy and Visvanathan 1990; Priya 2012; Sadgopal and Sagar 2007; Sathyamala, Nalini, and Nirmala 1986). This has created an alienated health service that reflects social class and expert–layperson hierarchies based on hegemony of a singular worldview.

Each of these explanations incorporates the previous one, so that the third incorporated both the first and the second. While the first is based on a liberal democratic analysis and the second on a dialectical materialist analysis, the third adds a politics of knowledge framework to economistic analyses. This framework combines a materialist explanation with the analyses of bureaucratic power and cultural hegemony dis-privileging large sections of the population, demonstrating continuity between the pre- and post-1990s periods. This is the lens through which we will examine the relationship of the state, community, and PHC as evidenced in HSD in India.

Alternative visions and models to the colonial-technocratic-capitalist one did emerge but had limited impact. It is important to examine why.

The Bhore Committee report with its plan for HSD in India (Government of India 1946) and PHC (WHO-UNICEF 1978a, 1978b) were alternatives that were adopted by the national and international health establishment. Therefore their articulation requires greater scrutiny.

EARLY DEVELOPMENTS

State's View of Community and Primary Health Care

The Indian state has been described as a 'modernizing interventionist state' that did not have the characteristics of the classical liberal-welfare states of Europe (Jayal 1999). While it did attempt to deal with poverty, disease, and inequalities through its constitutional arrangements for political processes of affirmative action and planning for socio-economic development, it did not ensure provision of social services to all citizens. It has been argued that the model of development adopted by the ruling elite was a mechanical imitation of that existing in the Euro-American industrialized societies, with the promise of modern science and technology, a 'modern' secular society, and a democratic polity. The processes of modernization and provision of the benefits of science and technology to the masses, first by the colonial government and later by the government of independent India, were part of a 'civilizing mission'. The masses were characterized as backward and superstitious, who needed to be transformed for the adoption of the scientifically legitimized lifestyle and a secular European worldview (Nandy 1988). This vision was therefore intolerant of the diverse ways of knowing and mostly treated allopathy as the only system of valid medical knowledge. This is well illustrated in Foucault's examination of the links between state power and the modern scientific medical establishment which sheds light on the dominance of medical knowledge and organized practice through the 'expert gaze', and laboratory-based indicators over patient's experience and voice (Foucault 1973).

Three broad phases of HSD can be discerned—first under the British Empire, then in the initial three decades of Independent India, and since the end of 1980s a third phase located under the rubric of 'economic globalization'. Elements of PHC, including a prominent role for 'the community', have been present in all the three phases of HSD in India, but with varied perspectives and content.

A brief description of the post-Independence development of health services will suffice here since much has been written about them (Banerji 1985; Baru 2006; Duggal 2005; Jeffery 1988; Priya 2005; Qadeer, Sen, and Nayar 2001). Only the strengths and limitations of the model proposed by the BC relevant to the questions in this chapter will be highlighted.

The Bhore Committee blueprint drew from the various HSD approaches adopted in the first and second worlds. Its basic premises were its strengths, namely, the public provisioning of free health services to all, and its view of health services as one among several other dimensions to be planned to improve the health of the population. The design for HSD was three-tiered, from primary units to the district hospital, each modelled as hospitals with additional preventive activities. While the population norm for number of facilities has been more or less achieved, only a fraction of the bed strength and human resource envisaged (see Table 1.1) has been possible.

The Bhore Committee took a considered position that only the state-of-the-art 'fully trained' doctors were good enough to serve the masses (GoI 1946, vol. 2). This one policy has had long-lasting negative impact on shaping of health care in the country. At that time, the country had a doctor:population ratio of 1:6,300. The Bhore Committee wanted the ratio to move to 1:2,000, and yet recommended the banning of licentiate education and the gradual elimination of this category, which at that time constituted two-thirds of all practising doctors. This created the urgency to enhance the capacities of medical graduate education, in the British mode, rapidly.

While adopting this model, the government rejected the bottoms-up approach recommended by the Indian National Congress' Health Planning Sub-Committee (Sokhey Committee). It had recommended

TABLE 1.1   The Long-Term Programme Personnel

	Medical officers	Non-Medical staff	Hospital beds	Population per institution
Primary Unit	6	78	75 beds	20,000
Secondary Unit Headquarters	140	358	650 beds	6,00,000
District Hospital	239	1,398	2,500 beds	30,00,000

Source: GoI (1946) cited in Bhore Committee, Volume 2:24.

that youth be trained as health workers in each village, with the best among them provided higher education as graduate doctors (National Planning Committee 1948). The chosen policy was in keeping with the Nehruvian internationalist model of modernization, as against the bottoms-up Gandhian vision of development (Priya 2005).

With medical colleges for the production of doctors getting priority, little attention was paid to the primary and secondary levels of public health service delivery institutions especially in rural areas. Few jobs were created in the system, therefore newly minted doctors inevitably went into private practice. Over the years, private doctors became an organized interest lobby that acquired power to orient policies. This sector was already garnering state support long before the liberalization and privatization perceived as products of globalization (LPG). The health systems development did not materialize as planned; mainly because only 3–5 per cent of the government budget was allocated to health whereas the BC had proposed that 15 per cent of the budget be allocated.

What then was the normative rationality of the hospital-based, doctor-centred model given its poor effectiveness, especially in the context of the country's human and knowledge resources and its expansive basic needs priorities?

The Bhore Committee took a conscious position against the inclusion of other systems of knowledge. This proved untenable since the sociopolitical pressures ensured that the traditional systems were officially recognized and supported. However, they were allocated only 2–3 per cent of the total health budget against 90 per cent to modern medicine, reflecting what has been termed as 'undemocratic pluralism' (Priya 2012). An even more step-daughterly treatment was reserved for folk knowledge by the state which chose to ignore it completely, demonstrating the hierarchy in the official imagination—from modern medicine to codified traditional systems to folk knowledge (Hardiman and Projit 2012; Shankar and Unnikrishnan 2004; Sujatha and Abraham 2012).

Health Sector Reforms

1980s–90s

Health sector reform (HSR) has been a major policy concern from mid-1980s—privatization, commercialization, and corporatization of health care advanced rapidly during this period. (Baru 2000; Qadeer, Sen, and Nayar 2001). Selective rather than Comprehensive PHC (SPHC and CPHC) was much in evidence, with the Reproductive Child Health (RCH) and disease control programmes. The World Bank's prescriptions for 'Investing in Health' further medicalized public health and commodified health care (Rao 1999). Epidemiological concepts and tools brought into use during this period have been acknowledged to be misplaced, for example, in estimating the extent of HIV prevalence (NACO, WHO, and UNAIDS 2007; Priya 2008), and the use of DALYs (Barker and Green 1996; Priya 2001b; Qadeer, Sen, and Nayar 2001). The outcome of such distortion of priorities has led to the increasing resort to private sector services, and growing disparity in access to health care (MoHFW 2007).

2000s

By 2000, there was wide recognition of market failure in health care (Rice 2013) causing a return of strengthening public systems to the agenda as reflected in the WHO Annual Reports over the decade. However, the approach adopted continued with the over-medicalizing spree instead of going back to the Alma-Ata PHC (Government of India 2002). The National Rural Health Mission (NRHM), initiated in 2005–06 (Government of India 2006) and the setting up of a High Level Expert Group on Universal Health Coverage (HLEG) in 2011, were two important initiatives by the central government to accommodate the demands of health activists and the international pressure for strengthening public services and UHC. Both involved civil society and health movement groups in their formulation with wide consultations. Their objectives included the improvement of access of services to all sections, community participation at all levels from village to secondary institutions, and a focus on addressing inter-sectoral linkages for health. Thus, NRHM and HLEG seem to hark back to Alma-Ata. Significantly, though they do not mention 'appropriate technology' and 'self-reliance'.

Although the Indian state viewed the provision of universal health care as its responsibility, the model of HSD it adopted created a 'logic' that tilted the system towards provisioning by the private sector through a doctor and institution-centred system, to the detriment of the objectives of PHC. These trends in public health planning have been analysed as attempted welfarism, in the 1950s to 1970s, its limitations being recognized and correctives instituted over the 1980s but allowing for HSR of the 1990s and 2000s to take over and destroy whatever had been built as public health services over the previous decades. The narrative above suggests continuity across these phases, since HSR can be viewed as an intensification of the capitalist and technocratic, commodifying logic of the previous period.

Over the years, there have been social, political, and professional perspectives that have resisted such trends (MFC Bulletin 1976–2015). The discourse and campaigns on issues related to strengthening public services, making them accountable to the communities they are meant to serve—on rational drug-use and generic drugs at reasonable prices, on the right to health care—have been strengthened with evidence to support the policy advocacy. Although by and large unsuccessful in shaping the direction of HSD, these pro-poor strands have managed to restrict, and in some states, reverse anti-poor policies, such as the introduction of user fees in public institutions or the conversion of public services into public–private partnerships. Thus, these campaigns have served to slow down the pace of commercialization of health services.

Through this whole process, there have also been efforts at creating other models of HSD (Government of India 2006; JSS 2015).[1,2] Public health scholars, civil society and movement groups, policymakers, and administrators have worked at developing ideas that are more conducive to universal access, self-reliance, cost-effectiveness, less commercialization and medicalization (Banerji 1986, 1993; Government of India 2011; Phadke and Shukla 2011; Priya 2011). Community participation and pro-poor health care models have been the hallmark of these efforts. 'Demystification' of modern medical knowledge and the legitimization of traditional and folk knowledge are two approaches that address issues of the politics of knowledge.

COMMUNITY IN HEALTH SYSTEMS DEVELOPMENT

The definition of 'a community' has been a contested issue in public health. The most commonly understood use of the word, that is, 'a group of people living in the same place or having a particular characteristic in common', does not take into account the existing social diversity and hierarchy.

A more acceptable definition is as 'a social unit of any size that shares common values or interests'. Since the 'group with commonality of values and interests' may vary depending on the purpose of coming together as a community, demarcating the community can be at various levels, from each caste/tribe or 'pada' in a village being considered a community, for example, when deciding location of hand pumps, to the village being one community—as in case of getting a health centre in the village—to the district or region being perceived as one's 'desh', to the 'Indian community' among the diaspora.

Geographically located rural and urban communities are divided into caste/tribe/religion-based subcommunities that may have differential access to health resources and be very insular in that specific knowledge and information is shared only within the family or caste group. However, the great divide is the significant health differentials between the poor and the economically better off since conditions of life are starkly different, epidemiological needs and priorities tend to be different, thereby the class background of those in power and the constituencies they cater to influence policy priorities (Banerji 1985; Qadeer 1985a). Finally, there is the multiplicity of intersecting identities across social groupings, for example, of women of a particular caste, who could simultaneously be mothers, adolescents, women workers, and so on (Priya 2006).

What has been called the 'Bharat–India divide' represents two different kinds of cultural capital. 'Bharat' notionally represents forms of social capital that are largely indigenously rooted, socialized in traditional ways of life, and relating to local ecosystems. 'India' represents the more globalized, modernized form of cultural capital. This is not so much an economic divide as one of legitimacy of ways of life and worldview (Nandy 1988; Nandy and Visvanathan 1990). Another variation that is significant to this analysis is of a mindset with a centralizing, homogenizing, controlling tendency and the other that tends to support diversity, openness, contextualization, and autonomy. Both are found within *both*—the Bharat and the India segments (Heredia 2009).

Common interests and social cohesion for 'an Indian community', or communities seem to emerge when we compare Indian data sets with those of other countries, on aggregate and across socio-economic categories (Priya 2006; Upadhya 1998). Social capital in India is strong in its various forms—bonding, bridging, and linking—but with the caveat that given the level of diversities, conflicts of interest are also likely to surface in the context of an environment of competition (Kesharvani 2007). Thus, it is the complexity of community groups and their societal interactions, the cohesion, and conflicts that have to be kept in mind.

Communities and the State

The state has attempted to involve communities, most often geographically located populations with administrative units creating boundaries, such as a village, block, or district. The BC recommended Village Health Committees to enlist the community's cooperation in health programmes. In the 1950s and 1960s, HSD at the primary level was incorporated in the Community Development Programme. With its limited achievements, attempts were made by civil society and health activist groups to strengthen primary-level services through active community participation. The official Community Health Volunteer scheme was initiated in 1978, the local elected bodies in rural and urban areas were given greater powers over primary-level services, especially in the 1980s–90s in wake of the 73rd and 74th constitutional amendments. Communitization of services was adopted through an Act in the state of Nagaland in 2002, and the NRHM included a basket of measures for it. Implementation of these was confronted by the societal complexity, but was often not addressed within the services/programme design (Qadeer 1985b).

Community monitoring and planning under the NRHM remained at the pilot stage in seven of the nine states where they were initiated. However, in two, Tamil Nadu and Maharashtra, they were taken forward by non-governmental organizations (NGOs), who built systematic mechanisms to involve communities in monitoring services at the primary and secondary levels. These efforts have expanded to make dialogue with government health care providers possible and show visible impact on functioning of services (Gaitonde et al. 2015; Shukla, Scott, and Kakde 2011). These are undoubtedly important initiatives towards democratic engagement of communities. But they did not adequately question the prevailing over-medicalization of health.

Health interest groups such as 'People Living with HIV' and 'service user groups', have also begun to be acknowledged by public health initiatives since the 1990s. This chapter refers to them only in passing since they do not appear to have had salience as yet in the development of general health services in India.

The policy of affirmative action—reservations and special targeting of benefits to the historically deprived groups, the Scheduled Castes (SC) and Scheduled Tribes (ST)—has also configured affirmative action on reservations in education and jobs, and others. The SC, ST, and households Below Poverty Line (BPL) have received financial concessions for specific services. Medical care for workers/employees of the formal sector—constituted less than 10 per cent of all workers—has been provided through such entities as the Employees Social Insurance Scheme (ESIS), Central Government Health Service (CGHS), and the railways health services.

The greater resort of the poor to public services for institutional health care has been well documented. Studies point to a greater level of trust and higher assessment by laypeople of the knowledge and skills of government doctors. Until the 1990s when privatization took over the public imagination, it was the District Hospital and larger government hospitals that were largely preferred by all classes. However, by 2000s, it is largely the poor who approached public hospitals mostly because of their inability to pay for private sector services.

Across this great complexity in Indian society, we find some common patterns of health-seeking behaviour, of perceptions and knowledge. Medical pluralism is a common finding in medical anthropological studies (Gould 1967; Sujatha and Abraham 2012).

Studies of the 1950s and 1960s, mainly anthropological, focused on the 'resistance to use of modern medical services' (Carstairs 1955; Marriot 1955). Historical evidence even in the 1940s (cited in the BC Report) demonstrates otherwise, with reports of overcrowded hospitals and dispensaries. Other studies of the 1960s find a significant resort to modern medicine (Banerji 1973; Banerji and Anderson 1963). From the 1980s, studies (especially public health and health systems studies) have tended to focus on the resort to allopathic medicine to the exclusion of other forms of health care (Banerji 1982; FRCH 1994; MoHFW 2007; Zurbrigg 1984). Policy statements as well as civil society initiatives have incorporated other systems in community health programmes variously highlighting their role in health care (Antia and Bhatia 1993; Banerji 1979; Government of India 2002, 2011) and there has been a growing research interest in other systems of medicine. But only from the 2000s did public health researchers begin to examine them from a systems perspective (Lohokare 2012; Narayan 2008; Priya and Shweta 2010; Sadgopal and Sagar 2007).

The 'resistance to modern medicine' was shown to be a misinterpretation of the non-utilization of medical services by the villagers (Banerji 1973; Djurfeldt and Lindberg 1975; Gould 1967). However, what these and a large number of other studies demonstrate is the social alienation of the modern health care service structure and providers from the community. This arose from three health service factors—the contemptuous behaviour of the health care providers, commercialization of health care, and the experience of the limitations of modern medicine.

Data sets and studies showing the gradient of health status across the hierarchy of caste/tribe, class and gender, spatial location, and so on abound (IIPS 2007). They all show a dominant resort to modern medicine. But they tend to ignore a considerable continuing use of other forms of treatment (Priya and Shweta 2010; WHO 2005). This under-reporting of use of the 'other' forms of health care has resulted in a gap in public health data and literature on health-seeking behaviour and perceptions of 'the community'.

Democratizing struggles, such as of the women's movement, Gandhian, and environmental perspectives, have highlighted the issue of hegemony of the doctor over the bodies of people, and actively worked for alternatives that empower people to 'know their own bodies' and thus break the hegemony of the expert (Boston Women's Health Collective 1971; Gandhi 1954; Khattri and Joshi 2015). Studies on the politics of contraception, on the notion of 'default' by patients, on 'malingering' by workers, on bottom-up versus top-down planning, all relate to the 'rationality' of the lay people and the significance of this rationality for designing health systems and programmes (Banerji 1985; Priya 2001a, 2001b; Sathyamala 2005). This perspective has been widely available in sociological and anthropological literature but is yet marginal to public health and systems discourse. The greater resort of the poor to public services for institutional health care has been well documented and studies increasingly point to greater level of trust and higher assessment by laypeople of knowledge and skills of government doctors (Priya 2012, 2001a).

In according supremacy to the physician, Ayurveda is similar to the modern medical system's doctor-centred vision of health care (Sharma 2014). Yet, it needs to be noted that the organic link of folk medicine and the textual indigenous systems is remarkable in its continuity (Balasubramanian and Radhika 1990; Sujatha and Abraham 2012; Priya and Shweta 2010). Therefore, understanding the epistemology and principles of the textual systems is relevant for validation, legitimization, and promotion of the folk knowledge and practices.

The final section of the chapter examines why primary health care as a concept did not become mainstream despite its wide acceptance. Besides reiterating the role of the larger social and political system in determining the directions and extent of implementation of the policy framework, we contend that the articulation of the PHC approach itself contributed to non-implementation of its very spirit. We examine the Alma-Ata Declaration for the way it defined the state's role in health care, and of its vision of the 'community' in the PHC approach.

PRIMARY HEALTH CARE APPROACH: ALMA-ATA 1978

The principles of PHC were specifically enunciated and adopted in the 1970s in the Alma-Ata Declaration of 1978. It was defined as

> Primary Health Care is *essential* health care based on *practical, scientifically sound, and socially acceptable methods and technology* made *universally accessible* to individuals and families in the community by means acceptable to them, through *their full participation* and at a cost that the community and country *can afford to maintain* at every stage of their development *in the spirit of self-reliance and self-determination.* It forms an integral part both of the country's health system of which it *is the central function and main focus,* and of *the overall social and economic development* of the community.
>
> (WHO-UNICEF 1978a; emphasis added)

It incorporated outcomes of efforts in Russia, UK, and the Nordic countries in earlier years, as well as later developments in third world countries such as China and India. It was, however, evident that the alternative bottom-up models developed on the ground in the third world were mere mentions in the larger context of the continued advocacy of dominant modern medicine. As an illustration, the barefoot doctor in China and the three-tier health care service structure adopted for rural health services in India since 1950 are echoed in the PHC documents. However, the incorporation of traditional medical systems and practitioners in the public health care systems that had taken place in the two largest Asian countries found only a passing mention.

PHC, the State, and the Community

In a resolution of the UN member nation states, national governments accepted responsibility for implementing PHC. Yet, arguing that the state in developing countries could not afford the expense or adequately deliver PHC, community participation was considered necessary (WHO-UNICEF 1978b: 1).

The community was to be 'mobilized through appropriate education' to take the responsibility for its own health. This

> ... includes the acceptance by individuals of a high degree of responsibility for their own health care—for example, by adopting a healthy life-style, by applying principles of good nutrition and hygiene, or by making use of immunization services. In addition, members of the community can contribute labour as well as financial and other resources to primary health care.
>
> (WHO-UNICEF 1978b: 20)

This can only be read as a strategic 'use' of the community to implement what the state was not capable of doing on its own. On the other hand is the notion of empowering the community to be in control of developments related to its life concerns through its participation at every stage of planning and implementation (WHO-UNICEF 1978b: 20).

However, nowhere in the declaration is there an acknowledgement of the laypersons and the community's fund of knowledge, both traditional and contemporary experiential. Traditional practitioners are mentioned almost in passing:

> These community health workers, *including traditional practitioners where applicable,* will function best if they reside in the community they serve and are properly trained socially and technically to respond to its expressed needs.
>
> (WHO-UNICEF 1978a: 3; emphasis added)

> Traditional medical practitioners and birth attendants are found in most societies. They are often part of the local community, culture and traditions and continue to have high social standing in many places, exerting considerable influence on local health practices. With the support of the formal health system, these indigenous practitioners can become important allies in organizing efforts to improve the health of the community. Some communities may select them as community health workers. It is therefore worthwhile exploring the possibilities of engaging them in Primary Health Care and of *training them* accordingly.
>
> (WHO-UNICEF 1978a: 33; emphasis added)

Thus, at best, their role is conceptualized as of trusted informal influencers of community health behaviour, needing training in PHC while their own knowledge and skills are attributed little worth in contributing towards it. Incorporating home remedies and other lay practices based on traditional and experiential knowledge is then a far cry.

The Alma-Ata documents speak of 'appropriate technology' and that 'health care must be available as close to the community as possible' to check costs and dependence on high-end medical technologies. Here too 'appropriate technology' does not include consideration of traditional medicine and folk practices, situated within the homes and communities.

There are three versions of PHC: (*i*) Primary-level care with a feasible, affordable, 'essential health care' package that has become known as Selective Primary Health Care, based on primary-level care and 'community mobilization' through the campaign mode, as adopted for the RCH and Polio Eradication programmes (Chen and Cash 1988); (*ii*) Comprehensive Primary Health Care (CPHC) with primary-level care as central to HSD and appropriate secondary and tertiary care to support it, including medical and non-medical interventions that are preventive, promotive, curative, and rehabilitative; and (*iii*) The CPHC that includes the local folk knowledge-based home and community care at primary level, backed up by the institutional primary, secondary, and tertiary levels.

Even while promoting the role of non-medical personnel, the document offers no critique of prevailing medical practice. Missing in the PHC approach has been a consideration of ethics of the medical industry and profession. Concerns about professional medical ethics and lack of regulation in India had been raised earlier (Jesani 1995; Medical Action Forum 1983; Srinivasan 1995), but gained urgency in the late 1990s, with the crass commercialization of health care making unethical practices pervasive and the regulatory mechanisms paying scant attention to the violations (Bhat 1996).

Finally, these policy visions and blueprints do not address the issue of 'affordability' of all levels of the modern medical enterprise. The Bhore Committee to begin with pondered whether it should restrict itself to recommending a health service system limited by the resource constraints or should it create an 'ideal' blueprint unfettered by the question of financial outlay. It decided on doing the latter (GoI 1946), and found that this would require about 15 per cent of the total government budget (GoI 1946). Three decades later, PHC was offered as the solution to the unaffordability of the first world models of health care (WHO-UNICEF 1978a), promoting the role of a range of lesser trained providers of health care than the 'fully-trained doctor'. However, without a focus on people's empowerment, the language of appropriate technology, issues of feasibility and affordability have allowed the medical establishment to reassert (Walsh and Warren 1979), resulting in the well-known shift to 'Selective PHC' (SPHC).

Now, the HLEG provides a full blueprint for UHC but it is evident that only the primary level is implementable at the levels of financial and human resource presently available for the public system (much like the BC, see Figure 1.1). The NRHM attempted to operationalize CPHC, but it did not contend with the medicalized mindset, the commercialization of the sector, or the technocracy because of which it remained a top-down approach. The health systems development designing for people's empowerment through agency and space for community world views has been worked out by a third strand, but remains marginalized (Banerji 1986; ICSSR-ICMR 1981; Priya 2011).

Here too we need to examine the limitations of the discourse since the 1970s. Nearly all the focus of the civil society and health movement groups has been on how to design and implement primary-level services. A radical redesign of the secondary- and tertiary-level services in the spirit of PHC has not received much attention (Zachariah 2012). Secondly, the huge financial implications of modern health service systems have not been a major concern in the 1950s–80s. It is only the HSR that brought attention to these, first by shifting costs to the users, and, since the mid-2000s, through social insurance in the UHC

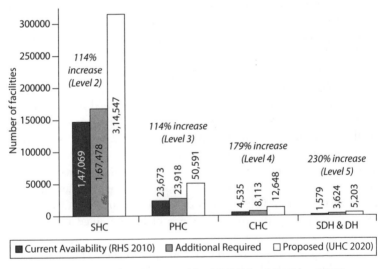

FIGURE 1.1   Plan Proposed by HLEG for UHC by 2020

Source: Government of India (2011: 206).

agenda (Prasad and Raghavendra 2012; Reddy et al. 2011). A spate of studies and policy discussions on financing has emerged in this period. But there is little thinking on how to design systems to check the ever-escalating irrational medical technology costs, or the iatrogenesis it inflicts (Illich 1977).

A critical analysis of the biopolitics and the political economy of health care development over the past century must thus consider five 'missing links' in the dominant discourse of HSD policy—the complexity of 'community' and disparities and diversities within; the validity of plurality of knowledge and its hierarchies; the culture and ethics of health care providers; the unaffordability of the Euro-American institutional model of medical technology-based health care; and the physical, social, and cultural iatrogenesis (Illich 1977). Negotiating this web poses a difficult challenge. There are no easy solutions. Policy choices will be made based on ideological predilections of the social forces wielding power. Answers can optimally come from creating structures that enable operationalization of the values of transparency in rational policymaking, democratic pluralism, bottom-up and dialogic processes for continuous shaping and reshaping of systems. This is the PHC agenda and spirit.

* * *

An expensive, commodified, and community-distant health service system was developed by an elitism that relied on colonial categories and dominance of expert knowledge (traditional and modern), through the collusion of the medical industry and the technocratic public administration. The primary health care approach was an attempt at course-correction, which influenced HSD globally, but could not redirect mainstream medical care that remained doctor and institution-centred. The primary health care approach paid little more than lip service to medical pluralism, lay knowledge, and self-care that had been delegitimized rendering communities disempowered.

Countervailing sociopolitical perspectives forced the mainstream to concede the role of communities. In the 1950s–60s, the Community Development Programme accommodated the Gandhian stream but the dominant Nehruvian approach adopted the BC plan for HSD. In the 1970s–80s the NHP–1983, ICSSR-ICMR report, and others, accommodated the dissent of that time but the medical establishment only grew in strength and the PHC implementation became SPHC.

In the 2000s, the NRHM and HLEG have again been initiatives to accommodate the dissent expressed through advocacy of the 'rights approach' and 'health systems strengthening', while the corporate private sector flourishes unregulated and the community becomes increasingly dependent on the profiteering and iatrogenic medical services.

The Bhore Comittee report was an excellent technical public health document. It espoused the universalist, singular knowledge of science, but was not purely medicalized in its paradigm for improving the population's health and did focus on building a strong edifice of a public system of health services. In hindsight three limitations in its model are evident—the expectation of high resource inputs into health care by an impoverished country, the explicit devaluing and rejection of other systems of knowledge, and the absence of any policy for the private sector in health care.

The PHC vision emerged as a negotiated document on primary health care as the Alma-Ata Declaration between the pro-poor and self-reliance streams and those in power within the international and national political economy. It focused primarily on the first of BC limitations. The need for low-cost 'affordable' health services perceived by the rulers to provide health care universally, coinciding with what the progressive health movement/activists of the time advocated. However, analysis of the outcome of the consensus declaration shows that the barriers to the declaration leading to self-reliance and community/people's empowerment are inherent in the articulation of the vision itself. My argument goes further to suggest that this is not merely because it is a negotiated document but also because even among those advocating the progressive view, the politics of knowledge is only weakly recognized as being important for the articulation of the vision of PHC. Unless the knowledge and choices of laypeople are valued, there is little possibility of 'community participation' especially in decision-making, which is essential for 'empowerment'. The analysis also identified four other major gaps in the Alma-Ata documents. Earlier critical analyses of the PHC document have found it to be too vague and open to multiple interpretations. Proposed here is a re-reading of the document as one that had inherent contradictions in its spirit, especially in relation to the community. We suggest here a redrafting of a PHC-II that draws upon and incorporates the experience of the last century.

Viewed from the community end, health care gets the most comprehensive vision, linking the environmental and social determinants as well as the continuum of health care from home remedies and preventive action to institutions providing outdoor and indoor care of allopathy and other systems. This, however, allows the political economy of HSD to be ignored.

The structural view of health care examines the political economy of HSD and the role of non-medical determinants of health, but it tends to be top-down and discounts the agency of communities and individuals. When converted into an operational vision for HSD, it has tended to undermine the communities of laypeople and their systemic role in health care.

The techno-managerial view of planning and implementation of health service systems tends to focus on the institutional infrastructure and its service efficiency, ignoring both the community's sociocultural dimensions and the political economy of health care. Attempts to incorporate these considerations in systems design, for example, by the NRHM and HLEG, without critically analysing the BC and PHC frameworks results in echoing the limitations of the latter, which had failed to consider the basic prerequisites for community agency in their model of health care.

Since all the three views have a valid and complementary role in HSD, the second challenge is to link the three views together in a holistic framework. Existing literature offers much data and several optional research designs. However, much more reflection seems necessary to contribute meaningfully to the constantly evolving health care system based on the dynamic relationship between the community, the state, expert knowledge, and the technologies available from home to hospital.

This is a challenge for health systems analysts and researchers as much as it is for planners and policymakers. Recent advances in health systems research have attempted to do so, but still tend to be focused on techno-managerial operationalization without according due significance to the agency of lay communities or to the political economy of health care. Since people are central actors in their own health, health systems studies and health systems designing need to take their knowledge and behaviour as important components of the health care system. Beginning at this end of the system and moving up the pyramid of health care is the bottom-up approach to understanding systems and planning that is likely to produce contextually suited health care. This is an area for much more scholarship, research, and action through holistic health systems studies and action research.

NOTES

1. See also IHST, Institute of Trans-disciplinary Health Sciences and Technology. Available at: http://ihstuniversity.org. Accessed on 2 October 2015.
2. See also ARSI, 2005. Introducing the Association of Rural Surgeons of India. Available at: http://www.arsi-india.org/. Accessed on 2 October 2015.

REFERENCES

Antia, N.H. 1981. 'Health for All: A Reaffirmation', *Economic and Political Weekly* 16(33): 1363–4.

Antia, N.H. and K. Bhatia. 1993. *People's Health in People's Hand: Indian Experiences in Decentralized Health Care.* Pune: Foundation for Research in Community Health.

Balasubramanian, A.V. and M. Radhika. 1990. *Local Health Traditions: An Introduction.* Madras: LSPSS.

Banerjee, M. 2009. *Power, Knowledge, Medicine: Ayurvedic Pharmaceuticals at Home and in the World.* Hyderabad: Orient Blackswan.

Banerji, D. 1967. 'Health Economics in Developing Countries', *Journal of Indian Medical Association* 49(9): 417–21.

———. 1969. 'Administration of the Family Planning Programme: A Plea for an Operation Research Approach', *Management in Government* 1(2): 46.

———. 1973. 'Health Behaviour of Rural Population in India: Impact of Rural Health Services', *Economic and Politcal Weekly* 8(51): 2261–8.

———. 1979. 'Place of the Indigenous and the Western System of Medicine in the Health Services of India', *International Journal of Health Services* 9(3): 511–19.

———. 1982. *Poverty, Class and Health Culture in India.* New Delhi: Prachi Prakashan.

———. 1985. *Health and Family Planning Services in India—An Epidemiological, Socio-Cultural and Political Analysis and a Perspective.* New Delhi: LokPaksh.

———. 1986. *Social Science and Health Service Development in India—Sociology of Formation of an Alternative Paradigm.* Delhi: LokPaksh.

———. 1993. 'A Social Science Approach to Strengthening India's National Tuberculosis Programme', *Indian Journal of Tuberculosis* 40: 61–82.

Banerji, D. and Anderson. 1963. 'A Sociological Study of Awareness of Symptoms Among Persons with Tuberculosis', *WHO Bulletin*: 665–83.

Barker, C. and A. Green. 1996. 'Opening the Debate on DALYs (disability-adjusted life years)', *Health Policy and Planning* 11(2): 179–83.

Baru, R.V. 2000. 'Privatization and Corporatization'. *Seminar* 489.

———. 2006. *Privatisation of Health Care in India: A Comparative Analysis of Orissa, Karnataka and Maharashtra States.* New Delhi: IIPA.

Bhat, R. 1996. 'Regulation of the Private Health Sector in India', *International Journal of Health Planning Management* 11(3): 253–74.

Bose, A. and P.B. Desai (eds). 1983. *Studies in Social Dynamics of Primary Health Care*. Delhi: Hindustan Publication House.

Boston Women's Health Collective. 1971. *Our Bodies Ourselves*. Boston: Boston Women's Health Collective.

Carstairs, G.M. 1955. 'Medicine and Faith in Rural Rajasthan'. In *Health, Culture and Community*, P.D. Paul (ed.), pp. 107–34. New York: Russell Sage Foundation.

Chen, L.C. and R.A. Cash. 1988. 'A Decade after Alma-Ata: Can Primary Health Care Lead to Health for All?', *The New England Journal of Medicine* 319(14): 946–7.

Djurfeldt, G. and S. Lindberg. 1975. *Pills Against Poverty: A Study of the Introduction of Western Medicine in a Tamil Village*. New Delhi: Oxford and IBH Publishers.

Drèze, J. and A. Sen. 2013. *An Uncertain Glory: India and its Contradictions*. Princeton, New Jersey: Princeton University Press.

Duggal, R. 2005. 'Historical Review of Health Policy Making'. In *Review of Healthcare in India*, L.V. Gangolli, R. Duggal, and A. Shukla (eds), pp. 21–40. Mumbai: Centre for Enquiry into Health and Allied Themes.

Foucault, M. 1973. *The Birth of the Clinic: An Archaeology of Medical Perception*. UK: Routledge.

FRCH. 1994. *Health Research Studies in India, A Review and Annotated Bibliography*. Bombay: FRCH.

Gaitonde R., K. Sheikh, P. Saligram, and D. Nambiar. 2015 (nd.). *Community Participation in Health: The National Landscape*. Available at: http://uhc-india.org/uploads/GaitondeRetal_CommunityParticipationinHealthTheNationalLandscapeinIndia.pdf. Accessed on 2 October 2015.

Gandhi, M.K. 1954. *Nature Cure*. Ahmedabad: Navajivan Publication House.

Government of India. 1946. *Report of the Health Survey and Development Committee* (Bhore Committee Report). Calcutta: Government of India.

———. 2002. *National Health Policy–2002*. Department of Health, New Delhi: Ministry of Health and Family Welfare.

———. 2006. *National Rural Health Mission. A Framework for Implementation*. Available at: http://nrhm.gov.in/.

———. 2011. *High Level Expert Group Report on Universal Health Coverage for India*. New Delhi: Planning Commission of India.

Gould, G.D. 1967. 'Implications of Technological Changes for Folk and Scientific Medicine', *American Anthropologists* 59(3): 507–16.

Hardiman, D. and B.M. Projit. 2012. *Medical Marginality in South Asia Situating Subaltern Therapeutics*. London and New York: Routledge.

Heredia, R.C. 2009. 'Gandhi's Hinduism and Savarkar's Hindutva', *Economic and Political Weekly* 44 (29): 62–7.

ICSSR-ICMR. 1981. *Health for All: An Alternative Strategy*. Pune: Indian Institute of Education.

IIPS. 2007. National Family Health Survey, (NFHS-3), 2005–6. Mumbai: International Institute for Population Sciences, Mumbai.

Illich, I. 1977. *Limits to Medicine: Medical Nemesis: The Expropriation of Health*. Harmondsworth: Penguin.

Jayal, N.G. 1999. 'The Gentle Leviathan: Welfare and the Indian State'. In *Disinvesting in Health–The World Bank's Prescription for Health*, M. Rao (ed.), pp. 39–47. New Delhi: SAGE.

Jeffery, R. 1988. *The Politics of Health in India, Comparative Studies of Health Systems and Medical Care*. Berkeley: University of California Press.

Jesani, A. 1995. 'Violence and Ethical Responsibility of the Medical Profession', *Medical Ethics* 3(1): 3–5.

JSA. 2000–15. 'People Health Movement–India'. Available at: http://www.phmovement.org/en/taxonomy/term/189. Accessed on 2 October 2015.

JSS. 2015. 'When Hospital Talks to Its People'. Available at: http://www.jssbilaspur.org/resource/index.php. Accessed on 2 October 2015.

Kesharvani, P. 2007. 'The Relevance of Social Capital for Public Health: Reviewing the Debate'. Unpublished MPhil Dissertation. New Delhi: Centre of Social Medicine and Community Health, Jawaharlal Nehru University.

Khattri, P. and P.C. Joshi. 2015. 'Bio-medicalization and Gandhi's Vision of Health: Observations from Sevagram', *Economic and Politcal Weekly* 50(10).

Lohokare, M. 2012. *Report of the Proceeding of the International Workshop-Integrating Traditional South Asian Medicine into Modern Health Care System*. Available at: http://www.jnu.ac.in/SSS/CSMCH/ITSAMMHCS.pdf. Accessed on 12 August 2014.

Marriot, M. 1955. 'Western Medicine in a Village of North India'. In *Health, Culture and Community*, P.D. Paul (ed.), pp. 239–68. New York: Russell Sage Foundation.

Medical Action Forum. 1983. 'Medical Ethics and Practice'. Letter to Editor. *MFC Bulletin*: 93.

MFC Bulletins. 1976–2015. Available at: http://www.mfcindia.org/main/bulletins.html. Accessed on 2 October 2015.

MoHFW. 2007. *Selected Health Parameters: A Comparative Analysis Across the National Sample Survey Organization 42th 52nd and 60th Round*. New Delhi: Ministry of Health and Family Welfare, Government of India in collaboration with WHO Country Office for India.

NACO, WHO, and UNAIDS. 2007. '2.5 Million People in India Living with HIV, According to New Estimates'. Available at: http://www.who.int/mediacentre/news/releases/2007/pr37/en/. Accessed on 23 February 2008.

Nandy, A. 1988. *The Intimate Enemy: Loss and Recovery of Self Under Colonialism*. New Delhi, New York: Oxford University Press.

Nandy, A. and S. Visvanathan. 1990. 'Modern Medicine and Its Non-Modern Critics: A Study in Discourse'. In *Dominating Knowledge: Development, Culture, and Resistance*, Frèdèrique Apffel Marglin and Stephen A. Marglin (eds), pp. 94–145. WIDER Studies in Development Economics. Clarendon Press.

Narayan, R. 2008. 'AYUSH and Public Health—Policy Review—Ideas and Mandates (1946–2006)'. Presentation at Stakeholders' Workshop on AYUSH Interventions in Public Health, FRLHT/CHC/Community Health Cell. Banglore, 8–9 February 2008.

National Planning Committee. 1948. *National Planning Committee—National Health (Sokhey Committee)*. Bombay: Vora and Co., Publisher Ltd.

Phadke, A. 2004. 'The Dismantling of Public Health System in India—What Should be Our Approach?', *Medico Friend Circle Bulletin* 304: 5–7.

Phadke, A. and A. Shukla. 2011. 'Toward a Regulatory Framework for Private Providers in UHC', *Medico Friend Circle Bulletin* 345–7: 1–8.

Prasad, N. Purendra and P. Raghavendra. 2012. 'Health Care Models in the Era of Medical Neo Liberalism—A Study of Aarogyasri in Andhra Pradesh', *Economic and Political Weekly* 47(43): 118–26.

Priya, R. 2001a. 'Study of Illness, Disease and Well-Being among a Group of Construction Workers in Their Ecological Context'. Unpublished PhD Thesis submitted at Centre of Social Medicine and Community Health. Jawaharlal Nehru University. New Delhi.

———. 2001b. 'Disability Adjusted Life Years as a Tool for Public Health Policy—A Critical Assessment'. In *Public Health and the Poverty of Reforms—The South Asian Predicament*, Imrana Qadeer, Kasturi Sen, and K.R. Nayar (eds), pp. 154–73. New Delhi: SAGE.

———. 2005. 'Public Health Services in India: A Historical Perspective'. In *Review of Healthcare in India*, L.V. Gangolli, R. Duggal, and A. Shukla (eds), pp. 41–74. Mumbai: Centre for Enquiry into Health and Allied Themes.

———. 2006. 'Towards Health Security for Women and Children: Exploring Debated and Options'. In *Health Security for All—Challenges and Possibilities*, Sujata Prasad and C. Sathyamala (eds), pp. 328–52. New Delhi: Institute of Human Development.

———. 2008. 'AIDS in Perspective: Between Exaggeration and Denial—Revisiting the Epidemiology of HIV Infection'. In *Dialogue on AIDS: Perspectives for the Indian Context*, Ritu Priya and Shalina Mehta (eds), pp. 29–81. New Delhi: Vasudhaiva Kutumbakam Publication.

———. 2011. 'UAHC with "Community Participation" Or "People Centre-stage"? Implications for Governance, Provisioning and Financing', *Medico Friend Circle Bulletin* 345–7: 9–15.

———. 2012. 'AYUSH and Public Health: Democratic Pluralism and the Quality of Health Services'. In *Medical Pluralism in Contemporary India*, V. Sujatha and Leena Abraham (eds), pp. 103–29. New Delhi: Orient Blackswan.

Priya, R. and A.S. Shweta. 2010. *Status and Role of AYUSH and Local Health Traditions (Report of a Study)*. New Delhi: NHSRC, NRHM.

Qadeer, I. 1985a. 'Health Services Systems in India: An Expression of Socio-Economic Inequalities', *Social Action* (35) July–September: 199–223.

———. 1985b. 'Social Dynamics of Health care: A Case Study of the CHW Scheme in Shahdol District'. *Socialist Health Review* II (2): 74–83, 97–100.

———. 2000. 'Health Care System in Transition III. India Part I. The Indian Experience', *Journal of Public Health Medicine* 22(1): 25–32.

Qadeer, I., K. Sen, and K. R. Nayar. 2001. *Public Health and the Poverty of Reforms—The South Asian Predicament*. New Delhi: SAGE.

Rao, Mohan (ed.). 1999. *Disinvesting in Health—The World Bank's Prescription for Health*. New Delhi: SAGE.

Reddy, K.S., V. Patel, V.K. Paul, A.S. Kumar, and L. Dandona. 2011. 'Towards Achievement of Universal Health Care in India by 2020: A Call to Action'. *The Lancet* 377(9767): 760–8. Available at: http://doi.org/10.1016/S0140-6736(10)61960-5. Accessed on 10 August 2014.

Rice, T. 2013. 'Market Failure in Health Care: Still Common After All These Years'. World Bank. Available at: http://go.worldbank.org/H7DCO95U70. Accessed on 10 August 2014.

Roy, B.C. 1982. 'Future of the Medical Profession in India: Reprint of the Presidential Address at the All India Medical Conference. Lahore. December 1929', *Journal of Indian Medical Association* 78 (1 and 2): 24–30.

Sadgopal, M. and A. Sagar. 2007. 'Can Public Health Open Up to the AYUSH Systems ... And Give Space for People's Views of Health and Disease?', *Medico Friend Circle Bulletin* 324–5: 45–50.

Sathyamala, C. 2005. 'Women's Health Movement in Independent India'. In *Maladies, Preventives and Curatives—Debates in Public Health in India*, Amiya Kumar Bagchi and Krishna Soman (eds), pp. 96–108. New Delhi: Tulika Books.

Sathyamala, C., B. Nalini, and S. Nirmala. 1986. *Taking Sides—The Choices Before The Health Worker*. Madras: Asian Network for Innovative Training Trust.

Sengupta, A. 2013. 'Universal Health Coverage: Beyond Rhetoric', *Occasional Paper no. 20*. IDRC.CRDI.

Shankar, D. and P.M. Unnikrishnan. 2004. *Challenging the Indian Medical Heritage*. India: Cambridge University Press.

Sharma, P.V. (translated). 2014. *Charaka Samhita*, Sutrasthana (verse 120–3). Volume 1. Varanasi: Chaukhamba Orientalia. Online version available at: https://archive.org/details/CarakaSamhitaEng.Vol.1.

Shukla, A., K. Scott, and D. Kakde. 2011. Community Monitoring of Rural Health Services in Maharashtra, *Economic and Political Weekly* 44(30): 78–85

Srinivasan, S. 1995. 'Ethical Issues in Low Cost Drug Manufacturing', *Medico Friend Circle Bulletin* 223–4.

Sujatha, V. and L. Abraham. 2012. *Medical Pluralism in Contemporary India*. New Delhi: Orient Blackswan.

Upadhya, C. 1998. 'Conceptualising the Concept of Community in Indian Social Science: An Anthropological Perspective'. Paper presented to National Workshop on Community and Identities: Interrogating Contemporary Discourses on India. Department of Sociology. Hyderabad: University of Hyderabad.

VHAI-ICDHI. 1995–2015. *Report of Independent Commission on Development & Health in India*. Available at: http://www.vhai.org/ceo/icdhi_backgound.php. Accessed on 2 October 2015.

Walsh, J.A. and K.S. Warren. 1979. 'Selective Primary Health Care: An Interim Strategy for Disease Control in Developing Countries', *New England Journal of Medicine* 301: 967–74.

WHO. 2005. *WHO Global Atlas of Traditional, Complementary and Alternative Medicine*. World Health Organization.

WHO-UNICEF. 1978a. *Declaration of Alma-Ata*. Geneva: WHO.

———. 1978b. *Primary Health Care (Report of the International Conference on Primary Health Care)*. Geneva: WHO.

Zachariah, A. 2012. 'Tertiary Healthcare within a Universal System', *Economic and Political Weekly* 47(1): 39–45.

Zurbrigg, Sheila. 1984. *Rakku's Story: Structures of Ill Health and Source of Change*. Madras: George Joseph.

2

Health Care Reforms

Do They Ensure Social Protection for the Labouring Poor?

Purendra Prasad

How do 35 crore people in India survive on Rs 32 per person per day in urban areas and Rs 26 per person per day in rural areas? The National Commission for Enterprises in the Unorganized Sector (NCEUS) data indicates that 79 per cent of workers in the unorganized sector live on an income of less than Rs 20 a day (Yadav 2014). The economic reforms in the post-1990s significantly resulted in heightened inequality among different classes, castes, and genders. Two recent reports substantiate the growing inequalities in India. One, a research paper by Chancel and Piketty (2017) indicated that the share of national income accruing to the top 1 per cent income earners is at its highest level since the creation of Indian Income Tax Act of 1922. The top 1 per cent of earners captured less than 21 per cent of total income in the late 1930s, before dropping to 6 per cent in the early 1980s and rising to 22 per cent today. Thus, the authors concluded that income inequality in India is at its highest level since 1922. Second, India Exclusion Report 2016 which examined 25 years of India's economic liberalization indicated that as India's economy grew rapidly, the inequality between the rich and poor increased, the number of landless farmers rose and employment generation was lowest in 2015. Crisis in agriculture has pushed nine million farmers out of the sector between 2001 and 2011. The report further said that economic growth has led to higher migration with 35–40 million labourers being seasonal migrants (Centre for Equity

Studies 2017). This raises several disturbing questions: what do these people do in contingencies of illness, old age, and death? How do they protect themselves from slipping further into poverty due to expenditure on ill health? The growing recognition of the devastating effect of illnesses on the capacity of the labouring poor to work, and the rising cost of medical treatment prompted the Indian state to propose a new set of reforms to provide social protection for the unorganized workers. How successful has the state been in designing and delivering such protection? This chapter provides a critique of these reforms focusing on the possible strategies of inclusion and greater access to vulnerable groups.

Three major trends in health care services stand out as crucial factors in analysing health care reforms initiated by the state in the last decade. First, there is a substantial change in the structure of health care services in the government sector, particularly the decline of primary and secondary services. Second, there is tremendous growth of private and corporate health care, which has emerged as the mainstay for tertiary health services in India. Third, there is significant rise in out-of-pocket (OOP) expenditure due to the decline of government spending or investments along with the rise in privatization of health care services. Keeping these factors in mind, this chapter, using a political economy perspective, critically examines the key reforms undertaken by the state post-2000 and analyses whether this new model of health care is moving towards individualizing and depoliticizing rather than collectivizing health care services.

The chapter is divided into four sections. The first section talks about the changing context in which health care reforms have been introduced in the last decade. The next section provides a discussion on 'health security' or 'social protection' initiated through publicly funded health insurance and also examines how social protection mechanisms have been conceived, designed, and executed by the central and state governments. Moving on, the third section raises questions on accessibility and social security by bringing in a case of workers from an informal sector in a slum of Bholakpur in Hyderabad. The final section provides a summary of the arguments in the paper for informed discussion on the state's discourse of health security for the labouring classes.

DYNAMICS OF GOVERNMENT AND PRIVATE HEALTH CARE

Although health care reforms started in India from the 1970s, the process intensified in post-1990s. These reforms have led to significant changes in the structure of health care services.

Structure of Government Health Services

In India, government health care services have gradually declined, public investments have come down, and health care costs have risen tremendously in the past few decades. In 2012, government expenditure on health was only 1.3 per cent of Gross Domestic Product (equivalent to USD 19 per capita), one of the lowest allocations of national income in the world, compared with 3 per cent in Thailand (equivalent to USD 164 per capita) (Das Gupta and Muraleedharan 2014). Workforce shortages in government health sector are also substantial.[1]

A review indicates that government health care system grew weak by 1990s and deteriorated further post-2000, with the retreat of a neo-liberal state. Despite growing health needs, the state did not increase its budgetary allocation, rather it introduced 'partial' user charges, created paying and non-paying wards in public hospitals, and so on. Also referral services, from primary to secondary and tertiary levels, became the weak links and hospitals increasingly levied charges for items such as drugs and surgical supplies. As a result, the cost of health care particularly for the labouring poor continuously increased. These processes also accelerated the flight to the private health care services and decline in the utilization of public services (Qadeer, Sen, and Nayar 2001).[2]

Growth of Private Sector

Most hospitals in India were run either by government or private charities and Trusts till late 1970s. In the early 1980s, the state encouraged private nursing homes and small and medium hospitals to supplement government health care. In 1991 there was a drastic cut in the central government budgetary allocation for health care, which favoured the establishment of private hospitals in India. Successive governments encouraged the growth of private sector, in various ways, such as releasing the prime building land at low rates, providing exemption from taxes and duties for importing drugs, high-tech medical equipment, and so forth. In 2000 the liberalization of foreign investment policy allowed Foreign Direct Investment (FDI) in hospitals and mobilization of capital through other forms like American Depository Receipts (ADRs) and Global Depository Receipts (GDRs), upto 49 per cent, which stimulated the establishment of corporate hospitals.[3] In 2002, the Insurance Regulatory Development Authority (IRDA) allowed Third-Party Administrators, which made medical insurance with cashless hospitalization more attractive. In 2007 the de-tariffing of general insurance allowed the creation of customized medical insurance products, which further accelerated this growth and enhanced the acceptance of medical insurance in India (Berman, Ahuja, and Bhandari 2010).

These reforms rapidly accelerated the expansion of private and corporate hospitals leading to commoditization of health in India. This reflected a shift towards the growth of curative (tertiary) services with a strong commercial focus at the neglect of primary health services. Public–private partnership (PPP) became one of the most appropriate models advocated by the state in the health sector. Subsequently, outsourcing of diagnostic, sanitary, and other services taking over hospital land for other purposes, non-renewal of land leases to charity hospitals, attempts to hand over primary health centres to private organizations, and so on, were some major reforms that occurred in the last two decades (Baru 2016). These measures have been justified by the state as being reform measures to increase the viability of health care services.

Out-of-Pocket Expenditure

Poor government spending on health, resulting in inefficient and inadequate services, is one of the reasons why people seek private health providers resulting in high OOP expenses. The National Accounts and Statistics data indicates that private expenditure on health care in India is about Rs 2,750 billion, of which 98 per cent is OOP spending. In addition, the public expenditure on health care is about Rs 600 billion. Together this adds up to a total health expenditure amounting to 5.7 per cent of GDP of which OOP expenses account for 78 per (Duggal 2007). Further, particularly OOP spending on medicines is the single largest item of expenditure for households. About 30 million additional people fall into poverty each year as a result of this expenditure (Balarajan, Selvaraj, and Subramanian 2011). Disaggregated data show that the share of OOP spending on private sector is relatively higher in India than in most other developing countries (Berman, Ahuja, and Bhandari 2010). Several research studies indicated that the cost of health care has become a major burden to the labouring poor, to the extent that seeking medical assistance to recover from illness or injuries is also forfeited (Ghosh 2014; Rao and Choudhury 2012; Srikant 2014).

Due to OOP expenditure and medical debts, it is widely reported that there is increased dependence on money lenders. As a result, more than 40 per cent of all patients admitted to hospitals borrow money or sell assets including inherited property and farmland, to cover expenses, and 25 per cent of farmers are driven below poverty line (BPL) by the cost of their health care (*British Medical Journal* 2005; Prasad 2015). Moneylenders charge exorbitant interest rates between 24 per cent and 60 per cent. One can imagine the catastrophic consequences on the labouring poor and society's productivity when these rates are applied to a major part of Rs 10,000 crore (Rs 100 billion) being spent every year on hospitalization of the poor through OOP expenditure.

The Government of India policy documents, particularly the Tenth and Eleventh Plans, also recognized the growing inequalities in access to health care and the rising OOP expenditure as a serious concern. The National Health Policy (2015) draft indicates that inequalities in access need to be addressed through policies that would ensure inclusion of the poor and other vulnerable sections of the population. This, in fact, pushed the government to develop stronger contractual arrangement with private sector providers in both the non-profit and for-profit sectors (Hodges and Rao 2016; Standing 2002). It also reflected a prevailing ideological view of the potentially greater quality and efficiency of the private sector and the virtues of using competitive contracting as a way of sharing public sector resources. This vision of the neo-liberal state proposes that gains from improved management could be obtained within a contracting framework. Hence, Indian state adopted contract-based models within a publicly set framework and expanded contractual relationships between public and private health sectors (MoHFW 2017). In pursuit of this model, public health budgets have been redirected to subsidize social insurance for those sections of the population (BPL) that have been judged to be unable to pay. Health insurance became one of the viable protection strategies of the state to address both growing cost of medical care and accessibility concerns.

Therefore, there have been three kinds of reforms in post-independent India. First, in the early 1980s, reforms were initiated to encourage private nursing homes and medium hospitals in order to supplement the existing public hospitals and facilities to meet the growing needs of the sick-poor. In 1990s, the State facilitated corporate health sector to establish tertiary-level super speciality hospitals to achieve 'high quality' care. Second, the government opened up, in 2000, FDI route in hospitals and mobilization of capital stimulating the growth of corporate hospitals. Third, Insurance Regulatory Development Authority allowed third-party administrators and customized medical insurance in the last decade, supposedly to provide greater access to the poor and social protection. What is common across these three sets of reforms is the gradual de-emphasis on public health care institutions (in terms of infrastructure, manpower, finances, services, and so on), and the promotion of private and corporate hospitals by effectively allocating government resources. A careful analysis is required to examine whether the above reforms are able to provide social security for the labouring poor.

STATE'S STRATEGIES TOWARDS SOCIAL PROTECTION/SECURITY

In 2003, the UN Commission on Human Security defined 'security' to encompass the protection and empowering of people, including a focus on factors such as health, education, and a social safety net. There is no simple definition of health security. It can mean variously—human security, the prevention and control of infectious diseases, revitalizing research and development to produce global public goods, attention to non-communicable diseases, dealing with substandard and spurious drugs, considering conflict and disaster settings, addressing international migration, and building stronger health systems through universal health coverage, and so on (Horton and Das 2015). The Indian state claims to provide health security through two mechanisms—one is health insurance coverage for employees in the organized sector and the other, community (targeted) health insurance for the workers in the unorganized sector.

The working class in the organized sector has some form of health insurance coverage, either through social security legislated schemes such as the Employee State Insurance Scheme (ESIS), the Central Government Health Insurance Scheme (CGHS), the maternity benefit scheme, and various others for mine workers, plantation workers, *beedi* workers, cinema workers, seamen armed forces, railway employees, and others, or through employer provided health services or reimbursements (Desai and Kamayani 2007). About 10–12 per cent of the country's population is estimated to have the right to health care at least during the working life of the main earner in the family. As part of health reforms in 1994, the government allowed employees' reimbursement of medical bills even through the private and corporate hospitals, supposedly to provide quality health care. This opened up the window for private health sector to effectively stake a claim in the health resources of the government.

By 2015, the Government of India, recognizing the low level of public spending and its uneven distribution, acknowledged the rising OOP expenditure on health as a major cause of the immiserization of the poor.

> Yet if health care costs are more impoverishing than ever before, almost all hospitalization even in public hospitals leads to catastrophic health expenditure, and over 63 million persons are faced with poverty every year due to health care costs alone, it is because there is no financial protection for the vast majority of health care needs. In 2011–12, the share of out of pocket expenditure on health care as a proportion of total household monthly per capita expenditure was 6.9 per cent in rural areas and 5.5 per cent in urban areas. (MoHFW 2017: 8)

Thus, Government of India and several state governments introduced community health insurance schemes at the national and state levels such as, Rashtriya Swasthya Bima Yojana (RSBY), Rajiv Aarogyasri, Rajiv Gandhi Jeevandayee Aarogya Yojana, and others. The government is indeed the sole contributor to health insurance premiums as the population covered is basically below poverty line. Eight states introduced health insurance programmes covering tertiary care. Over time, as expenditure increased, many of those states (Andhra Pradesh, Telangana, Maharashtra, Kerala, Rajasthan, and others) moved to direct purchasing of care through Trusts (MoHFW 2017). The current trend of governments purchasing health care from private health sector within the contracting model in India is recent and a new phenomenon. State discourse justifies this as a means to ensure equitable access to health care including expensive, surgical-based tertiary care to the vulnerable sick-poor that the government moved to purchasing health care. This chapter further examines this proposition critically through central and state government's specific social protection schemes below.

Rashtriya Swasthya Bima Yojana (RSBY)

In 2008, the central government under the Ministry of Labour and Employment launched the RSBY. In 2003–4, the population covered in terms of health security under various schemes was about 55 million people which, government claims, has been increased to about 370 million with RSBY in 2014 (almost one-fourth of the population). Nearly two-thirds (180 million) of this population are those in the BPL category. The Rashtriya Swasthya Bima Yojana was originally limited to BPL families but was later extended to construction workers, beneficiaries of Mahatma Gandhi National Rural Employment Guarantee Act (MGNREGA), street vendors, *beedi* workers, and domestic workers. Currently the scheme is implemented in 479 districts across 27 states and two union territories (Planning Commission 2013). The Rashtriya Swasthya Bima Yojana has become the prime national insurance initiative for reducing vulnerability of the labouring poor who are in need of hospital care for serious health problems. In contrast to the MGNREGA, which remained limited to the rural poor, the RSBY facility covers the labouring poor in the urban slums as well. The support covers the cost of hospitalization for an operation up to a maximum of Rs 30,000 per annum for a household consisting of five members. The scheme includes maternity benefits and the cost of childbirth. Promoted as a PPP, the premium of Rs 750 is paid to hand-picked private and some public-sector insurance companies, shared between central and state government in 75:25 ratio. A smart card is issued to the head of the household and a maximum of four other family members listed as beneficiaries by which, they can secure admission in any empanelled hospital of their choice. A summary analysis of the findings from previous studies is useful here.

First, the private sector is able to utilize RSBY funds to its optimum with some benefit to the sick-poor (Nandi et al. 2015). A report by the Public Health Resource Network, a voluntary network of public health professionals, found that private hospitals 'cherry pick' RSBY/ Mukhyamantri Swasthya Bima Yojna (MSBY) packages that are profitable while refusing to treat patients with general illnesses such as jaundice, malaria in the state of Chhattisgarh (Nandi et al. 2015: 135).

The lack of health infrastructure in rural areas is a stumbling block for RSBY. As a result in states like West Bengal, Bihar, Uttar Pradesh, Jharkhand, and Chhattisgarh new hospitals are set up by the private sector in urban areas with least trained medical staff. This leads to a huge proliferation of private training centres for paramedics and support staff. Students trained in anaesthesia from such centres can be found participating in the performance of complicated surgeries in hospitals. In fact the reports obtained by the union health ministry on forced sterilization in Chhattisgarh revealed that the deaths were caused by the use of non-sterilized surgical equipment and spurious drugs. Upto 2014, more than 250 hospitals have been de-empanelled from the scheme due to fraud (Jain 2014).

Second, private hospitals have been reportedly performing operations encouraging unethical practices including unnecessary and invasive procedures. For instance, Bagchi reports the case of two women from Abhanpur block, Sharada and Ramlal, who were made to undergo hysterectomy operations on the advice of doctors in private hospitals in Raipur who prescribed it in order to relieve stomach pain. Sharada was made to pay an extra Rs 20,000 despite using the RSBY card, which offers cashless hospitalization for up to Rs 30,000. 'We had to sell land to arrange for the money', she said. More than 20 women in her village had undergone hysterectomies for similar reasons. An estimate in 2012 found that nearly 7,000 women had got their uterus removed under the RSBY over a period of 30 months (Bagchi 2014).

Third, a major limitation of RSBY is that it covers only in-patient treatment. As two-thirds of the health expenditure is on OOP, RSBY fails to adequately protect the labouring poor (Shahrawar and Rao 2011). For example, a study conducted in Durg district of Chhattisgarh shows that more than one-third of the beneficiaries who utilized RSBY incurred OOP expenses. On an average, users spent Rs 686 with an average OOP expenditure of 309 in public hospitals and 1,079 in private hospitals (Nandi et al. 2015). There were similar findings in Delhi as well, where more than one-third of users interviewed had spent money out of their pockets. On an average, RSBY beneficiaries in Delhi spent Rs 1,690 (Mukherjee 2015). Another study on Andhra Pradesh, Karnataka, and Tamil Nadu indicated that due to weak RSBY scheme, its poor administration, and absence of accountability mechanism, OOP expenditures are high (Selvaraj and Karan 2012). Based on household-level panel data from Uttar Pradesh and Bihar, Raza, Poel, and Panda (2016) indicated that in-patient coverage in the absence of out-patient coverage might only lead to inefficient and unnecessary hospital care.

Similarly, a study by Palacious, Das, and Sun (2011) revealed that under RSBY, patients were asked to buy medicines from private medical stores. In addition, there are some deeper problems with the design of RSBY. For example, there are no standard treatment guidelines. So a case of fever can be conveniently labelled by the doctor as dengue fever and the patient gets admitted under fear. The patient is given IV fluids, undergoes unnecessary investigations, and the government pays bills in hundreds for a case which could have cost Rs 20. In such cases, primary-care patients become secondary care and patients are burdened with irrational and excessive medication.

Fourth, studies pointed out concerns regarding the supposed portability of the smart card. Although card holders are entitled to avail hospital services throughout the country, their claim for treatment is not provided when they are away from their home state/region. While RSBY was meant for BPL population, in some states such as Chhattisgarh, it was introduced for people above poverty line (APL) indicating the pressure on the government both from private sector as well as sick-poor. Also states such as Punjab are already experimenting to extend RSBY smart cards to Aam Admi Bima Yojana (AABY), a special scheme for delivering the life and disability insurance.

Arogyasri–Health Insurance in Andhra Pradesh and Telangana

Arogyasri, launched in 2007 by the Government of Andhra Pradesh, covers about 70 million people (BPL households). It provides an insurance coverage of Rs 2 lakh for specified health problems requiring surgical interventions, which is nearly seven times the coverage under RSBY. The Government of Andhra Pradesh justifies the health insurance in these terms:

> Rural population of state, majority of whom are farmers, are not having access to advanced medical treatments and are silent sufferers of ill health. This is true in case of diseases related to heart, kidney, brain, cancer, and injuries due to domestic accidents and burns. While the Government is in the process of adequately strengthening the health institutions for basic health care, lack of specialist doctors and equipment for treatment of serious diseases has created a wide gap between the disease load and the capacity of the Government hospitals to serve the poor. These facilities though available in corporate sector are catering mainly to the affordable sections of society and are beyond the reach of poor families living in villages. Because of this gap poor patients are constrained to go to private hospitals for treatment and in the process incur huge debts leading to sale of properties and assets or are, sometimes, left eventually to die. (http//www.aarogyasri.org)

In order to facilitate the effective implementation of the scheme, the government has set up Arogyasri Health Care Trust under the chairmanship of the chief minister. The insurance premium works out to about Rs 250 per family unit. The total reimbursement of Rs 1.5 lakh can be availed either by an individual or for the entire family. An additional sum of Rs 50,000 is provided as a buffer to take care of expenses if it exceeds the original allocation. As an exception, cost for cochlear implant surgery with auditory verbal therapy is reimbursed by the Arogyasri Trust up to a maximum of Rs 6.5 lakh for each case.

The official document describes Arogyasri as a unique PPP model in the field of health insurance, tailor-made to the health needs of poor patients providing end-to-end cashless services for identified diseases through a network of service providers from private and government sector. In 2007 when Arogyasri was launched, it identified 163 procedures. With the growing popularity of the scheme and demand, the list of procedures increased to about 938 in 2011. An analysis of this list of diseases indicates that out of total 938 procedures, 352 are under Star Health and Allied Insurance Company and 586 managed by Arogyasri trust. Star Health Insurance which was a loss making and unknown private insurance company was chosen for Arogyasri scheme. Government insurance companies such as General Insurance Corporation, National Insurance Co., New India Insurance Co., United India Insurance Co., and so on, which were already dealing with health and family insurance schemes were kept out. Of course, today Star Insurance Company is a profitable company.

I draw here from my field research (Prasad 2015) to illuminate the critical analysis below:

> As in RSBY, Arogyasri is also heavily loaded in favour of private insurance companies and private hospitals. A total of 491 hospitals have been empanelled by Arogyasri Trust in Andhra Pradesh and Telangana. Out of 491, nearly 80 per cent of them are in private sector while remaining 20 per cent in the government sector. Although Arogyasri is meant for sick-poor in rural areas, there is not even one private hospital in the rural areas while the distribution of government hospitals recognized under the empanelled hospitals in rural and urban areas is almost even. Going by the Arogyasri Trust data, government health sector is in a better position to serve the rural sick-poor compared to the private health sector.

Arogyasri health card to BPL families as per the government officials entails the freedom to avail the best quality surgical facility in any hospital across the state. However, we found that this is one mechanism by which superspecialty hospitals located in urban centres gained access to the sick-poor both in rural and urban areas. Moreover, the insurance company and private health sector has devised direct control over scrutiny and case referral of patients through, Arogyamitras, a cadre of private health workers. These Arogyamitras act as the first contact located in primary health centres (PHCs), community health centres (CHCs), and district/state hospitals to facilitate the BPL patients from rural to urban areas. The study revealed that Arogyamitras functioned as parallel administrative workers with no accountability to the local health administration, also helping to divert cases from government to private hospitals (Shukla, Shatrugna, and Srivatsan 2011: 39). A discussion with doctors in Osmania Government Hospital in Hyderabad indicated that these are not new choices; rather, they are new ways of invoking surgical interventions without adequate rationale. There is a spurt of unnecessary surgeries after Arogyasri was initiated. For instance, in Warangal district of Telangana, there are thirteen private hospitals and five government hospitals. Out of the total 38,090 surgeries till 2010, 3,346 operations were reported to be hysterectomy cases. As there is scope for more surgeries and quick money, private hospitals used rural medical practitioners (RMP doctors) to refer poor women with some gynaecological problems such as hysterectomies. Similarly, in the case of neurosurgeries, kidney stones in adults, and ulcers more patients were encouraged to go for surgeries.[4] Our study indicated that there is widespread culture of commissions, irrational investigations, unnecessary surgical procedures, excessive influence of pharmaceutical companies on prescribing doctors through medical representatives, inflation of patient bills, holding the patients longer or shorter time so as to claim higher amounts, and so on, in various hospitals both in Andhra Pradesh and Telangana. These unethical practices have been so rampant that state government stopped payments and launched punitive action against 66 hospitals for committing irregularities under Arogyasri in 2011 (*The Hindu* 2011).

While private hospitals redirect and reject 'unwanted' cases, government hospitals take up all cases under Arogyasri regardless of whether they are expensive or inexpensive procedures. In the words of a doctor in Osmania hospital, 'government hospitals have become "dump yards" of high-risk, low-cost procedures, hugely complicated cases, under Arogyasri'. There is tremendous pressure in government hospitals to provide free food, medicines, longer hospital stay, and post-operative follow-up, among others, under Arogyasri scheme along with the surgery. Denial of any of these services and any lapses in prescribed practices are immediately reported to the higher hospital authorities through their local political leaders including their MLA/MP. They also immediately come to the attention of the media.

Similarly, the political pressure is exerted on Nizam Institute of Medical Sciences (NIMS), an autonomous government hospital to accept all the Arogyasri cases including those cases that exceed the actual cost of procedure as per the defined code. The NIMS records indicated that additional financial burden in such cases is to the tune of 20–25 per cent above the actual allocation. As the chief minister is the chancellor of NIMS, and the fact that several cases are recommended by chief minister's secretariat (*peshi*), health minister, and other political leaders, these cases will have to be treated. However, there is no scope for any political pressure in case of private and corporate hospitals. Given that several non-BPL households also procured Arogyasri eligibility card (white card) in rural areas through their social and political connections, their ability to exert pressure on government hospital network is also comparatively high. The existing structure of empanelled hospitals under Arogyasri in public and private sector indicate a clear trend. The government hospitals have been more vulnerable to public pressure and are able to provide health services at a lower cost to a large proportion of patients whereas the private and corporate hospitals have effectively used and manipulated Arogyasri to extract surplus.

Finally, despite the implementation of Arogyasri, OOP payments among all the hospitalized families remained very high at around Rs 280,000 in 2012, financed through loans and sale of assets. As outpatient care and common diseases are not covered under Arogyasri, poor families are often compelled to spend on health care beyond their capacity. Arogyasri card does not entail the members to use it outside the state. This significantly limits the advantages of the scheme, since many of the card members are workers who migrate outside the state for work and remain vulnerable outside their home state (Jain 2014).

Rajiv Gandhi Jeevandayee Arogya Yojana (RGJAY) in Maharashtra

The Government of Maharashtra introduced RGJAY, a free medical care scheme for the poor in 2011, committing Rs 800 crore in the first phase to benefit nearly 50 lakh families earning below Rs 1 lakh per annum in eight districts. This scheme facilitates 972 surgeries/therapies/procedures along with 121 follow-up packages in 30 identified specialized categories.[5] For 2014–15, according to the RGJAY, the premium was paid for 21.9 million households. The insurance company hires private firms known as third-party administrators (TPAs) to carry out all the administrative work of the scheme such as hospital empanelment, hospital grading, preauthorization, checking claim documents, and so on. The RGJAY has empanelled 142 hospitals in eight districts, majority of which are private hospitals. The findings from RGJAY indicate the following:

First, a few studies indicated that more than three-fifths (63 per cent) of the beneficiaries incurred OOP payments for health services even when admitted in the hospital under RGJAY. And significantly higher proportion of BPL families (88 per cent) reported paying for diagnostics, medications, or consumables. The predominant reason cited for paying for services in private hospitals (30 per cent) were 'procedure was not covered under RGJAY' followed by 'lack of knowledge' (18 per cent). A notable finding was that the mean OOP spending in private hospitals was more than twice compared with public hospitals (Ghosh 2014; Rent and Ghosh 2015).

Second, RGJAY does not have a mechanism in place to check whether the hospital is charging the patient despite already receiving funds, courtesy insurance, leading to double billing. The studies also indicated that diagnostics and medications together accounted for almost 80 per cent of the total OOP expenditure (Rent and Ghosh 2015: 9).

Third, it has been reported that the most vulnerable—migrant workers, street children, deserted women, and others—did not get health cards and were excluded from the benefits. The analysis revealed that almost half of the RGJAY beneficiaries actually belonged to non-eligible category whose family income is higher than Rs 100,000. A large number of vulnerable households are actually not in possession of any of the cards, which proved their vulnerability status. Hence, they will not be reached by the health insurance-based health system unless the targeting approach is abandoned by the government and a universal approach is adopted (Dréze and Sen 2014).

Bhamashah Health Insurance in Rajasthan

The Government of Rajasthan launched a health insurance scheme for the families covered under the National Food Security Act from April 2015 to provide coverage between Rs 30,000 to 50,000 in not-so-serious ailments and up to Rs 3,00,000 for very serious ailments. It is supposed to benefit 11 million families covering 47 million people. The state government allocated Rs 3.7 billion annually. This is justified by the government on the grounds that this will lessen the strain on district and medical college hospitals of the state and reroute them to the private sector (Dhar 2015). Some of the findings on Bhamasha Insurance indicate the following:

While the scheme is intended to benefit the patients from lower income categories to obtain quality health care from private hospitals, private hospitals are reportedly charging patients and their families over and above the insurance coverage by showing one part of the treatment not covered under the scheme. To inflate medical bills, private hospitals levy superfluous charges and overheads on the patients (Dhar 2015: 17).

The government claims that the insurance scheme would not cut into the existing free medicines and free diagnostic schemes. However, private health care providers are not bound to prescribe medicines by generic names and adhere to the state essential drug list. Civil society organizations have pointed out that the insurance-based model of health care actually compromises and sidelines the immensely successful free medicines and free diagnostics schemes already operational in the state under the National Food Security Act. Jan Swasthya Abhiyan, a people's health organization, argued that on the one hand there is complex socio-economic structure and accessibility issues while on the other hand, there is complete non-adherence to standard treatment protocols by the doctors and the presence of a vast unregulated private health care system. Therefore, an insurance-based model of health care in Rajasthan will only turn out to be more of a barrier in making health services available to all rather than making it more accessible.

Third, the government claimed that the insurance scheme will be a level playing field for both public and private hospitals. But this is not evident given the fact that while the total number of procedures for which claim rates have been fixed at 1719, government institutions can only make 170 claims. Jan Swasthya Abhiyan said that in order to increase the number of claims, there will be over-medication and unnecessary surgical procedures, and patients will be subjected to unwarranted medical risks. Therefore, critiques point out that the scheme is carefully conceptualized and meticulously crafted to essentially promote more opportunities for the private health care sector (Gupta and Pachauli 2015).

The Comprehensive Health Insurance Scheme in Kerala (CHIS)

In Kerala, the RSBY and CHIS are jointly implemented by the Labour and Rehabilitation Department, Health and Family Welfare Department, and the Local Self-government Department. A separate agency, Comprehensive Health Insurance Agency of Kerala (CHIAK), was entrusted with the implementation of the scheme. During the first year of implementation, 135 hospitals in the public sector, and 165 in the private sector, including hospitals in the cooperative sector were part of the scheme. In the government sector, all the hospitals at the level of CHC (community health centres) and above were empanelled. In addition, five medical colleges from different districts were also empanelled. The insurer for the first and the second year was United India Insurance Company. A third party administrator, a private company from Pune, is given the responsibility of deploying the field staff, upkeep of the software and electronic interface, and mediate between insurer and the service provider. Unlike RSBY, CHIS expanded its coverage to include APL families as well. The findings on CHIS indicate the following:

First, private hospitals have gained as the scheme emphasized production of receipts as an indicator of service delivered. The utilization pattern of those covered by CHIS suggests that since a large percentage are choosing private hospitals for their treatment, public subsidies are largely benefiting the private sector. This resulted in small and medium hospitals seeking empanelment as a means to ensure regular patient supply (Jisha 2015).

Second, a private hospital empanelled under CHIS at Oachira in Kollam district had poor infrastructure; the operation theatre was in a bad condition but still minor operations were being carried out. Certain procedures as outpatient services helped the private hospital augment its resources. A few empanelled hospitals were found to have no qualified doctors but doctors from outside were roped in for the period of inspection and were sent off after the hospital got its accreditation. These incidents point to the absence of any regulation before empanelment (Jisha 2015: 166).

To conclude this subsection, publicly funded health insurance (PFHI) coverage for the employees in the organized sector and customized schemes for the BPL population in the unorganized sector is expected to provide social protection, greater access to tertiary care, and reduce health risk particularly by cutting down the OOP expenditure. Has this been the case in India?

The PFHI designed in the PPP model, allowed a relatively higher proportion of private hospitals than government hospitals in the empanelled hospital lists across the central and state government schemes benefitting the private sector at large. Consequently, there is also rise in unethical practices such as unnecessary surgeries, forced sterilization, unwanted hysterectomies, surgical interventions with untrained medical personnel, over prescriptions, high dose of antibiotics and drugs, and so on. On the other hand, government hospitals are put at a disadvantage, providing high-risk, low-cost procedures with these insurance schemes even as they are subject to 25–50 per cent cuts in their existing budget.

Simply put, in the existing framework, this is not a level-playing field where the government sector competes with private hospitals. This meets the needs of health care industry more than it does that of vulnerable groups.

Insurance schemes have negative consequences in states such as Kerala, Tamil Nadu, and Rajasthan, where public health care is relatively more accessible both in terms of services, free medicines, and diagnostics. Studies indicate that in these states the sick-poor are forced to move towards expensive branded drugs and private hospitals rather than reliable health care system. This, in fact, signals intense privatization and increased health care costs, further impoverishing the poor.

All the above tailor-made insurance schemes have been widely popular in policy circles and among the sick-poor. However, it has not resulted in reducing the OOP payments. Rather it has contributed to a further rise in health care costs.

Finally, it is evident that there is significant enrolment of non-eligible groups of people leaving out the most vulnerable such as migrant workers, deserted women, street children, and others, thus raising questions about success of social protection strategies of the state.

WORKERS IN INFORMAL SECTOR: CASE OF BHOLAKPUR, HYDERABAD

The National Commission for Enterprises in the Unorganized Sector (NCEUS) brought out a series of reports until 2009, which indicated that 86 per cent of the total workers are in the informal sector. Of the remaining 14 per cent workers, 46 per cent were employed as informal workers in the formal sector. Close to 90 per cent of informal sector workers belong to households who could be characterized as poor and vulnerable. Apart from low wages, conditions of employment are often abominable due to absence of basic amenities, exposure to hazardous materials and the employment of bonded and child labour in certain specific occupations in many parts of the country (Kannan and Breman 2012; Kannan and Jain 2012). The incidence of informal sector work is much higher among women than men workers as well as among the *dalits* than others, with pronounced wage disparities, compounded by a greater degree of illiteracy, low education, low skills, and so forth. Given this condition, a case study of Bholakpur slum is presented based on my own field work in the year 2013 to examine the issues of accessibility to health care.

Bholakpur is a municipal ward with a population of 72,000 located in Musheerabad which connects the twin cities Hyderabad and Secunderabad. It plays a vital role in the economic system of the city by connecting the two processes 'production of waste' and 'production from waste'. Bholakpur is densely populated by Muslims along with a small proportion of *dalits* who migrated to Bholakpur from neighbouring districts of Hyderabad several decades back. The major economic activity in Bholakpur is scrap trading. They deal with all kinds of leftovers starting from animal skins to electrical and electronic scrap. The other important economic activities in Bholakpur are eateries and cloth markets. Previous studies indicated that informal workers in the waste recovery sector subsidize risk and contribute to urban development (Kumar 2014).

Scrap trading in Bholakpur dates back to 150 years. Bholakpur was primarily a skin trading centre and there were also many tanneries located here. This was the main livelihood of the residents of Bholakpur. As Hyderabad transformed, tanneries at Bholakpur were gradually shut down due to environment and other government regulations. Now, there is not a single tannery in Bholakpur. All these old tanneries have transformed into function halls, cloth markets, or empty buildings. Following the closure of tanneries, skin trading was also heavily affected after semi-finished leather export was banned by Indian government in 1991. Skin traders and labourers found plastic and electrical scrap trading as alternative livelihood options.

Traders at Bholakpur claim that one needs immense knowledge to trade in plastics as there are more than 400 varieties of plastics and the price change is volatile. Plastic trade became attractive and one of the main livelihoods of the residents of Bholakpur after the slump in the leather trade in 1990s. In Bholakpur there are two kinds of plastic activity, one is segregation of plastic and the other is processing of plastic, mainly grinding. But grinding has largely reduced in the last few years due to various reasons, an important one being government regulations. The 2009 E. colitis incident reduced number of grinding units to marginal level of 10–20. According to the local plastic welfare association, there are 300 plastic industrial units located in Bholakpur.

Production of Risk and Diseases

Bholakpur is one of the few scrap processing sites situated in the middle of a city. The work of scrap processing, plastic recycling, and processing of 2000 animal skins a day involves a number of cleaning jobs. Salt is applied to the skins to prevent decomposition before being sent to Tamil Nadu and West Bengal for leather processing. All the wastage and dirty water flows into the drainage pipelines, because of which the pipes are frequently clogged, and it takes months to clear them. An overpowering decaying smell hangs in the air. The roads are narrow and pot-holed with perennially flowing drainage lines. Thus, on the one hand, it is an overcrowded slum with the labouring poor dependent on waste economy while on the other there is almost non-existent waste disposal system. Given this situation, the possibility of risk and disease production is very high.

The abysmal working conditions reinforce the equally unsatisfactory living conditions of people. The work they do is classified as 3-D work, that is, dirty, dangerous, and demeaning. 3-D is American neologism derived from a Japanese expression referring particularly to difficult work done involving high risk and low status. This 3-D work can impose severe physical and mental costs to workers. There is often a risk of not being able to work for a long time due to general depletion of health or mental fatigue. The respondents often reported problems such as hyperacidity, respiratory illnesses, jaundice, stomach-related ailments, injuries, dizziness, nausea, back pain, and other ailments.

In 2009, E. colitis killed 14 people and affected 300 people in Bholakpur. Municipal officials and media linked E. colitis to scrap processing and termed it as 'hazardous'. However, the local residents and activists argue that the spread of E. colitis was not because of scrap processing but due to municipal negligence that led to the contamination of water. Interviews with the municipal officials confirmed that water supply had been contaminated due to a mixing of drainage and water pipes in Bholakpur. The biological analysis of water samples from Bholakpur revealed abnormally high levels of E.coli making the water unfit for human consumption.

With the epidemic and deaths in Bholakpur, real estate developers, with an eye of the prime real estate, in collusion with the local state, have been attempting to persuade the slum people to relocate to the outskirts.

Existing Choices and Access to Health Care

While the slum residents bear the risk by engaging in the recycling sector, contributing to the clean and safe environment to the city, the municipal corporation does not even provide the basic facilities such as safe drinking water, sanitation, and other facilities, in carrying out their activities. Bholakpur is located in close proximity to two government hospitals—Gandhi Tertiary Hospital and Quarantine Fever Hospital along with two private nursing homes and eight private clinics. As all the labouring poor are BPL households, they also have Arogyasri health cards.

Slum residents indicated that they approach both government and private hospitals for various illnesses. But, most of them felt that Anjuman Tajiran-e-Chirm, a trust provides relatively easy accessible health services. The trust collects money from every skin transported out of the slum and other recycling units to run the free clinics. In general people have to spend more money in both the government and private hospitals, while they incur the least expenditure in community-run clinics.

Discussion with the respondents indicated that even those covered under the Arogyasri Insurance find it difficult to utilize the services. A few respondents said that the empanelled hospitals either declared that particular illnesses were not covered under Arogyasri or they would have to pay an additional Rs 5,000–10,000 as the insurance coverage has a ceiling. A women respondent said that that they see both hope and despair with Arogyasri. For instance, often Arogyamitras, the intermediaries, often suggest a particular surgery as a permanent solution, quite overlooking the fact that their own kin members who went through the particular surgery had a number of post-operative complications.

Clearly, accessibility to health care needs to be seen not only in terms of government, private hospitals, or health insurance. It encompasses a whole gamut of illnesses that affect the labouring classes due to occupational hazards, water contamination, as well as OOP expenses in hospitals, mischief by the touts, and Argoyamitras putting obstacles in availing Argoyasri scheme, and other reasons. In particular, women in Bholakpur faced further hardship as they are the last ones to seek health care, when they have to pay for it.

* * *

The Indian state initiated new reforms in the last decade to provide greater accessibility and social protection for the vast majority of workers in the unorganized sector. However, accessibility is a huge political agenda which needs deeper conceptualization than is usually defined in the policy debates. We argue that poverty reduction lobby on individual and household-level protection has in fact different priorities from that of public health agenda of preventive and primary health care which primarily benefits the poor people. Social protection implied not merely curative and surgical-based interventions but prevention and control of diseases as well. In the name of providing more choices to unorganized workers through empanelled hospitals, the state's social protection strategies are boosting health insurance markets and consequently leading to commoditization of health services. In fact policymakers expect the share of the health insurance, which is pegged at only 2 per cent, will rise to 20 per cent by 2020. The current health insurance-based health system has actually led to a provider–purchaser split where the government's role has been reduced to paying health care packages offered by the health insurance companies, thus promoting the interests of the corporate health industry over the needs of the vulnerable groups. However, in the long run there is no better insurance than investment in a health care infrastructure that is accessible to the poorer groups. It has been rightly pointed out by Amartya Sen (2015) that the neglect of education, health, and social safety net in the deeply rooted class structure of society has been foundational in creating inequality in India.

In brief, the reforms by the Indian state are based on two assumptions. One, the strategic purchasing of curative health services from health insurance market provided through public and private hospitals can enable India to achieve the goal of universal health coverage. Second, contingent upon the first one that the reforms will provide greater access to tertiary health care, reduce OOP expenditure, and contribute towards health security of the BPL population. This chapter based on health insurance studies in eight states and central government scheme argues that these assumptions are flawed and points out various contradictions in the very discourse of neo-liberal reforms. Despite the popularity of the health insurance models in policy circles, I argue that these reforms have created inefficiency, increased costs, and accelerated the expansion of a largely unregulated health care market. In fact the expert group on universal health coverage constituted by the Planning Commission of India also pointed out that publicly funded universal health care reduces the impact of ill health while insurance systems can increase inequalities in access to care. Countries such as Brazil and Thailand have invested heavily in strengthening the public health system rather than moving in the direction of health insurance which typically promotes delivery of services by the private sector. Health insurance is then an important contributor to the expansion of the health care industry, accelerating the process of predatory capitalism led by the private corporate sector and protected by the state.

NOTES

1. As of 31 March 2015, more than 8 per cent of 25,300 PHCs in the country were without a doctor, 38 per cent without a laboratory technician, and 22 per cent had no pharmacist. Nearly 50 per cent of posts for female health assistants and 61 per cent for male health assistants remained vacant. In CHCs, the shortfall is huge in the departments of surgery (83 per cent), obstetricians and gynaecologists (76 per cent), physicians (83 per cent), and paediatricians (82 per cent) (see Sharma 2015).

2. Several studies indicated that 66 per cent of the patients fall on private health services and only 33 per cent on government services (MoHFW 2017; Patel 2015) indicating the status and accessibility to government health system.

3. Some of the examples of the hospitals established through the FDI route include Apollo Gleneagles, Columbia Asia, and Max Healthcare.

4. Earlier there were some efforts to examine whether these cases can be addressed through non-surgical methods. But now, the easiest option is to direct them for major surgery.

5. These include general, ENT, ophthalmology, gynaecological and obstetrics, gastroenterology, cardiac, paediatric, and others; surgeries in a cashless manner.

REFERENCES

Bagchi, Suvojit. 2014. 'Public Health, Private Tragedy'. *The Hindu*, 26 November.

Balarajan, Y., S. Selvaraj, and S.V. Subramanian. 2011. 'Health Care and Equity in India', *The Lancet* 377(9764): 905–15.

Baru, R. 2016. 'Commercialisation and the Poverty of Public Health Services in India'. In *Public Health and Private Wealth: Stem Cells, Surrogates and Other Strategic Bodies*, Sarah Hodges and Mohan Rao (eds), pp. 121–38. New Delhi: Oxford University Press.

Berman, P., R. Ahuja, and L. Bhandari. 2010. 'The Impoverishment Effect of Health Care Payments in India: New Methodology and Findings', *Economic and Political Weekly* 45(16): 65–71.

British Medical Journal. 2005. 'The Private Health Sector in India is Burgeoning But at the Cost of Public Health Care', Editorial, *British Medical Journal* 331(7526): 1157–8.

Center for Equity Studies. 2017. *India Exclusion Report, 2016*. New Delhi: YODA Press. Accessed on 2 November 2017.

Chancel, Lucas and Thomas Piketty. 2017. 'Indian Income Inequality 1922–2014: From British Raj to Billionaire Raj', *WID. World Working Paper Series N 2017/11.* Accessed on 21 October 2017.

Das Gupta, Monica and V.R. Muraleedharan. 2014. 'Universal Health Coverage—Reform of the Government System Better Than Quality Health Insurance', *Economic and Political Weekly* 49(35): 29–32.

Desai, Mihir and Kamayani Bali Mahabal (eds). 2007. *Health Care Case Law in India: A Reader.* Mumbai: Centre for Enquiry into Health and Allied Themes (CEHAT) and India Centre for Human Rights & Law (ICHRL).

Dhar, Aarti. 2015. 'Activists Oppose Health Insurance Scheme'. *The Hindu*, 15 February.

Dréze, Jean and Amartya Sen. 2014. *An Uncertain Glory: India and Its Contradictions.* London: Penguin Books.

Duggal, Ravi. 2007. 'Poverty and Health: Criticality of Public Financing', *Indian Journal of Medical Research* 126: 309–17.

Ghosh, S. 2014. 'Publicly Financed Health Insurance for the Poor: Understanding RSBY in Maharashtra', *Economic and Political Weekly* 49(43–44): 93–9.

Gupta, Narendra and Chhaya Pachauli. 2015. 'Promoting Private Health Care', *Economic and Political Weekly* 50(50): 4–5.

Hodges, Sarah and Mohan Rao (eds). 2016. *Public Health and Private Wealth: Stem Cells, Surrogates and Other Strategic Bodies.* Delhi: Oxford University Press.

Horton, Richard and Pamela Das. 2015. 'Global Health Security Now', *The Lancet* 385(9980): 1805–6.

Jain, Nishant. 2014. 'Rashtriya Swasthya Bima Yojana: A Step Towards Universal Health Coverage in India'. In *India Infrastructure Report 2013/14*, IDFC Foundation (ed.), pp. 120–34. Hyderabad: Orient Blackswan.

Jisha, C.J. 2015. 'The Comprehensive Health Insurance Scheme (CHIS) in Kerala: an Exploratory Study in Kollam District', In *Medical Insurance Schemes for the Poor—Who Benefits?*, Rama Baru (ed.), pp. 151–68. New Delhi: Academic Foundation.

Kannan, K.P. and Jan Breman (eds). 2012. *The Long Road to Social Security.* New Delhi: Oxford University Press.

Kannan, K.P. and Varinder Jain. 2012. 'Historic Initiative, Limited by Design and Implementation: A National Overview of the Implementation of NREWG'. In *The Long Road to Social Security*, K.P. Kannan and Jan Breman (eds), pp. 33–80. New Delhi: Oxford University Press.

Kumar, Kishore S. 2014. 'Modeling Waste Recycling through the Lens of Joint Production System: The Case of Bholakpur Scrap Market in Hyderabad'. Unpublished MPhil dissertation, University of Hyderabad.

MoHFW. 2017. *National Health Policy 2017.* New Delhi: Government of India.

Mukherjee, A. 2015. 'The Rashtriya Bima Yojana—An Overview'. In *Medical Insurance Schemes for the Poor—Who Benefits*, Rama Baru (ed.), pp. 89–110. New Delhi: Academic Foundation.

Nandi, S., M. Nundy, V. Prasad, K. Kanungo, H. Khan, S. Haripriya, T. Mishra, and S. Garg. 2015. 'Implementing of RS. BY in Chattisgarh, India—A Study of the Durg District'. In *Medical Insurance Schemes for the Poor—Who Benefits*, Rama Baru (ed.), pp. 111–50. New Delhi: Academic Foundation.

Palacious, R.J., J. Das, and C. Sun. 2011. *A New Approach to Providing Health Insurance to the Poor in India: The Early Experience of Rashtriya Swasthya BimaYojana in India's Health Insurance Scheme for the Poor*. New Delhi: Centre for Policy Research.

Patel, Vikram. 2015, 'Health Insurance, Assurance and Empowerment in India', *The Lancet* 386 10011: 2372–3.

Planning Commission. 2013. *Twelfth Five Year Plan 2012–17*. New Delhi: Government of India.

Prasad, N. Purendra. 2015. 'State, Community Health Insurance and Commodification of Health Care: A Case of Arogyasri in Andhra Pradesh'. In *Medical Insurance Schemes for the Poor—Who Benefits*, Rama V. Baru (ed.), pp. 61–88. New Delhi: Academic Foundation.

Qadeer, Imrana, Kasturi Sen, and K.R. Nayar. 2001. *Public Health and Poverty of Reforms—the South Asian Predicament*. New Delhi: Sage.

Rao, Govinda M. and Mita Choudhury. 2012. 'Health Care Financing Reforms in India'. Working Paper No. 2012–100, March. New Delhi: National Institute of Public Finance and Policy.

Raza, Wameq, Ellen Van de Poel, and Pradeep Panda. 2016, 'Analyses of Enrolment, Drop Out and Effectiveness of RSBY in Northern Rural India'. Available at: https://mpra.ub.uni-muenchen.de/70081/MPRA Paper No. 70081. Accessed on 12 June 2016.

Rent, Priyanka and Soumitra Ghosh. 2015. 'Understanding the "Cash-Less" Nature of Government-Sponsored Health Insurance Schemes: Evidence from Rajiv Gandhi Jeevandayee Aarogya Yojana in Mumbai', *Sage Open*, 1–10 October–December.

Selvaraj, S. and A. Karan. 2012. 'Why Publicly Funded Health Insurance Schemes are Ineffective in Providing Financial Risk Protection', *Economic and Political Weekly* 47(11): 62–8.

Sen, Amartya. 2015. 'Amartya Sen: National Security Is One Component of Human Security'. Interview with G. Sampath, *The Hindu*, 24 December. Available at: http://www.thehindu.com/opinion/interview/interview-with-prof-amartya-sen-national-security-is-one-component-of-human-security/article8022388.ece. Accessed on 25 December 2015.

Shahrawar, Renu and Krishna D. Rao. 2011. 'Insured yet Vulnerable: Out-of-pocket Payments and India's Poor', *Health Policy and Planning* 27(3): 213–21.

Sharma, Dinesh C. 2015. 'India Still Struggling with Rural Doctor Shortages', *The Lancet* 386(10011): 2381–2.

Shukla, R., V. Shatrugna, and R. Srivatsan. 2011. 'Aarogyasri Healthcare Model: Advantage Private Sector', *Economic and Political Weekly* 46(49): 38–42.

Srikant, Nagulaplli. 2014. 'Burden of Out-of-Pocket Health Payments in Andhra Pradesh', *Economic and Political Weekly* 49(42): 64–72.

Standing, Hilary. 2002. 'An Overview of Changing Agendas in Health Sector Reformed', *Reproductive Health Matters* 10(20): 19–28.

The Hindu. 2011. 'Vasectomy Akramalu', 13 December.

Yadav, Anumeha. 2014. 'How Effective are Social Security and Welfare in India', *The Hindu*, 26 January.

3

Medical–Industrial Complex
Trends in Corporatization of Health Services

Rama V. Baru

The commercialization of health services and the consolidation of markets within it is an important feature of the Indian health care economy. The concept of commercialization acknowledges the role of markets within and outside the public sector. It emphasizes ' ... the provision of health care services through market relationships to those able to pay; investment in, and production of those services, and of inputs to them, for cash income or profit, including private contracting and supply to publicly financed health care; and health care finance derived from individual payments and private insurance' (Mackintosh and Koivusalo 2005: 3).

This definition allows us to examine the relationship between the market and the state as co-producers of health services. Further we argue that the role of the state in the growth of private sector is not a passive one, but that it has actively promoted the entry of markets in the health services. The consolidation and transformation of markets in the Indian health service system now presents the features of a medical-industrial complex. Drawing on the analogy of the military-industrial complex, Arnold Relman, the former editor of *The New England Journal of Medicine*, characterized the rise of diverse business interests in medicine as a medical-industrial complex in the US during the 1980s (Relman 1980). He, along with several other scholars who were critical of private interests in medical care, wrote extensively on the entrenched network of power relations, the rise of business lobbies, and their influence on policy. Several scholars studied the manner in which capital consolidated itself in medical services through pharmaceutical, medical devices, insurance, and provisioning corporations in the US (Starr 1982). Starr highlighted the pathways through which market forces actively engaged and furthered their interests in the policy arena. Examples of their entrenched interests was reflected in their active lobbying and backroom deals[1] to ensure that public health reforms were diluted during the Clinton and Obama regimes and the interests of corporate American medical care remained largely protected.

This chapter seeks to examine the transformation and consolidation of markets in the health service system over the last three decades in India. The complex architecture of the private sector involves a range of actors and institutions, which are arranged hierarchically. This produces a complex network of power relations. These power relations actively engage with the political processes at the local, state, and central levels. The extent of leverage of power among these actors with the government varies. In recent times, Indian and foreign capital has entered into alliances and are firmly entrenched within the health service system. These have been asserting their power over health policy-making.

Much of the scholarship on the Indian private health sector has tended to focus independently on the pharmaceutical products, medical devices, medical education, and the provisioning aspects of the private sector in health services. In reality, these subsystems are not independent of one another but interrelated. Markets have a significant presence in all the above and have penetrated the public sector through the introduction of public–private partnerships (PPPs). This has resulted in the blurring of boundaries between the public and the private sectors.

Some writing on the pharmaceutical sector has pointed to the power wielded by the corporate sector, domestic, and overseas, as compared to the small- and medium-scale enterprises (Ray and Bhaduri 2012). These studies have also shown the influence of the corporate sector on drug policy in terms of pricing and production (Ray and Bhaduri 2012). A lesser body of work exists on the medical devices industry and how it has played an important role in transforming hospitals from small-scale enterprises to the status of an industry (Baru 1998; Chakravarthi 2013a). The private sector has received attention through the analysis of utilization surveys that show a growing reliance on a range of providers, high out-of-pocket (OOP) expenditures for treatment leading to the impoverishment of households.

This paper is divided into three sections. The first section provides an overview of the nature of markets in medical technology that includes pharmaceuticals and medical devices. The second section discusses the characteristics of markets in provisioning, and the final section analyses how the state has accommodated and facilitated the rise of markets in health services.

MARKETS IN MEDICAL TECHNOLOGY

At the time of Independence, medical technology was dependent mainly on multinational corporations and import of devices. During the first three decades after Independence, the pharmaceutical sector had four distinct categories based on ownership that included multinational pharmaceutical companies (MNCs), public sector units, Indian-managed large-scale companies, and small-scale private enterprises (Santhosh 2011). Among the various categories, the MNCs had the largest presence soon after Independence. There was a small presence of Indian entrepreneurs during this period and it is only in the 1950s and 1960s that public sector units were set up. During the late 1960s and 1970s the government sought to protect Indian markets and privileged the growth of the private sector, large and small. However, this did not lead to the desired results because, as Santhosh (2011: 105) observes, 'The dependency over for technology and capital investment compelled both the state and private manufacturers to compromise in many ways. With this dependent relationship the MNCs could ensure that the drugs and pharmaceutical industry in India would not be a monopoly of the state'.

It may be argued then that the state has aided the process of accumulation of private capital in the pharmaceutical sector since Independence. With liberalization and globalization, the Indian large-scale companies and MNCs, gained the most. By this time, the public sector units had weakened resulting in the closure of some during this period (Santhosh 2011).

Medical Device Industry

At the time of Independence, the Bhore Committee observed that while the pharmaceutical industry was dominated by multinational corporations, there was an excessive reliance on import of medical devices ranging from syringes, autoclaves, scalpels, and so on (Baru 1998;

Chakravarthi 2013a). The Bhore Committee (BC) recommended that India must acquire self-sufficiency in the production of pharmaceuticals and medical devices through investments in the public sector and also create conducive conditions for private manufacturers. This idea was given a more concrete direction by the Mudaliar Committee which argued that Indian entrepreneurs must be encouraged to manufacture medical and surgical instruments, hospital appliances, laboratory equipment, and the like. This resulted in the growth of a domestic devices industry in the production of X-ray machines and other electromedical instruments during the 1950s and 1960s (Chakravarthi 2013b). However, the volume of production was very small and did not significantly reduce India's dependence on import of devices. There was an expansion of the industry during the 1970s to include ultrasound scanners, a range of laboratory equipment, and other devices. During this period, specialized technology was being imported and introduced in government hospitals. Given the high cost of specialized technology, the small and medium private hospitals were not in a position to make the required investments to acquire it. By the 1980s there was a dramatic change in the global markets for medical devices. Due to the recession in the US health industry, medical device companies were seeking newer markets (Baru 1998). These companies with their large volume of production were able to sell their devices at attractive prices in other countries (Chakravarthi 2013a). India, with its slow pace of growth and low volume of production of medical devices, was unable to compete with the MNCs which consequently had access to a large market for these devices in both the public and private sectors. During the 1990s, as a part of the Structural Adjustment Programme, loans from the World Bank were used to upgrade infrastructure and technology in the public health services. The conditionalities attached to these loans required state governments to import drugs and medical devices from the private sector through a process of international tendering and competitive bidding. In sum, markets for technology did not observe boundaries between the public and private sector.[2]

The medical equipment industry is an important avenue for Foreign Direct Investment (FDI). The growth of the domestic medical equipment market is singularly dependent on collaborative arrangements with international companies. According to a 2007 projection by a consulting company, the medical equipment market was slated to double between 2006 and 2012. This is closely related to the growth in the tertiary private hospital sector during the same period (Chanda 2007).

COMING OF AGE OF CORPORATE HOSPITAL

The private sector is structurally plural[3] and hierarchical in its organization. The primary level of care is dominated by individual practitioners in rural and urban areas who can be classified as those who are formally and informally trained across systems of medicine. The secondary level is occupied by small and medium nursing homes promoted by a single owner or partnerships, mostly among doctors. The spread of these institutions is marked by interstate and rural–urban variations. The states of Punjab, Gujarat, Maharashtra, Andhra Pradesh, Karnataka, Tamil Nadu, and Kerala have a higher proportion of 'for-profit' institutions than public institutions than other states in India (Baru 1998). These states may be exhibiting a higher growth because of a variety of factors. Importantly, the entry of the upper- and intermediate-castes investing in professional education and the agrarian prosperity of these regions due to green revolution helped to create surpluses. These surpluses were invested in a variety of entrepreneurial activities that included medicine and engineering. In medical care—hospitals, diagnostic facilities, and laboratories—are also seen as areas of returns for investments.

Structure of Private Sector in Medical Care

A large proportion of the private sector continues to be dominated by independent practitioners, formal and informal, followed by small and medium enterprises and a small segment, which is private and public limited. Independent practitioners in the private sector include those who have received formal training in allopathy, ayurveda, unani, homeopathy, and siddha. It also includes a range of informally trained practitioners who are sought out for primary-level care. Their numbers are difficult to estimate since there is no system of registration for these independent practitioners.

Several studies on utilization of health services in rural and urban areas show a high dependence on these various practitioners for out-patient services (Dilip 2010; Sen, Iyer, and George 2002; Sundararaman and Muraleedharan 2015). The secondary level of care in the private sector consists of small and medium nursing homes that are promoted by single owners or partners, mostly doctors. These nursing homes are located in urban, semi urban, and rural areas. The economically better developed states and districts have a higher concentration of these nursing homes. Across income quintiles, these nursing homes are being used for out-patient and in-patient services.

The tertiary sector is mostly dominated by the private- and public-limited hospitals. A majority of these enterprises, around 80 per cent, were established in the western and southern states with investments from non-resident Indian (NRI) doctors from the US (Chanda 2007). The corporate sector that initially provided only tertiary and specialist services has now diversified its operation to secondary- and primary-level care leading to a vertical integration of the market.

Another distinguishing feature of the private sector is that it is dependent on the public sector in terms of a variety of subsidies, sharing human resources, especially government doctors, who practice privately and contracting in and out of clinical and non-clinical services in public hospitals. Based on the complex nature of the interrelationships between the public and private sectors, it is apt to characterize it as a mixed economy in health services. Understanding the dynamic relationship between the two sectors is important to explain how and why the private sector has managed to gain power and influence over health policy. The interrelatedness of the private and the public sector and the power dynamics result in competition, contradictions, and conflicts within and across the two sectors.

Up until 1980s, the private sector can be characterized as a cottage industry. But soon a significant shift in government policy led to the recognition of hospital as an industry. The liberalization policy and health sector reforms provided opportunities in the health care markets for local and international corporations (Lefebvre 2010). The policy to support growth of corporate sector continued through the 1990s and 2000s. The Health Policy 2002 and the subsequent Union Budgets gave a number of tax concessions to encourage the setting up of 100-bed hospitals in tier two cities. This also led to the phenomenon of medical tourism in the tertiary sector. Medical tourism was seen as a revenue generation proposition contributing to economic growth. Corporate hospitals started actively soliciting patients from abroad for treatment in India.

These policies found their echo in the attitude of the political class and large sections of bureaucracy whose trust in the public sector was eroding. Both the Congress governments of Indira Gandhi and Rajiv Gandhi played a significant role in effecting several policy changes for hospitals to be recognized as an industry; facilitated access to finance; offered concessions for infrastructure; and slashed import duties on high technology equipment. These public subsidies were meant to boost FDI and attract professionals back to India (Gupte 2013). The liberalization of the health sector is reflected in the Health Policy, 1982 which actively sought to engage the for-profit and non-profit sectors. The establishment of Apollo Hospital in Chennai marks the rise of corporatization of health care in India. Prathap Reddy, a cardiologist professional long practising in the US, returned to India in the late 1970s and lobbied with the Indian political class and bureaucracy to create conducive business conditions for corporate hospitals. Reddy's Apollo Hospitals project symbolizes the integration of the professional diaspora and the social and political networks to redefine the determinants of what constitutes modern, scientific, and good quality in medical care.

The real push for liberalizing import duties and including designating hospitals as an industry came from Reddy when he set up the first corporate hospital in India. He modelled the Apollo hospital in the image of American multi-speciality hospitals that required high-end equipment like CT scanners which had to be imported. For this, Reddy had to get the necessary permissions from the central government. He used social, political, and bureaucratic networks to bring about the changes in the import policy for medical equipments. Hodges argues that this is how the myth of Apollo and Prathap Reddy was created and further developed by the media (Hodges 2013). She suggests that the climate for liberalization already existed and the political class were ideologically in sync with Reddy's project. However, it is important to acknowledge Reddy's considerable lobbying with Indira Gandhi and Rajiv Gandhi to effect changes in rules relating to finances and imports.[4]

Pranay Gupte's adulatory biography of Prathap Reddy describes the vital role played by him in bringing about changes in legislation. The 1980s was an important period of change in the mindset of the political class and the bureaucracy towards private industry. Reddy lobbied with several ministers and specially acknowledges the role played by Pranab Mukherjee and R. Venkatraman, who supported the Apollo project.

He (Pranab Mukherjee) championed so many significant changes in the country—each leading to transformational impact in India. The very first support I would cite is the urgent assistance that he extended in 1981. At this point there was tremendous scarcity of steel and cement and that was holding up the construction of Apollo, Madras. Pranab Mukherjee was so impressed with our project that he sanctioned an allotment of 500 tons of steel at the price of Rs 1,850 per ton and 1,500 bags of cement at the highly subsidised government price of Rs 18—the market price for each item was at least three times more. The second support which I would refer to is that although R. Venkatraman, as finance minister, granted corporate status for Apollo and allowed listing of the company, he could not succeed in amending the existing rules for hospital funding. (Gupte 2013: 205)

Pranab Mukherjee continued his support for relaxing rules for hospital financing. Reddy had lobbied with Indira Gandhi and as she was convinced that 'Dr Reddy will bring international doctors and establish world class health care in our country' (Gupte 2013: 205).

While there are descriptions of Apollo hospitals as a business model, there is not enough analysis of how changes were effected at the policy level that facilitated the shift to recognizing hospitals as an industry— the role of banks in financing, the relaxation of import duties, and the availability of subsidized land. Did the government have a well-articulated vision for all of the above and the emergence of the hospital industry, or was it due to lobbying by an individual, in this case Prathap Reddy? In what manner does a professional returning from the US harness his cultural capital to influence the political class? What were the networks he used to build these links and persevered to effect the required changes in policy that would make his project work? These are questions that need further exploration.

What is certain is that the political class played an important role in providing the support and public subsidies to the Apollo project. It gained legitimacy when the Apollo hospital was inaugurated by the then President, Giani Zail Singh. Apart from receiving subsidies for infrastructure, the other issue for which Reddy actively lobbied for was the elimination of various conditionalities in the import of medical equipment at concessional rates of duty. With P.V. Narasimha Rao as Prime Minister, the Finance Minister, Manmohan Singh, announced in his 1995–6 Budget Speech in Parliament:

> For promoting health care, last year I had simplified the import duty structure on medical equipment, exempted many types of life-saving equipment from payment of duty, and abolished the certification procedure for availing of the exemption for charitable hospitals. In order to help manufacture and maintenance of medical equipment, I am extending the benefit of full exemption from import duty to all parts of exempted life-saving and sight-saving equipment. (Government of India 1995)

Health being state subject, efforts were needed to engage with politicians in Tamil Nadu and Andhra Pradesh while setting up hospital projects. Lobbying with the central government had its place but negotiations around acquisition of land, building rights, infrastructure clearances, and transfer of finances was under the control of the respective states. Hodges describes how Reddy lobbied with the then Chief Minister, M.G. Ramachandran, for the various requirements to build a hospital.[5]

Following closely on the Apollo experience, several corporate hospitals were established mainly in southern and western India. Some like Wockhardt, which was primarily a pharmaceutical company, diversified into the hospital industry. Other corporate hospitals included Fortis, Max, Care, Rockland, Paras, and several others were established. During the 2000s, several of these hospitals entered into partnerships with state governments and municipalities.

The hospital industry is a capital-intensive project. While the industry lobbied for public subsidies, this was clearly inadequate for sustaining these projects. The liberalization of the insurance sector, which allowed 100 per cent Foreign Direct Investment (FDI) in health, gave a further fillip to the hospital industry. Partnerships with insurance companies like Apollo-Munich and Max BUPA are some prominent examples. Foreign Direct Investment came in the form of venture and private equity firms investing in these hospitals.[6] The International Finance Corporation (IFC), the private sector lending arm of the World Bank, has granted loans to several hospital projects that include Max Healthcare, Rockland, Artemis, Apollo, and Duncan Gleneagles. More recently international private equity firms like AIG, JP Morgan Stanley, Carlyle, Blackstone Group, Quantum, and Blue Ridge have been investing in hospital projects (Lefebvre 2010).

Foreign investments in the hospital sector are in the form of collaborative ventures between hospital companies and Indian partners. There are a variety of collaborations that include capital investments, technology tie-ups, hospitals, medical education, and training (Chanda 2007). The major international health care companies are from Singapore and the US. Others from the UAE, Australia, and Canada are also important players in the market. An important area of collaboration is in the area of diagnostic services. Chanda's analysis shows that foreign investments came mostly from the US followed by Singapore, UK, UAE, Australia, and Canada. These investments were mostly in the southern states of Kerala, erstwhile Andhra Pradesh (Hyderabad), Karnataka, Tamil Nadu, and Gujarat. These were not corporate hospitals but private limited enterprises. The only exception was Max Healthcare with investment from Mauritius (Chanda 2007).

Professional Networks

Professionals and their social networks play a very important role in the hospital industry. During the 1980s, the small- and medium-sized hospitals drew on professional expertise from the public sector as consultants. The government doctors used their position in the public hospitals to refer cases to these private hospitals. Some of the promoters of corporate hospitals were NRI doctors based mostly in the US and the UK. They tapped into the various forms of cultural capital that they had built through their practice. As treating physicians they interacted with the Indian social and political elite who went abroad for specialized treatment. This gave them access to their social and cultural capital which proved to be useful when they returned to India to set up speciality hospitals.

Regional, caste, and political networks play a very important role in the building of cultural capital. Access to other professionals was also facilitated through the alumni networks of medical colleges in India and the US. The Association of Physicians of Indian Origin, based in the US, the American Association of Physicians of Indian Origin (AAPIO), and the UK-based British Association of Physicians of Indian Origin (BAPIO) provide a valuable platform for recruiting doctors to come back to India as consultants in corporate hospitals. There is an element of the personal relationship that a doctor builds with his patient. If the patients are politically and socially influential, doctors are able to gain access to influence policy decisions.[7] These networks play an important role in exercising professional power nationally and globally. These networks give rise to institutions that are capable of giving direction to policy and ensure that their interests are protected. In 1998, the Confederation of Indian Industry (CII) set up the National Committee on Health Care and the Indian Health Care Federation. These two committees have lobbied with the central and state governments for subsidies and concessions for the large private hospitals. They have also played an important role in showcasing Indian hospitals in the Middle East, East, and South East Asia for medical tourism.

POWER OF MARKETS AND RECONFIGURATION OF PUBLIC SECTOR

The transformation of the private sector has led to the partnership of big capital, domestic, and overseas, in financing, provisioning, medical education, pharmaceutical, and medical devices in the health service system. Holistically, they represent and fulfil the idea of a medical–industrial complex. The different actors have exerted power and influenced health policy over the last three decades. The extent of their influence is determined by the relative power that they are able to exercise depending on their size and access to capital across different levels of care. The power to influence policy is graded across the hierarchy with individual private practitioners having the least power, small and medium nursing homes exercising their power and influence through district- and state-level bodies of the Indian Medical Association (IMA) to lobby for their interests. The corporate hospitals use the platforms of the CII and Federation of India Chamber of Commerce to collectively articulate their needs and put forth vision documents. At all these levels the various actors are engaged with political parties at the local, state, and central levels.

In several states, politicians set up educational trusts that include private medical colleges. As Baru (2016: 128) observes:

> The growth of private medical colleges is part of a larger process of the movement of regional private capital into higher education, especially engineering, IT and medicine. These institutions were promoted by the intermediary castes like the Marathas in Maharashtra, Reddys and Kammas in Andhra Pradesh, Chettiars, Mudaliars and Gounders in Tamil Nadu and the Patidars in Gujarat.

There is a growing nexus between politicians, real estate, liquor lobby, and religious bodies in private higher education. A large number of these are seen in Maharashtra, Karnataka, Andhra Pradesh, Tamil Nadu, and Kerala. There are fewer in the north than in the south of India.[8] The power that they derived from this nexus has made it possible for them to receive public subsidies and influence the Medical Council to grant licenses.[9]

The informal private practitioners who are the least powerful in the hierarchy have also formed associations across states and are aligned to political parties. For example, in Khammam district the association was aligned to the Communist Party of India (Marxist) (CPI[M]). Similar associations are found in other states. Moves to ban or regulate private practice by the IMA are consistently resisted. The Indian Medical Association, dominated by private interests, systematically opposes all efforts by the government at regulating quality care. The poor uptake and implementation of the Clinical Establishments Act is due to resistance by the IMA. The Medical Council and Nursing Council too show the nexus between professional power and local politics.

Several scholars have commented on how commercialization undermines the values that the public sector represents (Mackintosh and Koivusalo 2005). The values that the public sector embodies are based on the principles of social solidarity and ethical dimensions like fairness and equity (Sandel 2012). Social solidarity helps to build 'ownership' of public facilities across classes and brings in the crucial dimension of moral responsibility in an unequal society. Thus the collective need is privileged over individual need.

A study of retired doctors of the All India Institute of Medical Sciences (AIIMS), Delhi, captures the gradual erosion of values in the public sector. This erosion is contributed by several factors that include under-investment, political interference, poor infrastructure, and poor working conditions in public hospitals. Simultaneously, the growth of an unregulated private sector has transformed medicine into a commodity (Baru 2005).

It is well recognized that an inclusive and universal health services ensures a better standard of care since those who use the services belong to different socio-economic groups. However, when the fabric of social solidarity gets weak it leads to the more powerful sections exiting from public services. This leads to a process where marginalized sections, along the multiple axes of religion, caste, class, and gender rely more on public services. Given their relative powerlessness in society, these sections are unable to exercise power to demand accountability from the public services. The majority of doctors who wield the maximum power within the health services also reinforce market ideology in their practices (Baru 1998).[10]

In this context, the growth of markets in the health services, within and outside the public sector, has far-reaching implications because it reconfigures the structure and behaviour of institutions and professionals who provide health services. There are several examples of the reconfiguration of the public sector with the introduction of market principles. When user charges, contracting in and out of diagnostic services, and hiring of contract workers are introduced into the public sector, the personnel and the institution starts behaving like a private sector entity. At this stage, the process of further devaluation of the public sector gains momentum with policymakers who are convinced about power of markets.

NOTES

1. Steven Brill's (2015) book, *America's Bitter Pill: Money, Politics, Backroom Deals, and the Fight to Fix our Broken Healthcare System*, was reviewed in *The Economist*, 17 January 2015.

2. For a detailed analysis, see Chakravarthi (2013b).

3. By plural we mean that different systems—formal and informal form a part of the private sector.

4. In a conversation, Dr Badrinath, founder of Shankara Netralaya, mentioned that Dr Reddy used to make several visits for changing rules to import medical devices. Dr Badrinath himself met Rajiv Gandhi when he needed to import a specific medical device for an eye surgery that the religious leader Shankaracharya needed. Rajiv Gandhi immediately agreed to reduce import duties for the same.

5. Gupte's biography of Prathap Reddy has references to the role of state chief ministers in Tamil Nadu and Andhra Pradesh in the establishment of Apollo, Chennai and Hyderabad. There are also references to the heads of banks, religious leaders, and bureaucrats who played the role of facilitators in his various projects. Dr Reddy got social and political access through influential patients.

6. Schroder Ventures group was run by Anil Thadani, who started his private equity business in 1981 and had major investments in the hospitality sector. By the late 1980s he decided to invest in health care. In 1994, Dr Reddy offered 25 per cent equity interest in the Indraprastha Apollo hospital in Delhi. Thadani started investing in several projects in South East Asia, the leading one among them being Parkway Holdings in Singapore. Malaysian wealth fund, Khazanah, was one of the early investors, still invested in the hospital chain, which picked up 5.5 million shares during 2005 for USD 44.23 million from TWL Holdings, an investment fund advised by Singapore-based PE firm Symphony Capital Partners. Khazanah had started consolidating its shares in AHEL in 2011 and currently holds 10.85 per cent share. Oppenheimer Funds, a subsidiary of Massachusetts Mutual Life Insurance Company, has another 8.39 per cent stake. Apax Partners has reportedly sold 19 per cent stake in AHEL for Rs 2,240 crore through several transactions in the open market, giving it a three-fold return over a six-year period. It started picking up stake in 2007, starting from the acquisition of 11.5 per cent shares in AHEL for USD 104 million (Rs 420 crore at that time). Later, it increased its stake. In October 2013, US-based PE firm, Kohlberg Kravis Roberts, infused around Rs 550 crore in the holding company—PCR Investments—which was expected to be used to repay the promoters' debt (Narasimhan 2015).

7. There are several such examples in Reddy's biography. Treating relatives of influential politicians gave him access socially. This became an important aspect of accessing political networks for policy influence.

8.   Details of the nexus was observed while the author was a member of the Ethics Committee of the Medical Council of India.

9.   Many of these colleges flouted all the required norms for recognition by Medical Council of India.

10.   Baru documents the role of commissions offered to doctors by diagnostic centres and labs for referring patients. Also see Nagral (2002).

REFERENCES

Baru, R. 1998. *Private Health Care in India: Social Characteristics and Trends.* New Delhi: Sage Publications.

————. 2005. 'Commercialisation and Public Sector in India: Implications for Values and Aspirations'. In *Commercialization of Health Care: Global And Local Dynamics And Policy Responses*, M. Mackintosh and M. Koivusalo (eds), pp. 101–16. New York: Palgrave Macmillan.

————. 2016. 'Commercialisation and the Poverty of Public Health Services in India'. In *Public Health and Private Wealth: Stem Cells, Surrogates and Other Strategic Bodies*, Sarah Hodges and Mohan Rao (eds), pp. 121–38. Delhi: Oxford University Press.

Brill, Steven. 2015. *America's Bitter Pill: Money, Politics, Backroom Deals, and the Fight to Fix our Broken Healthcare System.* New York: Random House.

Chakravarthi, I. 2013a. 'Medical Technology in India: Tracing Policy Approaches', *Indian Journal of Public Health* 57(4): 197–202.

————. 2013b. 'Medical Technology in India: Production, Procurement and Utilisation', *Indian Journal of Public Health* 57(4): 203–7.

Chanda, R. 2007. 'Foreign Investments in Hospitals in India: Status and Implications', IIMB in collaboration with WHO India Country office and WHO cell, Ministry of Health and Family Welfare, Government of India. September.

Dilip, T.R. 2010. 'Utilization of In-patient Care from Private Hospitals: Trends Emerging from Kerala, India'. *Health Policy Plan* 25(5): 437–46. September. doi: 10.1093/heapol/czq012. Epub 2010 28 March.

Government of India. 1995. 'Budget Speech of 1995–96 by Finance Minister Dr. Manmohan Singh'. Available at: indiabudget.nic.in/bspeech/bs199596.pdf. Accessed on 20 September 2016.

Gupte, P. 2013. *Healer: Dr Prathap Chandra Reddy and the Transformation of India.* India: Penguin Books.

Hodges, S. 2013. '"It all changed after Apollo": Healthcare Myths and their Making in Contemporary India', *Indian Journal of Medical Ethics* 10(4): 242–9.

Lefebvre, B. 2010. 'Hospital Chains in India: The Coming of Age?', published by *Centre Asie ifri*. Available at: www.ifri.org. Accessed on 30 January 2015.

Mackintosh, M. and M. Koivusalo (eds). 2005. *Commercialization of Health Care: Global and Local Dynamics and Policy Responses*. New York: Palgrave-Macmillan.

Nagral, S. 2002. 'General Practice: Some Thoughts', *Issues in Medical Ethics* 10(2): 7–8.

Narasimhan, E. 2015. *Business Standard*, 22 January.

Ray, A.S. and S. Bhaduri. 2012. 'The Indian Pharmaceutical Industry in a Changing Global Landscape: Competing Through Technological Capability', CSSP Electronic Working Paper Series, Paper No. 3, September. Jawaharlal Nehru University, India.

Relman, A.S. 1980. 'The New Medical-Industrial Complex', *The New England Journal of Medicine* 303(17): 963–70.

Sandel, M.J. 2012. *What Money Can't Buy: The Moral Limits of Markets*. New York: Farrar, Straus and Giroux.

Santhosh, M.R. 2011. 'An Enquiry into the Implications of Liberalisation on the Indian Drugs and Pharmaceutical Sector' (1991–2010). Unpublished PhD thesis, School of Social Sciences, Jawaharlal Nehru University.

Sen, G., A. Iyer, and A. George. 2002. 'Structural Reforms and Health Equity: A Comparison of NSS Surveys of 1986–87 and 1995–96', *Economic and Political Weekly* 37(14): 1342–52.

Starr, P. 1982. *The Social Transformation of American Medicine*. New York: Basic Books.

Sundararaman, T. and V.R. Muraleedharan. 2015. 'Falling Sick, Paying the Price: NSS 71st Round on Morbidity and Costs of Healthcare', *Economic and Political Weekly* 50(33): 17–20.

4

Social Roots of Medical Education

Neha Madhiwalla

India has one of the largest numbers of medical colleges in the world. In 2016, there were 426 recognized medical colleges offering undergraduate allopathic medical education in India. An estimated 60,000 undergraduate and postgraduate medical students are currently enrolled in these colleges.[1]

The introduction of western/allopathic medicine in India was deeply embedded in colonialism. At the beginning of the nineteenth century, when the East India Company was consolidating itself in India, the needs of the European population, both its military and civilians, was met through the Indian Medical Service, which recruited European-trained doctors. The colonial government made some attempts to impart additional training to existing indigenous practitioners through schools and institutes, such as the School for Native Doctors, established in Calcutta in 1822 (Jeffery 1979). However, indigenous systems of medicine were viewed as resources, to be examined and subsumed into scientific medicine, rather than as complete independent systems of legitimate knowledge and practice (Guthrie 1963). Moreover, with the adoption of English as the exclusive language of higher education and the privileging of western education over all other existing traditions, the integration of indigenous systems with Western medicine became increasingly difficult. State funding was exclusively reserved for the establishment and development of western medical institutions, whether in education, research, or practice.

The first medical colleges were established in Calcutta and Madras in 1835, and ten years later, in Bombay. In 1860, another medical college was established in Lahore. Surprisingly, Indian elites—upper-caste Hindus, Parsees, Christians, and Muslims—took to medical education quite keenly showing no reluctance to learn anatomy or surgery, undertaking dissection, touching the bodies of patients, and handling bodily fluids, and so forth, which violated religious rules regarding ritual pollution (Gorman 1988). The Indian elite also supported the colonial government in establishing a dominant role for Western medicine through financial aid and patronage.

Europe remained the reference point for Indian allopathic medical institutions and practitioners. Medical colleges in India were modelled on existing schools in Europe. Faculty from European schools was brought in specifically to establish institutions and departments along similar lines. Western medical education in India not merely imbibed the 'natural sciences essentials', but also the social and cultural 'over coatings' of a colonial Europe (Banerji 1973). Subsequently, members of the Indian Medical Service, who were exclusively European, automatically assumed leadership positions in the medical colleges and research institutes (Power 1996).

The first generation of graduates from the medical colleges remained in the Presidency towns, where there was an English-educated, westernized middle-class, which would patronize their services. The most privileged students invariably sought further training in Britain (Jeffery 1979).

By the beginning of the twentieth century, Western medicine had established its dominance in the urban areas. Between 1906 and 1926, six more medical colleges were established in Lucknow, Delhi, Calcutta, Bombay, Vizagapatnam, and Patna, respectively. Missionary institutions also established a few medical colleges, notable among them, the Christian Medical College, Vellore; Christian Medical College, Ludhiana; and St John's Hospital, Bangalore.

As medical services managed by the government and philanthropic bodies expanded, giving rise to a demand for trained personnel, a shorter course of training—known as 'Licentiates'—was instituted. There were 27 licentiate training schools by the end of the 1930s. Initially, these were exclusively employed as subordinate staff in government hospitals but in time a section of them also set up private practice.

With the devolution of powers to Provincial governments after 1930 and the subsequent transfer of the management of health institutions to local bodies there was a further expansion of health infrastructure in some provinces prompting a new demand for health care workers. This expanded employment opportunities for licentiate practitioners. However, their demand for professional status was never fulfilled. While provincial medical councils accepted them on the medical register, the Indian Medical Council which was formed in 1933, refused to recognize them (Muraleedharan 1992). Eventually, about ten years after Independence, the licentiate course was abolished.

This move was in sharp contrast to China's approach towards universalizing health care, through 'barefoot doctors'. India did not adopt either of the innovations taken up in China—training professionals with a specific objective of providing primary care with a rural orientation and the integration of traditional systems of medicine and allopathy (Singh 2005). Arguably, the Western medicine practitioners, though fewer in numbers and marginal to the provision of primary care to the population at large, had the political influence to maintain their monopoly over the health care system.

At the time of Independence, there were 17 medical colleges in India. By 1957, these had rapidly expanded to 42 (Woodruff 1957). Following Independence, the central government offered financial assistance to the state governments for setting up more medical colleges. As a result, there were 81 medical colleges by 1964. Another feature of the early post-Independence era was the establishment of institutes exclusively for postgraduate training. These were located at Chandigarh, Calcutta, and Pondicherry. By a special Act of Parliament, specialized institutes, such as the All India Institute of Medical Sciences and Sri Chitra Tirunal Institutes of Medical Sciences and Technology were also established. These institutions were expected to focus on research and training of medical teachers.

Some of the more developed states, such as Maharashtra, Karnataka, Tamil Nadu, and Kerala expanded their network by establishing medical colleges attached to several of the district hospitals. These states, incidentally, also have the highest number of private medical colleges (Ananthakrishnan 2010). The concept of medical education as a lucrative business emerged in the 1980s, at a point where private practice had become viable. There was a substantial middle-class willing to make large investments for professional education and there was a slowing down of state investment in higher education. Today, private medical colleges have come to outnumber government and philanthropic hospitals: of the 310 recognized institutions, 157 are private colleges.[2]

ISSUES AND CONCERNS

At the time of Independence, medical colleges were state-sponsored and education was heavily subsidized. Existing non-governmental institutions too were managed by philanthropic organizations, which largely funded students' education and patient care through donations and grants. Even at that time, certain problems were becoming apparent: the lack of full-time faculty (Wahi 1956), the shortage of infrastructure and the difficulty of ensuring that students receive adequate clinical training (Pandit 1958). Later commentaries point to a growing frustration with the inability of colleges to attract high quality full-time teachers. The shortage of teachers is particularly acute for non-clinical subjects. Mismatches in terms of the number of teachers for clinical subjects and the total number of students admitted to each course, and the unwillingness of graduates to join faculty of medical colleges are some of the reasons of this problem (Ananthakrishnan 2007).

Many of the new private medical colleges have been established in non-metropolitan areas, but these are not accessible to local students because of their high fees. Private medical colleges have also been characterized by corruption, shortage of teachers, and poor standards of teaching (Davey et al. 2014).

Apart from the problem of finding good faculty, the orientation and goal of medical education whether private or public, has not significantly changed. It remains exclusive and disconnected from the health care needs of the population, at large. Nearly 30 years ago, in an analysis of American medical schools, Bloom (1988) had remarked that, since their establishment in the early twentieth century, there had been relatively little change in their orientation, despite numerous attempts to instill progressive educational values and a community perspective. He attributed this to the fact that research had taken precedence over teaching, the ascending dominance of technology and the rise of specialism at the cost of general practice. This analysis is strikingly applicable to present medical education in India. Medical colleges in India, typically, are organized under separate health universities rather than multidisciplinary universities. This insulates them from new ideas and social influences, thereby perpetuating existing hierarchies and biases (Lempp 2009).

The rampant commercialization of medical education has led to a palpable deterioration of standards and institutionalization of corruption, devaluing the process of medical training and the profession itself.

Private colleges have triggered a local brain drain, drawing away faculty and staff from government medical colleges (Amin et al. 2010). Some commentators have noted that the quality of education is also declining due to pervasive corruption and violation of norms in these colleges. There is a prevalent practice of private practitioners being paid an exorbitant fee to present them as teachers for a few days when inspections by the medical council are being carried out (Ananthakrishnan and Shanthi 2012). It has been pointed out that the accreditation process emphasizes primarily on the infrastructure and human resources availability, rather than measures of quality and outcomes. Moreover, this information is sought only from the college administration and no effort is made to elicit the views of faculty, students, or patients in this process (Supe and Burdick 2006).

Policy measures to reform medical education have not been complemented with actual changes in practice. For example, while centralized admissions on the basis of a single competitive exam has helped to equalize opportunities for all students, it has also given rise to several challenges. Few students gain admission in the hometown or even home states. Thus, students are cut-off from the family and support systems and thrust into unfamiliar cultural environments (Mavani 2007). Medical colleges rarely focus on orienting students to the local culture and milieu. Nor are students trained to understand social, emotional, and ethical aspects of practicing medicine. They are not taught how to communicate with patients and take into account the background and circumstances in which their patients live.

There is an absence of focus on ethics in the medical curriculum, except the teaching of 'bedside manners' and a few lectures on medical jurisprudence (Chattopadhyay 2009). The difficulty of teaching ethics to students in institutions tainted by corruption, which seemed to have lost their 'moral compass' has also been discussed (Chattopadhyay 2009: 93). A routine prescription for reforming medical education has been the introduction of teaching modules on ethics, communications, and psychomotor skills at the undergraduate level. In practice, because, students do not have any contact with patients at this level, these topics are also being taught through textbooks, like all the others, rather than in conjunction with patient care (Mavani 2007).

There is not much reflection in literature on the structural and historical factors that shape medical education. As a result, policy proclamations on reforming medical education tend to emphasize specific changes in teaching methodology and content, without much reference to the overall context in which medical education is delivered. For example, recommendations to make rural service compulsory are made frequently by various states, but are never fully implemented because nothing in the medical education system orients students to understand and appreciate the challenges of delivering health care to rural populations. Similarly, the report of the Task Force on Medical Education for the National Rural Health Mission, in a move to decentralize medical education, suggested the adoption of district hospitals by private medical colleges without any comment on improving conditions of government medical colleges that are attached to district hospitals in small towns (Ministry of Health and Family Welfare 2007). This is despite the fact that medical colleges attached to district hospitals have inadequate teachers and poor standards of teaching.

CONTENT, CULTURE, AND SOCIAL CONTEXT

India had medical schools when the vast majority of the population had not even achieved literacy. Thus, it was a profession largely reserved for the elite. As we have noted earlier, the first few generations of Western medicine doctors were drawn predominantly from the upper castes (Brahmins and the 'writing castes') and the more privileged minority groups, such as Parsees and Christians (Jaggi 1979; Ramanna 2002). The first medical colleges were established in the metropolitan areas, drawing local urban students who would settle down to practise where they had trained, leading to a concentration of medical practitioners in these cities. Although Indian doctors started out as an underclass to European doctors within the profession (Arnold 2000; Forbes 1994), by the time of Independence, Indian doctors had assumed comparable positions of authority and influence subsequently. The political power and influence of these practitioners was in sharp contrast to their actual contribution to health care. Only 2.5 per cent of the villages had a modern medicine practitioner at the time of Independence (Mehta 1965). Modern medicine was largely intended to serve the needs of the European population and, by extension, a section of the Indian elite. Hence, the evolving subculture of medicine was deeply embedded in the culture of the Indian elite.

The outcome of this particular history was the consecration of an aristocratic, intellectual, paternalistic, but benevolent man as the archetype of the ideal doctor (Kamath and Karmarkar 1993). The prevailing culture of medicine reflects the persistence of a bias towards the culture of the urban elite. The informal leadership of the profession continues to rest with the metropolitan, private practitioners, as they head professional associations and figure prominently in the 'speaking circuits'. More resources and a conducive academic environment enables faculty and administrators of premier metropolitan medical colleges to do more research and to publish, perpetuating their intellectual dominance. Prominent doctors practicing in the metropolitan areas are more likely to be inducted into government committees, where they are able to influence decisions about curricula, development of new specialties, and research priorities. This is reflected in the institutional culture of medical education and practice. Thus, instruction continues to be primarily in English and in the lecture mode.

Medical educationists are preoccupied with updating curricula to keep abreast with developments in hi-tech medicine and 'cutting-edge' fields, such as genetics, while there has been virtually no movement to revitalize disciplines such as preventive and social medicine. Students are socialized into a professional culture that privileges employment in the highly capital-intensive, technology-focused, and corporatized medical industry, rather than comprehensive primary care or public health. Consequently, there is a glaring mismatch in the stated objectives of medical education, that is, to provide universal access to health care and the orientation and training being provided to students. Relatively few graduates of allopathic medical colleges seem to enter general practice. The dissonance between practising 'scientific' medicine and 'practical' medicine is mentioned frequently in the accounts of professional practice. A dilemmatic situation has arisen within medical education where students are eager to train in government medical colleges because they offer abundant 'clinical material', but do not intend to practice in the public sector (Ghoshal 2011).

The process of diversifying the student body of medical colleges has also been slow. Despite the institution of various policy measures to increase diversity in medical colleges, entry of marginalized students is still quite restricted. Relying on available secondary information, we find that, despite the existence of quotas for backward caste, scheduled caste (SC), and scheduled tribe (ST) students there were very few students admitted from these categories (Table 4.1). On the basis of information provided by universities and medical colleges, in contrast to Master of Science (MSc) students, among whom more than one-fourth belonged to the other backward castes and a little more than 10 per cent to the SCs, their representation among medical students, both at the undergraduate

TABLE **4.1** Proportion of Enrolled Students by Social Category
(as per information submitted by institutions)

	Scheduled castes	Scheduled tribes	Other backward classes
MSc—Master of Science	10.14	3.09	26.73
MD—Doctor of Medicine	6.56	3.17	13.94
MS—Master of Surgery	6.02	3.73	16.22
MBBS—Bachelor of Medicine and Bachelor of Surgery		3.46	14.72

Source: Ministry of Human Resource Development (2014).
Note: Based on actual responses submitted by institutions participating in
the survey.

and postgraduate levels was lower (a sizeable number of private medical
colleges did not respond to the query).

Between 1970 and 2004, there was 900 per cent increase in private
medical colleges, which now account for 45 per cent of all medical
colleges in the country (Mahal and Mohanan 2006). Thus, when the
gaps in data are taken into account, the proportion and actual number
of students from socially disadvantaged backgrounds, appears to be quite
small. On all counts, not enough underprivileged students appear to be
able to avail of the benefits of the constitutionally guaranteed provision
for the reservation of seats.

Students who are not urban-, middle-class, and upper-caste feel
the challenges of professional education keenly. Studies indicate that
this is especially the case for SC and ST students in higher education,
especially professional institutions. These students are less prepared
for the intensive nature of professional training largely because of the
poorer quality of basic education that they have received, their poorer
English skills, and lack of academic support (Kirpal et al. 1985). They
typically have poorer scores, take longer time to complete their course of
training, and have higher rates of stagnation and wastage. These students
report less satisfaction with the institution than their peers (Verma and
Kapur 2010).

These overall figures are likely to obscure regional differences in
trends. In certain states, where social and economic development
has been more rapid, it is likely that the present body of medical
students may be more culturally diverse, reflecting the overall changes

in the caste/location character of the Indian middle class. There is some evidence that medical colleges in Maharashtra, for example, are admitting more first-generation medical students and more students with a rural/semi urban upbringing (Dandekar 2013). There has been a general expansion of higher education among the lower castes, minority groups, and women particularly in regions with higher concentrations of urban and urbanizing regions (Basant and Sen 2013). There has been a gradual linking of aspirations to social mobility and status to professional education among groups that have not so far accessed higher education. For castes, which primarily engaged in agriculture, trade, or craft, producing professionals such as doctors has assumed a significance much beyond the material returns that can be derived from it. For traditionally marginalized groups, medicine continues to have value as a means of gaining status and a secure, middle-class life. Apart from the prestige of being engaged in an intellectual, technology-invested occupation, medicine retains its association with service and public life, imparting prominence and influence to successful entrants and their communities (cited in Dandekar 2013). In states, such as Maharashtra, where the health market has expanded rapidly, extending to the semi-urban and rural areas, there is more incentive for new entrants to return to their hometowns to practice. However, as few of these practitioners have long-term plans of serving in the government health care system or in primary care, practitioners of Indian system of medicine and unregistered practitioners continue to meet much of the demand for primary health care in the rural areas (Ashtekar and Mankad 2001; Sheikh and George 2012).

* * *

The concentration of Western medicine practitioners in private practice, largely in the urban areas and in specialized medicine, creates a paradoxical situation where a significant proportion of the population is unable to access essential clinical services despite an increase in the number of doctors and specialists produced. Trained allopathic doctors and specialists seem to be disappearing from the public health system (Pandav 2006). There is an increasing tendency to plan public health programmes that take for granted the unavailability of doctors at the primary-care level and specialists at the secondary-care level. Thus, strategies such as decentralization and task-shifting are being deployed to devolve service delivery and health planning tasks to nursing staff,

Indian Systems of Medicine (ISM) practitioners, and community health workers at the primary level and non-specialist doctors at the secondary level.

The reservation policy, complemented by the rising aspirations of backward castes and other disadvantaged groups, may hold the prospect of a larger number of doctors motivated to practice in rural and semi-urban areas. However, this is unlikely to happen if medical training and its orientation continue to replicate the technologized, capital-intensive, and commodified metropolitan model of medicine. In this form of medical practice interpersonal skills, clinical acumen, insight into local culture and practice, and greater understanding and empathy with patients has less relevance than mastery of technology, acquisition of entrepreneurial skills, and entry into elite professional networks. The conceptualization of medicine as service, intended to meet the needs of the entire population, appears more untenable and alien. Thus, the promise of the cultural change in medicine held out by the entry of relatively less elite students into the profession will be belied by the increasingly distorted model of medical practice. This disjunction between the stated goals of medical education and its actual orientation and training renders graduates not merely unwilling, but also unfit to practice where they are needed. Thus, the present attempt by several states to compel graduates to spend some time serving in the public health care system are not likely to have any sustainable impact, even while the health market expands and colonizes the entire country.

India has one of the highest outmigration rates for medical personnel in the world. It is estimated that about one-third of the allopathic doctors, graduating each year migrate abroad (Supe and Burdick 2006). The artificial pressure of competition created by the private sector makes migration appear as a viable option, despite the financial costs and additional training/qualifying exams required to gain admission to postgraduate training or employment abroad. In some African and smaller Asian countries, the local health services have been left virtually devoid of any professionals due to migration. In India, because it produces a large number of doctors and specialists, migration does not necessarily lead to that kind of crisis (Mullan 2005). However, physician migration still represents a complete loss of returns from the large public investments made in medical education. While graduates from government medical colleges have received direct state support through heavily subsidized medical education, private medical colleges also absorb public resources, either by availing of land and infrastructure at concessional rates, subsidies, tax concessions, or the use of government hospitals for clinical training.

There appear to be divergent tendencies in the development of medical practice in India, which simultaneously move it towards democratization and elitism, autonomy, and subordination. (*i*) On the one hand, Western medicine's claim to science and the class position of its practitioners has enabled it to mobilize both material resources and political influence and retain its autonomy from state/societal control, conferring a high social status to its members. On the other hand, its high dependence on private capital and integration into the market means that its substantial resources and political power are not actually utilized for fulfilling the needs of the people. (*ii*) While affirmative action policies, greater participation of girls in higher education, and the rising aspirations of the backward classes brings greater numbers of non-elite students into government medical colleges in some regions, the growth of a large number of private medical colleges has led to greater commercialization and created another elite class of doctors. Thus, students from underprivileged backgrounds may be able to gain entry, but will find it increasingly difficult to cope with the competition and establish practice.

NOTES

1. See http://www.mciindia.org/Inform.
2. Available at: http://www.mciindia.org/InformationDesk/ForStudents/ ListofCollegesTeachingMBBS.aspx. Accessed on 13 August 2016.

REFERENCES

Amin, Z., W.P. Burdick, A. Supe, and T. Singh. 2010. 'Relevance of the Flexner Report to Contemporary Medical Education in South Asia', *Academic Medicine* 85(2): 333–9.

Ananthakrishnan, N. 2007. 'Acute Shortage of Teachers in Medical Colleges: Existing Problems and Possible Solutions', *National Medical Journal of India* 20(1): 25.

————. 2010. 'Medical Education in India: Is It Still Possible to Reverse the Downhill Trend?', *National Medical Journal of India* 23(3): 156–60.

Ananthakrishnan, N. and A.K. Shanthi. 2012. 'Attempts at Regulation of Medical Education by the MCI: Issues of Unethical and Dubious Practices for Compliance by Medical Colleges and Some Possible Solutions', *Indian Journal of Medical Ethics* 9(1): 37–42.

Arnold, D. 2000. *Science, Technology and Medicine in Colonial India*. United Kingdom: Cambridge University Press.

Ashtekar, S. and D. Mankad. 2001. 'Who Cares? Rural Health Practitioners in Maharashtra', *Economic and political Weekly* 36(5–6): 448–53.

Banerji, D. 1973. 'Social Orientation of Medical Education in India', *Economic and Political Weekly* 8(9): 485–8.

Basant, R. and G. Sen. 2013. 'Access to Higher Education in India: An Exploration of Its Antecedents', *W.P. No. 2013-05-011*. Ahmedabad: Indian Institute of Management.

Bloom, S.W. 1988. 'Structure and Ideology in Medical Education: An Analysis of Structure Resistance to Change', *Journal of Health and Social Behaviour* 29(4): 294–306.

Chattopadhyay, S. 2009. 'Teaching Ethics in an Unethical Setting: "Doing Nothing" is Neither Good nor Right', *Indian Journal of Medical Ethics* 6(2): 93–6.

Dandekar, V. 2013. 'Reservations in Medical Education in Maharashtra: An Empirical Study'. In *Beyond Inclusion: The Practice of Equal Access in Indian Higher Education*, S. Deshpande and U. Zacharias (eds), pp. 95–144. New Delhi: Routledge.

Davey, S., A. Davey, A. Srivastava, and P. Sharma. 2014. 'Privatization of Medical Education in India: A Health System Dilemma', *International Journal of Medicine and Public Health* 4(1): 17–22.

Forbes, G. 1994. 'Medical Careers and Health Care for Indian Women: Patterns of Control', *History* 3(4).

Ghoshal, R. 2011. '"Hands on Learning" in Medicine: Who Benefits?', *Economic and Political Weekly* 46(42): 16–18.

Gorman, M. 1988. 'Introduction of Western Science into Colonial India: Role of the Calcutta Medical College', *Proceedings of the American Philosophical Society* 132(3): 276–98.

Guthrie, D. 1963. 'Medical History in Modern India', *Medical History* 7(03): 275–7.

Jaggi, O.P. 1979. *History of Science, Technology and Medicine in India (Vol. 15)*. Delhi, India: Atma Ram & Sons.

Jeffery, R. 1979. 'Recognizing India's Doctors: The Institutionalization of Medical Dependency (1918–39)', *Modern Asian Studies* 13(2): 301–26.

Kamath, M.V. and R. Karmarkar. 1993. *Untold Stories of Doctors and Patients*. New Delhi: UBS Publishers' Distributors Ltd.

Kirpal, V., N. Swamidasan, A. Gupta, and R.K. Gupta. 1985. 'Scheduled Caste and Tribe Students in Higher Education: A Study of an IIT', *Economic and Political Weekly* 20(29): 1238–48.

Lempp, H. 2009. 'Medical-school Culture'. In *Handbook of the Sociology of Medical Educationi*, C. Brosnan and B. Turner (eds), pp. 71–88. New York: Routledge.

Mahal, A. and M. Mohanan. 2006. 'Growth of Private Medical Education in India', *Medical Education* 40(10): 1009–11.

Mavani, P.S. 2007. 'Restructuring Medical Education', *Indian Journal of Medical Ethics* 4(2): 62–3.

Mehta, J.N. 1965. 'Medical Services in India', *Journal of the Royal Society of Arts* 113(5112): 995–1019.

Ministry of Health and Family Welfare. 2007. *Report of Task Force on Medical Education for the National Rural Health Mission*. New Delhi: Ministry of Health and Family Welfare, Government of India.

Ministry of Human Resource Development. 2014. *All India Survey on Higher Education 2011–12*. New Delhi: Ministry of Human Resource Development.

Mullan, F. 2005. 'The Metrics of the Physician Brain Drain', *The New England Journal of Medicine* 353(17): 1810–18.

Muraleedharan, V.R. 1992. 'Professionalizing Medical Practice in Colonial South-India', *Economic and Political Weekly* 27(4): 27–37.

Pandav, C.S. 2006. 'National Rural Health Mission: An Opportunity to Bridge the Chasm between Prescription, Practice and Perception of Medical Education in India', *Indian Journal of Public Health* 50(3): 153.

Pandit, C.G. 1958. 'Medical Education in India-A Challenge', *Academic Medicine* 33(3): 185–92.

Power, H. 1996. 'The Calcutta School of Tropical Medicine: Institutionalizing Medical Research in the Periphery', *Medical History* 40(02): 197–214.

Ramanna, M. 2002. *Western Medicine and Public Health in Colonial Bombay, 1845–1895*. New Delhi: Orient Blackswan.

Sheikh, K. and A. George (eds). 2012. '*Health Providers in India: On the Frontlines of Change'*. New Delhi: Routledge.

Singh, A. 2005. 'Restructuring Medical Education', *Economic and Political Weekly* 40(34): 3725–31.

Supe, A. and W.P. Burdick. 2006. 'Challenges and Issues in Medical Education in India', *Academic Medicine* 81(12): 1076–80.

Verma, R. and D. Kapur. 2010. 'Access, Satisfaction, and Future: Undergraduate Education at the Indian Institutes of Technology', *Higher Education* 59(6): 703–17.

Wahi, P.N. 1956. 'Medical Education in India', *Academic Medicine* 31(4): 249–54.

Woodruff, A.W. 1957. 'Medical Training and Research in India To-day', *British Medical Journal* 2(5044): 537.

5

Medical Education and Basic Health Care
Forging Connections

Anand Zachariah

The privatization of medical education, health care, and lack of government investment in public medical colleges and public health care facilities are generally regarded as having led to the lack of access to basic health care in India. A less recognized aspect of the problem is the nature and content of medical knowledge. This chapter argues that medical solutions developed in western countries (and passed on to successive generations of Indian medical graduates) were not designed to address the health problems of countries, such as India, with their cultural and socially specific disease profile and poor health care system. Transplantation of knowledge from a western setting to India is leading to high cost and inappropriateness. To understand the lack of access to health care we have to consider the relationship between medical knowledge, medical education, and the health care system in India.

The chapter is divided into three sections. The first section looks at the structure of medical knowledge that is contributing to the lack of access to health care. The second section addresses the lack of linkages between medical education system and the health care system. And the final section elaborates on medical curriculum and pedagogy and points out their inappropriateness and inadequacy in dealing with local health problems and the local context. The chapter further discusses possible ways of dealing with the structural problems of knowledge, medical education, and health care system that are leading to the lack of access to health care.

MEDICAL KNOWLEDGE AND LOCAL HEALTH PROBLEMS: THE MISMATCH

Modern medicine had its birth in eighteenth- and nineteenth-century Europe in the historical context of nation states needing to govern their populations. Medicine leap-frogged in its scale and scope during and after the Second World War, with the Beveridge Plan and the commitment of England and other European countries to providing health care as a basic right to every citizen. From this time on, a substantial part of Western state budgets have been channelled into health care and research. This has fuelled the development of health care systems, large hospitals, specializations, pharmaceutical, and equipment industries (Zachariah 2010a). The rapid and miraculous transformations in medicine over the last half a century have been underpinned by large-scale investment in health care by western governments. Many specializations have evolved around specific technologies.[1] The structure of science and technology were a response to the cultural and social milieu in these countries. The problems that were researched and the treatments that were developed were also a response to the needs of these countries. Hence, the knowledge and experience was in tune with their health care systems and was generally economically viable in their context.

Today modern medicine is the gold standard. It has become universalized and is widespread across cultures and societies worldwide. This universalization, however has its nuances and complexities. For instance, disease definitions and treatment strategies have been designed for particular socio-economic and cultural settings and lifestyles, and fit with the administrative technology and health care apparatus (for example, the National Health System in UK and welfare health systems in Europe and elsewhere). Knowledge developed within Western health systems when applied to non-Western settings that are socially and culturally different and do not have similar health delivery systems and patient support mechanisms, cause severe dissonance of various kinds (Zachariah 2010a). Unfortunately, there has been a significant poverty of development of knowledge for local health problems in countries like India.

The development of a universal primary health care system in India was envisaged at the time of Independence through the primary health centres (PHCs). However, the government did not have administrative will nor the financial resources to achieve this. From the 1960s, the trends in the development of academic specialization have led to specialist dominated and privatized health care system without adequate attention to the development of primary care as an important discipline in the Indian setting.

As early as the 1950s, Indian physicians trained in the US and Europe have returned to establish speciality departments in government medical colleges and non-profit medical colleges in India. From a historical perspective, a range of medical specializations have developed in India over the last 50 years: cardiology, thoracic surgery, neurology, and neurosurgery developed in the 1960s; gastroenterology, nephrology, and urology in the 1970s; haematology, pulmonology, endocrinology in the 1980s; and critical care and rheumatology in the 1990s. With the establishment of academic departments in teaching institutions, super-specialization training programmes were started in these medical colleges. Each of these specializations and teaching courses simply applied the framework designed for developed countries in the establishment of these programmes in India (Zachariah 2010a).

The growing pool of super specialists from these programmes were absorbed into the western-style corporate hospitals that began to be set up in cities in the 1980s, feeding the human resource need of the technology-centred hospitals. Simultaneously, changing human power and immigration policies in the US forced the return of large numbers of highly qualified medical personnel, which too prompted the setting up of even more tertiary care facilities. Not surprisingly, only the private sector had the resources, as for instance derived from the new diversification of agricultural capital in some regions, to invest in the expensive technology-driven tertiary care hospitals (Baru 1998). This historical development of academic specializations and training programmes has, in large measure, contributed to the growth of private tertiary hospitals. Simultaneously, training in primary and secondary care has remained underdeveloped and inappropriate. While super-specializations were developing, the discipline of family medicine, for example, was not even recognized in India.

There are severe shortfalls in the number of primary-care physicians at the PHC level and secondary-care physicians at the community health care (CHC) and district hospital level (GOI 2006). If primary care had been developed as a medical discipline with large number of trained family medicine doctors, this shortfall could have been well addressed.

It is estimated that 14,000 family physicians (3,000 in the government hospitals and 11,000 in the private sector) could provide for a feasible and effective model of universal access to health care in India (Zachariah 2014). An ameliorating trend in this otherwise bleak situation has been the starting of Family Medicine in few medical colleges, the launch of MD programmes in some colleges, and innovative training programmes in that discipline through distance education at the Christian Medical College (Velavan 2012).

The United Kingdom has been the model and flag bearer for development of primary care as an academic discipline. In UK the largest number of postgraduate training posts are in primary care and they support the needs of the health care system. This has been the model for a large number of western countries in Europe, Australia, and Canada. Western welfare states have supported tertiary care hospitals on a large backbone of universal primary care. Several middle-income countries such as Brazil and South Africa have been able to develop systems of universal access to health care by training a large number of multi-competent primary-care physicians (Rahman et al. 2014). In all these countries both health care and medical care education are government-run.

Moving on, we elaborate upon two developments to demonstrate how the mindless application of knowledge systems, structures, and practices derived from other socio-cultural contexts have impacted the emergence of appropriate knowledge and practices in India.

Case of Ischaemic Heart Disease

India is in the midst of a twin cardiovascular epidemic: one epidemic among the rich reflecting the epidemic in the west, and another among the poor. The epidemic among the poor is actually larger, reflecting the increase in slum population, high rates of hypertension, smoking, poor diet, sedentary life style, and high stress. Epidemiological studies have shown a reversal of cardiovascular risk factors across the socio-economic gradient with increasing rates of tobacco use, hypertension, and abdominal obesity among people from lower socio-economic background (Deepa et al. 2011; Gupta et al. 2003). The rates of heart attack and stroke are higher among people of lower socio-economic background with higher death rates (Pednekar, Gupta, and Gupta 2011; Xavier et al. 2008). It is thought that people from lower socio-economic background are at an increased risk of developing vascular accidents and strokes.

The discipline of cardiology developed around the problem of Ischaemic heart disease (IHD). Drug trials have shown their success in field of IHD with the development of evidence-based treatments: beta blockers, statins, aspirin, thrombolytic therapy, stenting procedures, and coronary artery bypass graft (CABG). When these treatments are applied for the epidemic of IHD among the lower socio-economic classes in India, there are problems of cost and inappropriateness (Zachariah 2010c).

The elite are able to access and afford the expensive treatments of IHD provided by the private and corporate sector. Today there are over 500 cardiac catheterization labs spread across most metropolitan cities, predominantly in the private sector, performing more than 70,000 cardiac procedures every year (Kaul and Bhatia 2010). Very few government medical colleges have these facilities. To man these centres, medical colleges admit 265 Doctor of Medicine students in cardiology every year, the largest super specialty training programme in India.[2] In contrast, there are a negligible number of cardiologists in rural locations as evidenced by a study of eight middle-sized districts across the country (MoHFW 2005). The government is unable to provide cardiac tertiary care facilities for IHD in the majority of the government medical colleges due to lack of specialist posts and high costs of the required equipment. The management of patients with drugs, bypass surgery, and stenting is extremely expensive. So, the current standard of treatment for coronary artery disease is unavailable for the vast majority of patients with coronary artery disease in this country.

When poor patients are admitted to private hospitals for heart attacks, the cost of treatment can lead to immiserization of families. In some states, such as Tamil Nadu, the government is providing universal access to tertiary care by state insurance paying private hospitals for stenting and CABG. On the other hand, initiating primary prevention for slum dwellers in cities is difficult, because of the high cost of good quality food and the lack of opportunities for increased physical activity. The only feasible approach as advocated by the WHO is treatment of IHD with beta blockers, aspirin, and statins using generic drugs, and secondary prevention by screening and treating cardiovascular risk factors (WHO 2002). Studies show that the universal primary health care programme in Brazil focusing on cardiovascular disease prevention, care, and follow-up can contribute towards reduced hospitalizations and deaths due to heart attacks and strokes (Rasella et al. 2014).

The development of the knowledge of cardiovascular medicine in India has not occurred in a manner that takes account of the epidemic in India. The unreflective transfer of knowledge, developed in a western population and for the western health systems, to the Indian setting has led to a mismatch between the structure of the health problem and that of the knowledge that is being used to address it. These have led to lack of access and inappropriate care of coronary artery disease. In effect, the lack of access and inappropriateness are because of the profit orientation of super-specialty cardiovascular medicine that does not consider the accessibility and affordability of this treatment for those falling prey to the epidemic of cardiovascular disease among the poor.

Let us contrast the problem of management of ischaemic heart disease to that of rheumatic heart disease (RHD), which is the other main cardiovascular disease in India. Rheumatic heart disease declined in western countries even before cardiology became a specialty. Not surprisingly, the Western discipline of cardiology has not focused as much attention on rheumatic fever and RHD as it has on coronary artery disease. Today we should have been in a situation where our wards and OPDs should be free of chronic rheumatic heart disease. However, cardiac surgery centres are still full of cases of RHD requiring valve replacement, and RHD is still the cardiovascular case for the final MBBS examination, reflecting its clinical importance, notwithstanding the fact that rheumatic fever is declining and better treatments are available for mitral stenosis such as Balloon mitral valvotomy (Kumar and Tandon 2013). A more sustained academic focus on prevention and treatment of rheumatic fever could have led to a virtual eradication of the RHD today in India (Zachariah 2014). Rheumatic heart disease is an example of the lack of development of medical knowledge to address local health problems.

The argument here is not that that the government should not be providing state-of-the-art acute coronary care with primary Percutaneous Transluminal Coronary Angioplasty, or that medical teachers should not be advocating evidence-based guidelines for IHD management to medical students. The public health importance of IHD as a cause of morbidity and mortality, mandated research into cost-effective strategies for IHD prevention and treatment in India. However such treatment should be provided as part of a rational approach to integrated prevention and treatment. These should include: (*i*) primary prevention: affordable options for a widened food basket of vegetables and fruits and coarse cereals, space and options for physical exercise in slums, and educational approaches to tobacco cessation; (*ii*) secondary prevention programme through screening for diabetes, hypertension, and hypercholesterolemia and use of low cost generic drugs for effective risk factor management; and (*iii*) tertiary prevention or treatment: establishment of cardiac care in CHCs and district hospital with adequate equipment and trained personnel for quick ambulance transfer, appropriate triage, and interventional treatment of cardiac emergencies. A good example of the latter is the STEMI (ST-elevation myocardial infarction) project in Tamil Nadu in which ECGs are performed on the 108-strength ambulance system and electronically transferred to a control centre where decisions are immediately made regarding triage to a tertiary centre for coronary interventions (Alexander et al. 2013).

Case of Poisoning and Snakebite

Today suicides are the second most common cause of death among the young adults, after road traffic accidents (Manoranjitham et al. 2010; Prasad et al. 2006). In India, the deliberate self-harm (DSH) epidemic manifests as pesticide, rodenticide poisonings, drug overdoses, and plant poisonings. The epidemiology of deliberate self-harm in India is not the same as in the West, with impulsive episodes and low rate of psychopathology and low reattempt rates (Manoranjitham et al. 2010). It is generally thought that the epidemic of DSH is due to young people being exposed to acute or chronic stress in the context of easy access to highly toxic pesticides (Zachariah 2010b).

In the case of organophosphate poisoning, there are a few effective treatments (atropine, Intensive Care Unit (ICU) care, and mechanical ventilation). Aluminium phosphide poisoning has no known antidote. The only treatment for Yellow Oleander poisoning is Fragment antigen binding antibody (FAB antibody) against Digoxin, which are too expensive for regular use. Sri Lanka has shown that banning of Class I pesticides has led to fall in suicide death rates without affecting agricultural production (Gunnell et al. 2007). In India, however, pesticide restriction to reduce suicide death rate has not received public health policy attention.

Snake bite is an important public health problem in rural areas contributing to an estimated 50,000 deaths per year (Mohapatra et al. 2011). There is no diagnostic test available to identify the species of snake that has bitten the patient. Polyvalent anti-snake venom (ASV) produced in India is highly allergic and has variable efficacy. There has been no dose findings study to determine the exact dose of ASV for snake envenomation (Warrell 2011).

These issues indicate the lack of research and underdevelopment of knowledge in the field of toxicology (poisonings) and toxinology (envenomations) in India. The main poisons in the West are drug overdoses, with low morbidity and mortality, and the field of toxicology has developed around these problems. There is little government support and research money in India for developing improved treatments for organophosphate poisoning or snake envenomations. Pharmaceutical companies have not evinced interest in these diseases that affect people from lower socio-economic status and where treatment is provided mainly in the public health system.

There is clearly an under-investment in health care in India (1 per cent of Gross Domestic Product [GDP]) that is contributing not only to the lack of access to health care but also lack of research and development of appropriate care for India-specific medical problems. This lack of investment in provision of basic primary care is contributing to people having to access costly health care in the private sector. The result is that, on the one hand poor people are accessing expensive high technology cardiac care in private hospitals, and on the other, there is the lack of an effective treatment for poisoning and snakebites resulting in rising death rates.

POOR LINKAGES BETWEEN MEDICAL EDUCATION AND HEALTH CARE

Medicine is a field where education and practice are inextricably linked. To provide for the needs of health care, medical education needs to inform practice and influence the health care system. In India this chain is poorly developed.

The Department of Medical Education and the Department of Health Services function in silos, although they are under the administrative control of the health secretary (Zachariah 2012). In every state, the government medical college is the sole provider of tertiary care in the government health system; but, surprisingly, it is not linked to the health system. The referral system is planned only up to the district hospital. This means that the health system cannot make optimal use of the medical college. Training programmes for medical undergraduates and postgraduates occur almost exclusively within the medical college. Each medical college has two health centres, one urban and one rural, under the community health department operated by health service staff. The clinical teaching faculty of medical colleges is not involved in either service delivery or teaching at these centres. Medical colleges are not required to research local current health problems and be involved in health system research or policy planning.

Medical colleges have not been planned keeping in mind the human resource needs of the state. The five southern states have the majority of the medical colleges, while many of the states with the poorest health indices and health services have the fewest medical colleges (Sabde et al. 2014). The numbers of undergraduate or postgraduate seats in medical colleges are not tailored to the needs of the health system. In some states—Punjab, Assam, and Tripura—service in the health system after graduation is mandatory. Service quotas for selection to postgraduate course is another strategy for encouraging graduates to work in the health system. These do not, however, systemically address the problem of mismatch between the number of doctors produced and the human resource requirement in the government health system.

Private medical colleges have even weaker links to the health service than government medical colleges. Many private colleges heavily rely on retired medical college teachers as faculty and delay the setting up of hospitals even after they have been opened. Nor do they have adequate links to rural and urban health centres. All of which means that the clinical component of training is poor and the clinical load is, in general, low. Moreover, given that students pay high fees or large capitation amounts, in general their interest is in seeking lucrative careers rather than employment in the health system or in areas of need.

Content of Medical Education and Training

Globalization and Homogenization of Medical Education as a Discipline

Medical education, that is the pedagogy and content, is today an independent academic discipline with its own journals, textbooks, conferences, and postgraduate training programmes (Grant, Abdelrahman, and Zachariah 2013). Western medical institutions are exporting medical education methods such as problem based learning, skills trainers, training in communication, ethics and professionalism, and curricula such as problem-based and competency-based curricula in a revenue generation mode. The Foundation for Advancement in International Medical Education (FAIMER), the sister body of ECFMG (the US licensing board), has persuaded the Medical Council of India (MCI) to mandate that all medical colleges should have a medical education department headed by postgraduate trained medical educators and all medical college teachers have to complete medical education training. The rationale of this strategy is that the poor standards of medical education are due to medical college teachers, who have not received training in teaching. Such medical education training programmes for teachers focus on formats and methods that are primarily based on 'imported' ideas without a thought about the cultural contexts in which these ideas have emerged. For instance, skills training, standardized patients, and OSCE (objective structured clinical examination) emerge from settings where patient loads are small and therefore morbidities are thinner. Clinical skills including history taking and physical examination have been de-emphasized in Western medical centres because of diagnostic reliance on laboratory tests and imaging. In the context of depersonalization of Western medicine, communication, ethics, and professionalism modules have become necessary to bring back humanistic aspects of care. Competency-based curricula have emerged in the context of breaking down tasks for quality assessment required for managed care. Medical education ideas from the west are being implemented in standardized forms as solutions to the problem of medical education in India.

The Medical Council of India graduate regulation is oriented to train a global doctor (Grant, Abdelrahman, and Zachariah 2013; Zachariah and Grant 2015). The Medical Council of India, as the regulatory body for medical education lays down the guidelines and requirements for medical education. The curriculum for undergraduate medical education has been largely static with some minor changes over these years. Some of these changes include:

1. Under the Reorientation of Medical Education (ROME) initiative implemented in the 1970s, all medical colleges were recommended to set up rural and urban health centres for community health postings. The planned reorientation has been poorly implemented.
2. In 1993, the MCI shortened the preclinical phase from one and a half years to one year to increase integration in the preclinical, paraclinical, and clinical phases. While the shortening of the preclinical phase took place, the coursework of one and a half years was compressed into one year and the expected integration did not take place.
3. Other changes include changes in the duration of internship postings, OSCE as an assessment method, and inclusion of paediatrics as a full subject.

The Medical Council of India's vision of the doctor has been a world class doctor who can work anywhere in the world. This has unfortunately meant that graduates are not equipped to practice in rural areas or small towns. They cannot tailor their care to the local social and economic context. They end up seeking post-graduation and/or going abroad. The Medical Council of India's recognition of medical colleges is mostly based on fulfilling requirements regarding infrastructure, equipment, and staffing and not on the quality of education. In consequence neither private nor government medical colleges are interested in innovating beyond these requirements.

How is the health care system and medical education to be remodelled so that not only are there dynamic links between training and the system, and the content and pedagogy of medical training is appropriate and responsive to the needs of the people?

RE-INVENTING MEDICAL EDUCATION AND TRAINING

Linking Medical Education and Health Care Systems

To address the structural problem of the lack of linkage of medical college to the health system, it is necessary for each medical college to involve itself in four aspects: clinical care, teaching, research, and outreach towards the larger goal of improving health care (see Figure 5.1) (Grant, Abdelrahman, and Zachariah 2013). They are discussed as follows:

1. Clinical services: Medicals colleges should form the tertiary referral base for a health system.
2. Teaching: Medical colleges should orient their training to the needs of the health system in terms of intake and courses. Training may occur mainly in the tertiary-care hospital. However the medical college can use the entire health system and its personnel for training its students. It can offer CME and distance education to provide training support for the staff of the health system. In sum, the medical college and the health system can play a reciprocal role in training.
3. Research: Medical colleges can conduct research into the priority health problems and operational research issues of the health system. Students can be involved in research projects in the community.
4. Outreach: Medical colleges can support primary and secondary care through the community health and family medicine departments.

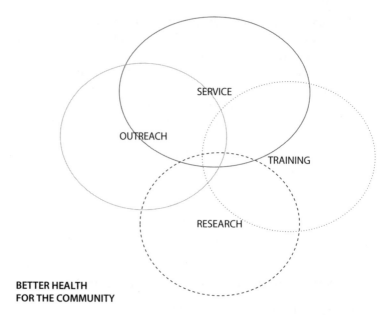

FIGURE 5.1   Roles That a Medical College May Play

Source: Author.

The following steps may be suggested to correct the lack of linkage between medical colleges and the government health care system based on the model (Figure 5.2) (Zachariah 2012). In this model, medical colleges should be responsible for providing tertiary care services in liaison with district health services for a given geographical area (one district or a set of districts).

The model is discussed as follows:

1. Medical colleges must be strengthened to provide tertiary care for each district. This should include the development of tertiary services for the common public health conditions (for example cardiac care, dialysis facilities, gastrointestinal endoscopy, trauma care, ICU facilities, and radiotherapy). The medical college should support secondary and primary level services through referrals and training.
2. The district health system will, in turn, offer the medical college an opportunity to expand its training base. Undergraduate and postgraduate students could be trained not only in the medical college, but also at the district hospital, taluk hospital, and PHC.

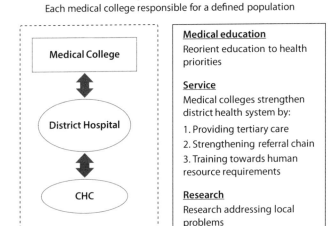

Proposed Model
Each medical college responsible for a defined population

FIGURE 5.2   Proposed Model

Source: Author.

3. The functioning of this referral system would require referral guidelines, training, referral linkages between secondary and tertiary care, and mechanisms for ensuring quality and accountability.

4. When medical colleges are responsible for a functioning health system, the priorities for medical education will need to change. Specialists now dominate the MCI board and postgraduate boards, which means there is undue emphasis on specialist courses. Integration of medical colleges with the health system will require a reorientation of medical training. It will have to change from a medical education system based on western requirements to one that will meet the human resource requirements of the health system.

5. This may require an expansion of paramedical training (village health nurses, nurse practitioners, physician assistants, paramedics, and so on) and the setting up of family medicine departments in every medical college to train multicompetent general practitioners (GPs). The specialist training requirements should be based on the needs of the health system.

Developing a Contextual Curriculum

Curriculum should be living document that is created and recreated so that education is alive. For education to address health care needs, it requires a contextual curriculum to train doctors in the local morbidity profiles, social determinants of illness and practical skills, and with opportunities to practice and solve problems within the health system (Grant, Abdelrahman, and Zachariah 2013). To do all this, requires an active planning process at the level of the medical college that converts the minimum MCI regulation into a curriculum that explores the full potential of developing doctors who can meet the needs of the health system.

A suggested approach to developing a contextual curriculum for a medical college are: (*i*) Prioritizing health problems; (*ii*) knowledge appropriate to local setting; (*iii*) practice of medicine; and (*iv*) linkages to the health system (see Figure 5.3).

They are discussed as follows:

1. *Knowledge and emphasis on the common diseases, local clinical presentations, local approaches to investigation and management*: Textbooks that students use are western textbooks written for western clinical problems. A contextual curriculum has to capture the differences in morbidity profiles and clinical presentations in India and variations within the country. For example, Table 5.1 shows the 10 most common causes of death in India as a whole. Such knowledge is important in the planning of the syllabus, to ensure weightage of these conditions in the curriculum.

The curriculum has to be cognizant of the differences in morbidity profiles between states and local presentations and the reasons for these.

Steps for the curriculum planner:
- Review the content of the curriculum to ensure adequate weightage and priority for the common diseases in your country.
- Each medical college should ensure that the curriculum has the focus on particular conditions which are local to the area and region and the differences in the local presentations of the disease and how these affect diagnosis and management.
- The curriculum should emphasize knowledge about health status of the people, the social determinants of health and interventions that can address these.

DESIGNING A CONTEXTUAL CURRICULUM

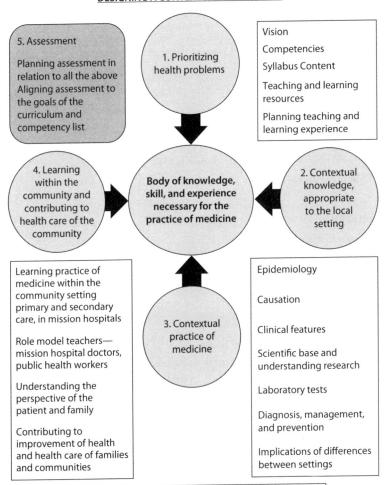

5. Assessment

Planning assessment in relation to all the above Aligning assessment to the goals of the curriculum and competency list

1. Prioritizing health problems

Vision

Competencies

Syllabus Content

Teaching and learning resources

Planning teaching and learning experience

4. Learning within the community and contributing to health care of the community

Body of knowledge, skill, and experience necessary for the practice of medicine

2. Contextual knowledge, appropriate to the local setting

Learning practice of medicine within the community setting primary and secondary care, in mission hospitals

Role model teachers—mission hospital doctors, public health workers

Understanding the perspective of the patient and family

Contributing to improvement of health and health care of families and communities

3. Contextual practice of medicine

Epidemiology

Causation

Clinical features

Scientific base and understanding research

Laboratory tests

Diagnosis, management, and prevention

Implications of differences between settings

Being involved in the practice of medicine

Learning by managing common problems in outpatient and emergency setting

Performing essential procedures competently

Being involved in communicating with patient and family

Addressing issues of cost, access, social, cultural, and health system issues in the process of care

FIGURE 5.3 Designing a Contextual Curriculum

Source: Grant, Abdelrahman, and Zachariah (2013: 22).

TABLE 5.1   Causes of Death in India, 2002

Causes	Deaths	
	[000]	*%*
All causes	105	100
Ischaemic heart disease	153	15
Lower respiratory infections	110	11
Cerebrovascular disease	771	7
Perinatal conditions	762	7
Chronic obstructive pulmonary disease (COPD)	485	5
Diarrhoeal diseases	456	4
Tuberculosis	364	4
HIV/AIDS	361	3
Road traffic accidents	189	2
Self-inflicted injuries	182	2

Source: http://www.who.int/entity/healthinfo/statistics/bodgbddeathdalyestimates.xls.

The social determinants for health such as socio-economic status, sex, maternal education, urban/rural location, SC/ST status need to be emphasized and their importance in addressing disparities in providing good health and health care.

2. *Skills required for a doctor to manage common problems at the level of primary and secondary care:* MBBS doctors are not competent to manage common problems at the PHC and CHC level as they are not trained in the skills required to handle these problems.

Steps for the curriculum planner:
- The curriculum planner should identify the skill level of the graduate at the end of the training based on the role of basic doctor in the health system.
- They should ensure that the curriculum offers graduated learning towards skills development.
- Practical training through skills laboratory, workshops, clerkship training, and internship are essential to developing such skills.

TABLE 5.2   Procedural Skills Required for Primary
and Secondary Care

Incision and drainage	Spinal anaesthesia
Lymph node biopsy	Regional anaesthesia
Excision of subcutaneous swelling	Ketamine anaesthesia
Plaster of Paris application	Normal delivery
Taking an ECG	Episiotomy and suturing
Pleural aspiration	Pap smear
Paracentesis abdomen	Intrauterine contraceptive device insertion
Lumbar puncture	Tubectomy
Urinary catheterization	Neonatal assessment and resuscitation
Nasogastric tube insertion	Lumbar puncture for meningitis
Intravenous cannulation	Oral rehydration solution administration
Basic and advanced life support	Intraosseous insertion

Source: Zachariah (2007).

A contextual curriculum requires identifying and training the
students in the skills required for a doctor within the health system.

For example, the procedural skills required for primary and
secondary care are as in Table 5.2.

3. *Practice of medicine and linkages with the health system:* A contextual
   curriculum requires that teachers in the medical college should
   analyse the strengths and weaknesses of the curriculum and make
   plans to address these problems. In analysing the curriculum the
   teachers should figure out how students can be exposed to authentic
   practice sites outside the medical college, including the choice of
   cases, the settings of learning, and appropriate teachers. They should
   see how linkages with the health system can be enhanced to expand
   opportunities for learning.

Case Study of a Government Medical College

Here is a case study of a government medical college in a small town.
The college enrolls 150 medical students every year. The medical college
faculties were involved in a planning process to assess their strengths and
weaknesses and to plan a set of educational innovations to address these
problems. A summary of the analysis is provided in Table 5.3.

TABLE 5.3 Analysis of Strengths and Weaknesses

Strengths	Weaknesses
1. Good clinical load	1. Infrastructure for patient care and teaching
2. Well trained and competent faculty	2. Poor quality of patient care
3. Some interested teachers	3. Low motivation of faculty
4. Functioning rural and urban health centres	4. Private practice
5. Interested students	5. Lack of involvement of community medicine department in the peripheral health centres
	6. Poorly planned clinical postings
	7. Ineffective internship

Source: Grant, Abdelrahman, and Zachariah (2013).

The faculty planned the following curricular innovations:

1. Clerkship posting: Active involvement of medical students in clinical care under supervision of PGs and faculty.
2. Strengthening of community health postings: By involvement of peripheral centre doctors in teaching, community health department teachers in visiting peripheral centres, and students planning research projects in the community.
3. Strengthening internship postings by more active involvement of interns in clinical work and posting of interns to a local voluntary hospital.

The processes of globalization and homogenization of medical education as a discipline are focusing on method and format. The real problems of medical education are structural problems related to orientation of medical knowledge, the privatization of medical education, and the lack of linkage of medical education with health care (Grant, Abdelrahman, and Zachariah 2013). As the above example shows it may be possible to enable medical colleges to develop a contextual curriculum that can strategically engage with these difficulties towards an education that can address health problems.

The lack of access to health care is structurally linked to the mismatches between medical knowledge and health problems on the ground, the development of specialty disciplines and underdevelopment of primary care, the development of a medical education system that is not aligned with the health care system, and the homogenization of western curricular approaches that focus on training a global doctor. The developments in medical science, the private business of medical education, and the increasing withdrawal of the government from publicly funded medical education are likely to exacerbate the current situation.

Given the complexity of the problem and its varied nature, we suggest that it may be possible to push along certain lines of cleavage that may work against the current structural forces such as:

1. Fostering the development of primary care and family medicine as disciplines for the Indian setting.
2. Encouraging experiments in medical colleges of educational linkage with the health systems.
3. Encouraging medical teachers to think critically about their education towards a pedagogy and curriculum of context.

NOTES

1. Some examples of specialties that have developed around specific technologies are: cardiology around bypass surgery and angiography, neurology and neurosurgery around CT scan and MRI, nephrology and urology around dialysis and kidney transplantation, gastroenterology around the gastroscopy and colonoscopy, critical care around ventilators, pulmonology around bronchoscopy, and haematology around bone marrow transplantation (Zachariah 2010a).
2. See Medical Council of India website (https://www.mciindia.org/).

REFERENCES

Alexander, Thomas, Suma M. Victor, Ajit S. Mullasari, Ganesh Veerasekar, Kala Subramaniam, and K. Brahmajee, Nallamothu for the TN-STEMI Programme Investigators. 2013. 'Protocol for a Prospective, Controlled Study of Assertive and Timely Reperfusion for Patients with ST-Segment Elevation Myocardial Infarction in Tamil Nadu: The TN-STEMI programmeme', *BMJ Open* 3(12): 1–8.

Baru, Rama V. 1998. *Private Health Care In India—Social Characteristics and Trends.* New Delhi: Sage Publications.

Deepa, Mohan, Ranjit Mohan Anjana, Manjula Datta, K.M. Venkat Narayan, and Mohan Viswanathan. 2011. 'Convergence of Prevalence Rates of

Diabetes and Cardiometabolic Risk Factors in Middle and Low Income Groups in Urban India: 10-Year Follow-Up of the Chennai Urban Population Study', *Journal of Diabetes Science and Technolgy* 5(4): 918–27.

GOI. 2006. *Bulletin on Rural Health Statistics in India*, Ministry of Health and Family Welfare. New Delhi: Government of India.

Grant, Janet, Mohamed Y.H. Abdelrahman, and Anand Zachariah. 2013. 'Curriculum Design in Context'. In *Oxford Textbook of Medical Education*, Kieran Walsh (ed.), pp. 13–24. Oxford: Oxford University Press.

Gunnell, D., R. Fernando, M. Hewagama, W.D.D. Priyangika, F. Konradsen, and M. Eddleston. 2007. 'The Impact of Pesticide Regulations on Suicide in Sri Lanka', *International Journal of Epidemiology* 36(6): 1235–42.

Gupta R., V.P. Gupta, M. Sarna, H. Prakash, S. Rastogi, and K.D. Gupta. 2003. 'Serial Epidemiological Surveys in an Urban Indian Population Demonstrate Increasing Coronary Risk Factors Among the Lower Socio-economic Strata', *Journal of the Associations of Physicians of India* 51: 470–7.

Kaul, Upendra and Vineet Bhatia. 2010. 'Perspective on Coronary Interventions and Cardiac Surgeries in India', *Indian Journal of Medical Research* 132(5): 543–8.

Kumar, R. Krishna and R. Tandon. 2013. 'Rheumatic Fever and Rheumatic Heart Disease: The Last 50 years', *Indian Journal of Medical Research* 137(4): 643–58.

Manoranjitham S.D., A.P. Rajkumar, P. Thangadurai, J. Prasad, R. Jayakaran, and K.S. Jacob. 2010. 'Risk Factors for Suicide in Rural South India', *The British Journal of Psychiatry* 196(1): 26–30.

Mohapatra, B., D.A.Warrell, W. Suraweera, P. Bhatia, N. Dhingra, R.M. Jotkar, P.S. Rodriguez, K. Mishra, R. Whitaker, and P. Jha. 2011. 'Snakebite Mortality in India: A Nationally Representative Mortality Survey, Million Death Study Collaborators', *PLoS Neglected Tropical Diseases* 5(4): e1018.

MoHFW. 2005. *Report of the National Commission on Macroeconomics and Health*. New Delhi: Ministry of Health and Family Welfare, Government of India.

Pednekar, Mangesh S., Rajeev Gupta, and Prakash C. Gupta. 2011, 'Illiteracy, Low Educational Status, and Cardiovascular Mortality in India', *BMC Public Health* 11: 567.

Prasad, J., V.J. Abraham, S. Minz, S. Abraham, A. Joseph, J.P. Muliyil, K. George, K.S. Jacob. 2006. 'Rates and Factors Associated with Suicide in Kaniyambadi Block, Tamil Nadu, South India, 2000–2002', *International Journal of Social Psychiatry* 52(1): 65–71.

Rahman, M.F. Sajitha, Ruby P. Angeline, Kirubah V. David, and Prince Christopher. 2014. 'Role of Family Medicine Education in India's Step Toward Universal Health Coverage', *J Family Med Prim Care* 3(3): 180–2.

Rasella, D., M.O. Harhay, M.L. Pamponet, R. Aquino, and M.L. Barreto. 2014. 'Impact of Primary Health Care on Mortality from Heart and

Cerebrovascular Diseases in Brazil: A Nationwide Analysis of Longitudinal Data', *BMJ* (3 July, 349): g4014.

Sabde, Yogesh, Vishal Diwan, Ayesha De Costa, and Vijay K. Mahadik. 2014. 'Mapping the Rapid Expansion of India's Medical Education Sector: Planning for the Future', *BMC Medical Education* 14: 266. Published online: 17 December 2014. doi: 10.1186/s12909-014-0266-1.

Velavan, Jachin. 2012. '"The Refer Less Resolve More" Initiative: A Five-year Experience from CMC Vellore', *Journal of Family Medicine and Primary Care* (1 January–June): 3–6.

Warrell, D.A. 2011. 'Snake Bite: A Neglected Problem in Twenty First Century India', *National Medical Journal of India* 24(6, November–December): 321–4.

WHO. 2002. *WHO CVD-Risk Management Package for Low and Middle Income Countries.* Available at: http://www.who.int/cardiovascular_diseases/media/en/635.pdf.

Xavier, D., P. Pais, P.J. Devereaux, C. Xie, D. Prabhakaran, K.S. Reddy, R. Gupta, P. Joshi, P. Kerkar, S. Thanikachalam, K.K. Haridas, T.M. Jaison, S. Naik, A.K. Maity, S. Yusuf. 2008. 'Treatment and Outcomes of Acute Coronary Syndromes in India (CREATE): A Prospective Analysis of Registry Data', *Lancet* 371: 1435–42.

Zachariah, Anand. 2007. 'Course curriculum of the Postgraduate diploma in Family medicine for recent MBBS graduates of Christian Medical College (unpublished)', Department of Medicine. Vellore: Christian Medical College.

———. 2010a. 'Introduction: The Dilemmas of Medical Culture Today'. In *Towards a Critical Medical Practice*, Anand Zachariah, R. Srivatsan, and Susie Tharu (eds), pp. 1–34. Hyderabad: Orient Blackswan.

———. 2010b. 'Rethinking Organophosphate Poisoning/Suicide in India'. In *Towards a Critical Medical Practice*, Anand Zachariah, R. Srivatsan, and Susie Tharu (eds), pp. 176–86. Hyderabad: Orient Blackswan.

———. 2010c. 'Development of the Cardiovascular Epidemic in India and Inappropriate Tertiary Care Treatment Guidelines'. In *Towards a Critical Medical Practice*, Anand Zachariah, R. Srivatsan, and Susie Tharu (eds), pp. 187–200. Hyderabad: Orient Blackswan.

———. 2012. 'Tertiary Healthcare within a Universal System: Some Reflections', *Economic and Political Weekly* 47 (12): 39–45.

———. 2014. 'Discrimination in Health Care and the Structure of Medical Knowledge', *Medico Friendly Circle Bulletin* 41–50.

Zachariah, Anand and Janet Grant. 2015. 'Tailoring your Curriculum to the Local Context: Linking Medical Education with Health Care Delivery'. In *The Art of Teaching Medical Students* (3rd edition), Pritha S. Bhuiyan, Avinash Supe, and Nirmala N. Rege (eds), pp. 398–420. New Delhi: Elsevier- Saunders, Mosby, Churchill Publisher.

II

PHARMACEUTICALS AND EXPERIMENTATION

6

Globalization, Intellectual Property Rights, and Pharmaceuticals

Amit Sengupta

The impact of globalization[1] on access to affordable medicines needs to be seen in the context of the changing dynamics of the pharmaceutical sector in India, accompanied by major changes in the country's Intellectual Property (IP) regime. Proponents of globalization have long targeted Intellectual Property Rights (IPRs) as an important area requiring reform at a global level, in order to promote global integration and expansion of global trade. By the 1980s, the pharmaceutical sector in India was already one of the best developed among all low- and middle-income countries (LMICs). A major reason for the development of the sector in India was its IP regime, based on the Indian Patents Act of 1970, which had special provisions for the pharmaceutical sector. The Indian law did not provide for pharmaceutical product patents and thus supported the domestic industry's endeavour to introduce new medicines at a fraction of the global price, unencumbered by patent protection.

India led other LMICs in resisting the introduction of harmonized laws on IPRs at the Uruguay Round of negotiations that culminated in the formation of the World Trade Organization (WTO). Resistance was systematically broken down during the negotiations. India's capitulation to pressures by the developed countries—leading to its agreeing to include IPRs under the WTO—was also a consequence of the changing trajectory of domestic economic policies in India. With the initiation of neo-liberal economic reforms, India formally embarked on a path of economic development that embraced rather than opposed global integration and harmonized laws. As the chapter examines, shifts in the domestic policy environment have led to the Indian state to begin questioning its earlier stance of defending lower standards of intellectual property protection. This has had implications both in the formulation of India's revised Patent Act in 2005 and in subsequent experiences regarding the application of the Indian Patent Act to safeguard public interest.

The shifts in the global and domestic policy environment, as regards IP protection, have also impacted the domestic pharmaceutical industry. Significant sections of the latter see an advantage in aligning with the multinational pharmaceutical companies, rather than in opposing them. This chapter also describes the net result of these changes over the last three decades in the form of higher medicine prices for new drugs in the country and the undermining of the domestic industry as a secure source of low cost generic medicines.

ASCENT OF INTELLECTUAL PROPERTY RIGHTS IN WORLD TRADE ORGANIZATION

Negotiations at the Uruguay Round of General Agreement on Tariffs and Trade

In 1986 a new round of negotiations was initiated under General Agreement on Tariffs and Trade (GATT), known as the Uruguay Round of negotiations. In these negotiations, developed countries introduced on the agenda a number of issues, which were hitherto not considered as trade issues. Prominent among these were issues related to IPRs, investment, and services.

The attempt to introduce IPRs as a trade issue was motivated by the conception of the WTO agreement as a binding agreement with clear commitments made by contracting parties. The dispute settlement mechanism of the WTO allows member countries to use trade sanctions to enforce rulings against member states that fail to comply with its decisions. It is the binding nature of the WTO agreement that impelled developed countries to push through an agreement on IPRs within the purview of the WTO, thus ensuring compliance of a harmonized global patent system.

In the initial three years of negotiations, developing countries, through the 'group of ten' led by India and Brazil, were able to stall the introduction of these new issues (Shukla 2000: 14–15). The US, however, continued to press for the inclusion of these new issues in subsequent negotiations. By the 1980s, the US had lost its competitive edge in the manufacturing sector to Japan and Germany, and faced new challenges from Brazil, Taiwan, Singapore, and Mexico. Its agricultural exports were also being squeezed, mainly as a consequence of competition from state subsidized agricultural exports from Europe. The US, thus, was keen to open up the services sector to facilitate entry of US corporations—especially financial services. At the same time the US had an interest in protecting its IP-dependent industries where it still had an edge, specifically the pharmaceuticals, software, and mass media sectors (Shukla 2000: 20–21).

The importance of the pharmaceutical sector in global trade can be gauged from the fact that pharmaceuticals are the most important health-related products that are traded, accounting for 55 per cent of all health-related trade. The top 20 transnational corporations, based in the US, the UK, Germany, Switzerland, and France, each have an average of more than 100 foreign affiliates in more than 40 countries (including 19 LMICs), with average sales of over USD 20 billion in 2008–09 (Smith, Correa, and Oh 2009).

India's Interest in Defending Domestic Industry

India's pharmaceutical sector had flourished in the wake of its 1970 Patent Act, which did not allow product patents in the case of medicines and agrochemicals. The Indian Patent Act exempted 'food or medicine or drug' from product patents (Chaudhuri 2002) and only allowed a seven-year patent on new processes to develop a new product.

The 1970 Patent Act, accompanied by other measures to encourage domestic manufacture of medicines, had a dramatic effect on India's pharmaceutical industry and on access to new medicines. The research capacity of public sector research institutions was harnessed to develop new processes for manufacture of medicines that were not already patented. As a consequence, though the patent term for medicines was 20 years, in India new drugs were introduced within 2–5 years of their introduction in the global market (see Table 6.1).

Not only were new drugs introduced in India much before the expiry of patents on these drugs, they were also significantly cheaper. Table 6.2 contrasts prices of generic equivalents of patented drugs in India with

TABLE **6.1**   Impact of 1970 Patents Act on Introduction
of New Drugs in India

Drug	Patented drug introduced in global market (year)	Generic equivalent introduced in Indian market (year)
Ranitidine (anti-ulcer)	1983	1985
Cimetidine (anti-ulcer)	1976	1981
Norfloxacin (anti-bacterial)	1984	1988
Astemizole (non-sedating anti-histamine)	1986	1988
Acyclovir (anti-viral)	1985	1988
Salbutamol (bronchodilator)	1973	1976
Mebendazole (anti-helmintic)	1974	1978
Ibuprofen (anti-inflammatory)	1967	1973
Lorazepam (anxiolytic)	1977	1978

Source: Bidwai (1995: 203).

TABLE **6.2**   Comparative Drug Prices in 1991–2: Impact of Generic
Production of Patented Drugs (All Prices Calculated in Indian Rs)

Drug	Year of patent expiry	Dosage and pack	Price in India	Price in Pakistan	Price in the US	Price in the UK
Norfloxacin (anti-bacterial)	1996	400 mg × 10	39.36	125.50	626.15	252.77
Ranitidine (anti-ulcerant)	1995	300 mg × 10	29.03	260.40	744.65	481.31
Enalapril Maleate (cardiovascular)	2000	5 mg × 10	9.00	37.20	230.83	147.97
Acyclovir (anti-viral)	1997	5 per cent cream × 5 g	33.75	363.32	356.74	577.68
Ketaconazole (anti-fungal)	1999	200 mg × 10	43.00	221.96	673.67	157.98
Fluoxetine (anti-depressant)	2001	2 mg × 10	29.00	618.76	517.83	562.41

Source: Bidwai (1995: 204).

prices in Pakistan (which did not have a Patent Act similar to that in India) and in the countries of origin (US and UK) of these drugs.

The post-1970 growth of a generic industry in India was to have far-reaching effects, not just in India, but also across the world. At the turn of the millennium the HIV/AIDS epidemic was at its peak. In 2000, HIV/AIDS was not a death sentence anymore and a combination of anti-retroviral drugs allowed patients to lead a normal life. These drugs, however, were beyond the reach of patients in most developing countries as they were protected by patents and cost about USD 10,000–15,000 for a year's treatment (UNAIDS 2011). The Indian generic company Cipla, changed the entire landscape of HIV/AIDS treatment in 2001 when it offered the same combination of anti-retrovirals at USD 350 for a year's treatment (Torbett 2001). Soon many other Indian generics were to enter the market and push the cost of treatment even lower. Figure 6.1 shows how the entry of generic anti-retrovirals manufactured in India changed the face of HIV/AIDS treatment and saved millions of lives.

The US, during the Uruguay Round of negotiations, had clearly anticipated the trajectory of the Indian generic industry and its potential to challenge the domination of US-based companies in the global pharmaceutical market. By the early 2000s India came to be termed the 'Pharmacy of the South' and Indian generics were supplying affordable medicines to over 100 countries in Africa, Latin America,

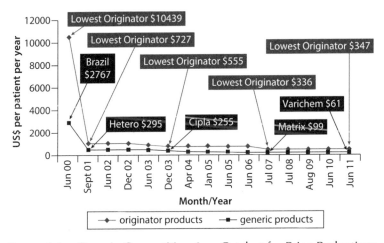

FIGURE 6.1   Generic Competition As a Catalyst for Price Reductions

Source: Medecins sans Frontieres (2011).

and Asia. In 2007–08, 92 per cent of patients on anti-retrovirals in LMICs were using generic drugs mostly from India (Yamey 2009). Further, approximately 50 per cent of the essential medicines that UNICEF distributes in developing countries come from India and 75–80 per cent of all medicines distributed by the International Dispensary Association (IDA) are manufactured in India (Medecins sans Frontieres 2007).

India's Capitulation and Growing Popular Resistance

By the beginning of 1989 the resistance by developing countries was breaking up. Both Brazil and India were plagued by domestic economic problems, and bilateral pressure from the US resulted in the two main holdouts changing their position with regard to the inclusion of IP issues in the negotiations. India went to the extent of replacing its chief negotiator at GATT, S.P. Shukla, because of his strong opposition to the inclusion of IP issues in the negotiating agenda (Marcellin 2010: 87).

In contrast to the very large popular mobilizations that took place in later years against the WTO, the significance of the Uruguay Round of negotiations was not clear to most popular movements and civil society groups in different parts of the world. The powerful 'Access to Medicines' campaign was to appear only in the late 1990s and India was perhaps the only region in the world where there was an attempt to build popular resistance. It was this popular resistance that resulted in India continuing to be the last holdout even after it agreed to put IP rights on the agenda of the Uruguay Round. India was the only country of significance that used the entire 10-year transition period available to developing countries, and agreed to fully amend its Patents Act only in 2005.

FINAL AMENDMENTS TO THE INDIAN PATENT ACT

In 1991, the then Congress government embarked on a formal policy to introduce neo-liberal reforms (Chandrasekhar and Ghosh 2006). This led to a significant shift in public policy, which had its impact on the government's official view on IP rights. From an earlier position that India was forced to concede in the GATT negotiations, there was now an attempt to argue that strong IP protection would actually further domestic interests in India.

The Trade-Related Aspects of Intellectual Property Rights (TRIPS) Agreement, finally signed in 1994, required India, as a signatory, to provide for product patent protection in all fields of technology from 1 January 2005. As a developing country India had the option of using a 10-year transition period before becoming entirely TRIPS compliant (Raju 2004).

The principal opposition party, the Bharatiya Janata Party (BJP), had generally been opposed to strong IP protection. However, after assuming office, the BJP-led National Democratic Alliance (NDA) government was clearly subsumed by the neo-liberal logic while engaging with public policy in a range of issues (see, for example, Arulanantham 2004). The government then circulated the draft 'Third Patents (Amendment) Bill' in 2003. The Bill could not be discussed in Parliament because of the change in government in 2004 (Rangnekar 2005). The draft Bill, was entirely inadequate in addressing concerns relating both to health care and development of the domestic industry.

When the Congress-led United Progressive Alliance (UPA) Government came to power in 2004 there was a clear consensus between the Congress and the BJP on the need to continue and strengthen neo-liberal reforms. In consonance with this overall consensus, the UPA Government circulated an almost unchanged version of the NDA's Third Patents (Amendment) Bill draft (Rangnekar 2005).

In the political spectrum represented in Parliament, only the Left Parties, given their opposition to the ongoing neo-liberal reforms, (along with some regional parties) stood firmly against the draft Bill. However, given their poor strength in Parliament, they were not in a position to block the Bill in the House. Things, however, changed almost dramatically towards the end of 2004 as signals started coming from the BJP that they would not support the passage of the Bill in Parliament. While this is in the realm of speculation, BJP's volte face had little to do with any opposition to the substance of the Bill (given that this Bill was identical to the one they had circulated, this is a logical assumption). It had more to do with an intent to embarrass the Congress-led UPA government on the floor of the Parliament. With support for the Bill now unsure, the UPA government decided to beat the 31 December 2004 deadline by promulgating an ordinance on 26 December 2004 (The Patents [Amendment] Ordinance 2004).[2]

The Patents Amendment Ordinance of 2004, had it been ratified by the Parliament, would have made it impossible for Indian companies to continue producing cheaper versions of new drugs. In early 2005, it became evident that the Ordinance would not be ratified by Parliament given the BJP's attitude towards the UPA government. The Congress-led UPA government, now denied support from the BJP in spite of the latter's ideological commitment to neo-liberal reforms, was forced to seek the Left's support in Parliament. This provided the Left with an opportunity to introduce several amendments to the 2004 ordinance.

The deliberations in Parliament were held in the backdrop of protests across the country, as well as in different parts of the world—all demanding that the 'pharmacy of the South' should not be jeopardized. By 2005 the Global Access to Medicines campaign was a powerful force and organizations such as Médecins Sans Frontières (MSF) and others were able to organize support across the globe. Patient groups representing HIV/AIDS patients had also organized themselves and formed a vocal and visible opposition to amendments in India's Patent Act. Protest letters were sent to the Prime Minister including one where the co-signatories included Jim Yong Kim, the present World Bank Chief (then Director, Department of HIV/AIDS, World Health Organization) (Khor 2013). Concurrently, the Indian generic industry too put pressure on the government to incorporate amendments that would safeguard their interests.

Health Safeguards in the 2005 Act[3]

As a result of the rather fortuitous role that the Left parties were able to play, and aided by the pressures exerted by popular mobilizations, the Indian Parliament enacted a new Patent Act in March 2015. This law, at least partially alleviated the impact of a product patent regime. Several important amendments to the 2004 ordinance were included in the final Act and several of these 'health safeguards' in the Act have been applied to promote access to new medicines (see Box 6.1).

When the 2005 Act was endorsed by Parliament, the government gave an undertaking that two issues would be examined afresh by an expert panel: (i) the proposal that patents should be further restricted to only 'new chemical entities' or to 'new medical entities involving one or more inventive steps' and (ii) the proposal that microorganisms be entirely excluded from patenting.

Subsequently the government constituted a Technical Expert Group (TEG) under the chairmanship of R.A. Mashelkar, former Director General, Council of Scientific and Industrial Research (CSIR). The panel submitting its report in 2007, opined that both the restriction of

Box 6.1   Important Amendments Incorporated in 2005 Act

1. *Restrictions on Patentability:* There were concerns regarding 'ever-greening' of patents, which is a perpetuation of patents monopoly beyond the stipulated 20 years by repeated patent grants based on small changes made to the original molecule. The amendments restricted the scope for the granting of patents on frivolous claims. It clarified that 'inventive step' meant a feature of an invention that 'involves technical advances as compared to the existing knowledge or having economic significance or both'. The amendments also incorporated a new definition for 'new invention' by stating that it means 'any invention or technology which has not been anticipated by publication in any document or used in the country or elsewhere in the world before the date of filing of patent application with complete specification, i.e. the subject matter has not fallen in public domain or that it does not form part of the state of art'. The amendments also provide a definition for 'pharmaceutical substance' as being 'a new entity involving one or more inventive steps'. As part of the exercise to strengthen the possibility to deny patents on frivolous claims the amendments clarified that 'the mere discovery of a new form of a known substance which does not result in the enhancement of the known efficacy' (Section 3(d))[4] is not patentable. It was further explained that: 'Salts, esters, ethers, polymorphs, metabolites, pure form, particle size, isomers, mixtures of isomers, complexes, combinations and other derivatives of known substances shall be considered to be the same substance, unless they differ significantly in properties with regard to efficacy.'
2. *Restoration of Pre-Grant Opposition to Patents:* There had been widespread apprehensions that the 2004 Ordinance restricted oppositions to the grant of a patent. The 2015 Act restored all the original grounds for opposition that existed in the 1970 Act.
3. *Export to Countries without Manufacturing Ability:* The 2005 Act clarified that a country could import from India if it 'by notification or otherwise allowed importation of the patented pharmaceutical product from India'.
4. *Continued Manufacture of Drugs with Applications in 'Mailbox':* The new amendments clarified that Indian companies which were already producing these drugs could continue to produce them after payment of a royalty even if the drug was subsequently granted a patent.
5. *Time Period for Considering Compulsory License Application:* The concern about the 2004 Ordinance that the process of granting Compulsory Licenses to counter the patent monopolies was too cumbersome was

addressed by the 2005 Act. The Act specified that the 'reasonable' time period before the Patents Controller considers issuance of a Compulsory License when such a license is denied by the patent holder 'shall not ordinarily exceed six months'.

6. *Export by Indian Companies of Patented Drugs*: The 2005 Act provided that when patented drugs are produced under compulsory license in India by Indian companies: 'the license is granted with a predominant purpose of supply in the domestic market and that the licensee may also export the patented product, if need be in accordance with Section 84(7) (a) (iii)' (that is, where an export market exists).

patents to new chemical entities and the exclusion of micro-organisms from patenting would be incompatible with the TRIPS agreement. This report generated considerable controversy as evidence surfaced that the report had been plagiarized from a study by the UK-based think tank Intellectual Property Institute, funded by Interpat, an association of 29 drug companies including Novartis (Padma 2007). The report was withdrawn and press reports indicated that Mashelkar had resigned from the committee (Padma 2007). Yet, curiously, the same committee resubmitted a slightly amended version of the report, but with the same conclusions, in 2009. The government promptly accepted these recommendations.

The account of the tortuous process that led to the final enactment of India's Patent Law in 2005 has to be understood in the context of several conflicting interests. The Indian Government, at the beginning of the Uruguay Round of negotiations in 1986, held the position that product patent protection in the case of medicines is not desirable and runs counter to attempts to safeguard public health. This position was supported both by India's growing generic drugs industry and by popular movements and progressive sections within the country. However, India diluted its opposition to strong IP protection in the face of extreme pressure from developed countries led by the US. By the 1990s India embarked on economic reforms and introduced explicit neo-liberal polices in different parts of the economy. The government's interest in pursuing neo-liberal reforms now constituted a contradiction to its earlier policy of adhering to lower standards of IP protection. This was clearly manifest in the manner in which the two principal parties in India, both adherents of neo-liberal reforms, converged towards a position that supported stronger IP protection in 2003–04. Circumstances, some of them fortuitous, led to the enactment of a Patent Act in 2005 that incorporated a range of health safeguards and promoted access to medicines. However, there remains a continuing tension arising from the contradiction between the Indian government's (whether led by the Congress or the BJP) adherence to neo-liberal reforms and an IP law that provides relatively weaker standards of protection. As we shall see later this tension is reflected in less than enthusiastic use of health safeguards in the Indian Act. It is also reflected in recent initiatives by the government to develop a new IP policy.

APPLICATION OF THE AMENDED INDIAN PATENT ACT

We now have substantial experience regarding the actual application of health safeguards (or flexibilities) that were incorporated in the Indian Patent Act in 2005 to mitigate the impact of the introduction of product patents. We summarize below some important experiences.

Grant of Patents Post-2005 and Litigations Arising from Them

Provisions in the Indian Act that restrict patentability have been used quite extensively by Patent offices' while examining patent claims. They have also been used by the Patent office to reject patent applications and have also been instrumental in many patent applications being voluntarily withdrawn. These provisions, combined with the 'pre-grant' opposition clause have been used by Indian generic companies and by civil society groups to file pre-grant oppositions (Reddy 2010). Importantly, several civil society organizations (especially networks of HIV+ve people) filed pre-grant oppositions soon after the Indian Act was amended in 2005 (and a few post-grant) and have been successful in a number of cases (see Table 6.3 for a selection).

A high-profile patent litigation that attracted global attention pertained to a protracted legal battle conducted by Novartis to obtain a patent for its anti-leukaemia drug Gleevec (Generic name: imatinib mesylate) and further to challenge the legal validity of Section 3(d) of the Indian Act. The Supreme Court of India finally rejected the legal challenge by Novartis in 2013 (Chaudhuri 2013).

Similar to the Gleevec case, several other litigations involving Section 3(d) have been contentious and cases have run for several years. Multinational Corporations (MNCs) have brought in a range of infringement proceedings against Indian companies for manufacturing and marketing drugs on which they claimed patent productions.

TABLE 6.3   Pre-grant Oppositions by HIV+ve Patients Groups

Drug and usage	Applicant	Status of application
Zidovudine/lamivudine First-line ARV	GSK	Patent application withdrawn
Nevaripine Hemihydrate (syrup) First-line ARV	Boehringer Ingelheim	Patent application rejected
Valgancyclovir For opportunistic infections	Roche	Patent rejected (after being previously granted)
Abacavir– Second-line ARV	GSK	Patent application withdrawn
Zidovudine/lamivudine First-line ARV	GSK	Patent application withdrawn
Nevaripine Hemihydrate (syrup) First-line ARV	Boehringer Ingelheim	Patent application rejected
Valgancyclovir For opportunistic infections	Roche	Patent granted
Abacavir Second-line ARV	GSK	Patent application withdrawn

Source: Summarized from information available at https://www.patentoppositions.org.

Courts have also liberally issued injunctions against Indian manufacturers while cases have dragged on for several years. Table 6.4 provides a summary account of a few cases that have run over protracted periods.

Multinational Corporations have invested substantially in litigations to prevent generic production of new medicines. Different courts are still interpreting the amended Indian Patent Act of 2005, given that many provisions are seen as 'grey areas' and open to differing interpretations (Nair, Fernandes, and Nair 2014: 79). In this virtual war of attrition MNCs are much better placed, given their command over significantly larger resources. The ability of generic companies to continue to withstand the plethora of legal challenges mounted by MNCs is now suspect (see also further discussion in this chapter on the Sofosbuvir case). Only a few companies continue to systematically challenge MNCs in courts. Many more companies are engaging in mediations and out of court settlements (Chaudhuri 2014: 12). Civil society groups and patients organizations too are constrained by limited capacities and financial resources to continue mounting patent grant oppositions.

TABLE 6.4   Some Important Patent Litigations Post-2005

Drug and usage	Applicant	Course of litigation
Erlotinib *Cancers of lung,* *pancreas, and* *so on*	Roche	Roche was granted patent post-2005 but Cipla also started manufacturing the drug, leading to infringement procedures by Roche and a plea for injunction in 2008. Roche's case was dismissed by Delhi High Court while Cipla filed a case for revocation of Roche's patent. Roche filed a petition in the Supreme Court but was referred back to Delhi HC. Roche also initiated infringement proceedings against other generic manufacturers—NATCO, Reddy's Lab., and Glenmark. In 2012 Delhi HC upheld Roche's patent but also held that Cipla had not infringed Roche's patent as it was marketing a variant (polymorph B) whose patent had been rejected earlier. Both Roche and Cipla have appealed against the judgment and the case is still pending after a court ordered mediation between the two parties failed.
Sitagliptin *Anti-diabetic*	Merck	Merck granted a patent post-2005 but another patent application of a variant (phosphate salt) was denied. Glenmark launched a generic version of the phosphate salt. Merck filed an infringement case in Delhi HC which was rejected. Merck filed an appeal in Delhi HC in 2013, and in 2015 Delhi HC granted an interim injunction to Merck against Cipla, thereby restraining Glenmark from selling the drug. The final order on the case is still pending.
Dasatinib *Chronic Myeloid* *Leukemia*	BMS	Various cases in different courts are pending based on infringement procedures initiated by BMS in 2008 against Natco, Hetero, and BDR for commencing production of the drug. A compulsory license application filed by BDR in 2013 was rejected by the patent office. Final judgments pending in the infringement cases.

(Cont'd)

TABLE 6.4 (Cont'd)

Drug and usage	Applicant	Course of litigation
Sunitinib *Kidney and* *gastro-intestinal* *cancers*	Pfizer	Pfizer was granted a patent in 2007 but the grant was overturned based on a post-grant opposition by Cipla. Pfizer appealed against this order in the High Court and then in the Supreme Court. The SC referred the matter back to the Patent Controller who upheld the revocation of the patent. Pfizer challenged this order in the HC, who referred the matter to the Patent Appellate Board who in turn referred it back to the Patent Controller for fresh hearing. Decision is awaited. Concurrently infringement proceedings against Cipla are also pending.

Source: Nair, Fernandes, and Nair (2014: 82–6).

Availability and Cost of New Medicines

A key provision in the amended 2005 Patents Act allowed Indian generic manufacturers to continue production of medicines that they had introduced into the Indian market from 1995–2005. At least partially, this mitigated the impact of the introduction of a Product Patent regime in 2005. The momentum of this facility provided under the Indian law has meant that it is only in the last four or five years that the full impact of a TRIPS compatible regime is starting to be felt, that is, now that drugs patented after 2005 are starting to enter the global market.

A recent (2014) study identified 140 patented products that were being marketed in India. Of these, information about whether these were manufactured in India was available for only 92 products, largely because companies refuse to divulge this information. Of these four were manufactured in India and the rest were being imported and marketed in India (Chaudhuri 2014: 12–14). There is a growing trend of imported drugs forming a significant portion of the domestic market. Table 6.5 provides the cost data of a selected range of imported drugs being marketed in India.

The new Drug Price Control Order was notified in 2012. But this Order does not cover patented drugs. A Committee on Price Negotiation of Patented Drugs was set up to recommend ways in which prices of patented drugs could be controlled. The committee's report, submitted

TABLE 6.5 Cost of Patented Protected Drugs

Molecule	Brand/Unit	Clinical use	MNC	Unit price	Treatment frequency
Ixabepilone	*Ixempra* 45 mg Injection	Breast Cancer, being investigated for other cancers	BMS	71,175.00	1 unit weekly for 4 weeks; cycle may need to be repeated
Goserelin	*Zoladex* 10.8 mcg Injection	Cancer of Prostate	Astra Zeneca	28,320.00	Every 12 weeks
Zoledronate	*Aclasta* 5 mg Infusion 100 ml	To prevent fractures and bone pains in some forms of cancers	Novartis	19,516.00	Every 3–4 weeks
Pegylated Interferon Alpha 2a	*Pegasys* 180 mcg Injection 10 ml	Hepatitis C	Roche	18,200.00	1 unit every week for 8 weeks
Ibandronate	*Bondronat* 6 mg Injection	To prevent fractures and bone pains in some forms of cancers	Roche	13,950.00	Every 4 weeks
Erythropoietin Products	*Mircera* 100 mcg Injection 0.3 ml	Treatment of anemia in kidney failure	Roche	8,821.00	Every 2 weeks

(Cont'd)

TABLE 6.5 (Cont'd)

Molecule	Brand/Unit	Clinical use	MNC	Unit price	Treatment frequency
Sunitinib	*Sutent* 50 mg Capsule	Cancers of kidney and Gastrointestinal tract	Pfizer	8,714.78	Daily for 4 weeks; may need to be repeated after two weeks
Everolimus	*Afinitor* 10 mg Tablet	Cancers of kidney, breast and brain	Novartis	7,217.60	Daily for 24 weeks
Liraglutide	*Victoza* 6 mg Injection 3 ml	Diabetes	Novo Nordisk	4,315.00	9 units a month
Erlotinib	*Tarceva* 150 mg Tablet	Cancers of lung, pancreas	Roche	4,030.00	Daily for 3–4 months
Dasatinib	*Sprycel* 50 mg Tablet	Chronic Myeloid Leukemia	BMS	3,287.30	2 units daily
Long acting insulin (Ultra Lente)	*Novorapid* 100 IU Injection 10 ml	Diabetes	Novo Nordisk	2,211.65	Variable

Source: Chaudhuri (2014: 14).

in 2013, suggested that ceiling prices of patented drugs could be fixed by factoring in prices of these drugs in a select basket of reference countries (practice known as reference pricing) and the comparative per capita Gross National Product (GNP) of India and the reference countries.[5] No headway has been made since then as the industry, especially the Organization of Pharmaceutical Producers of India (OPPI)— representing drug MNCs in India—has opposed the formula suggested. Concerns have also been raised that reference pricing would push up costs enormously given that patented drugs are exorbitantly priced in all countries and have no relation to real manufacturing costs. There are also concerns that price negotiations will retard the process of issuing compulsory licenses—a concern echoed by the government's own Department of Industrial Promotion and Policy (DIPP) (Datta 2013). It would be logical to argue that the best method of controlling prices of patented drugs would be by breaking the monopoly of the patent holder. The Indian Patent Act has elaborate provisions that can be used to break the monopoly of patent holders by issuing compulsory licenses and thus introducing competition.

Compulsory License (CL) Provisions

This provision has remained virtually unused and only one CL has been issued in India till date to NATCO in 2012 for Sorafenib, an anti-cancer drug marketed by Bayer as Nexavar (Chatterjee 2013). NATCO's price for Sorafenib is Rs 8,800 for a month's treatment, in contrast to Rs 2,80,000 for Nexavar.

A partial reason for the relative disinterest shown by generic companies in filing CLs is that they, in the immediate aftermath of the 2005 amendments to the Indian Act, were engaged in securing markets for new drugs introduced between 1995 and 2005. Anticipating the imposition of a product patent regime, several domestic companies had started production of new (under Patent) drugs in the years just prior to the amendments of the Indian Act in 2005. They were protected from infringement procedures (as discussed earlier) by application of the provision in the amended Act that allowed them to continue production post-2005.

However, even after the effect of the above clause had run its course and several patented drugs started entering the Indian market, there have been few CL applications. Intuitively this would indicate a link between the new strategy of domestic Indian companies to 'collaborate' rather than to 'oppose' pharmaceutical MNCs. This is a cause for serious concern and shows that it is incorrect to assume that Indian generic companies will automatically file CL applications, just because the Indian law has liberal provisions in this regard. This also has implications for access to affordable generics in a number of LMICs that are served by Indian generic exports. Further, in 2008, the Indian generic company NATCO, withdrew an application for CLs to export Pfizer's anti-cancer drug Sutent to Nepal (Basheer 2008).

The lack of interest in the use of this provision points to two allied barriers that compromise access in LMICs through exports of drugs produced by use of CLs. The first, as noted earlier, is the general lack of interest in filing CLs. Second, as has been widely commented upon, the TRIPS council's mechanism to allow such exports is too cumbersome.

ACCESS TO NEW DRUGS: EMERGING SCENARIO

Our discussion has indicated multiple challenges towards introduction of new medicines in the Indian market at affordable prices. In addition to the legal challenges, which we detailed earlier, the biggest change that has taken place is in the business practices of the Indian generic industry. Denied support of the earlier Patent Act, many big players in the domestic sector are changing their tactics towards MNCs. The shift in position by Indian generic companies has implications not just for India but also for poor patients across the world. The following episode, involving a Hepatitis C drug called Sofosbuvir, illustrates this shift and its implications.

The Sofosbuvir Story

In 2013, the US-based company Gilead Sciences began to market its new Hepatitis C drug, Sofosbuvir (marketed by Gilead as Sovaldi). Sovaldi's sales in the first quarter of 2014 touched USD 3.48 billion and the 2014 sales of is projected to outstrip that of the biggest blockbuster drug ever, Pfizer's Liptor, whose sales touched USD 12.9 billion in 2006. Thus Sovaldi's 2014 sales are more than the entire domestic market for medicines in India.

Sofosbuvir is one of a new class of drugs that have been launched recently as treatment for Hepatitis C. Called 'Directly Acting Antivirals' (DAA), these drugs have the potential to radically change the lives of patients suffering from Hepatitis C. Cure rates are in excess of

90 per cent and may touch almost 100 per cent when two DAAs are combined. Typically, treatment duration is 12–24 weeks depending on the type of Hepatitis C infection.

Globally, an estimated 160–180 million people harbour the Hepatitis C virus and many of them will eventually die of the infection. Each year about half-a-million people succumb to Hepatitis C infection and Hepatitis C is the single largest cause of patients requiring a liver transplant. In India there are about 12–18 million people who are infected by the virus and about 100,000 are estimated to die each year because of the infection. Some countries have extremely high rates of Hepatitis C infection, with Egypt reporting that 14–22 per cent of its population as being infected.

Sofosbuvir is to Hepatitis patients what anti-retrovirals were to HIV/AIDS patients, two decades back. But for that to happen the new class of drugs must be accessible to all patients of Hepatitis C. But Gilead initially priced its drug at over USD 1,000 per tablet. In an influential paper by Hill et al. (2014), the authors estimated that the total treatment cost over 12 weeks with Sofosbuvir should be in the range of USD 68–USD 136. So, with a fair profit included, a tablet of Sofosbuvir should cost one dollar and not a thousand dollars.

Patients of Hepatitis C from across the world had reason to hope that Indian generic companies would provide them a lifeline by manufacturing and exporting low-cost generic versions of Sofosbuvir. Unfortunately 2014 is not 2001, when Cipla launched anti HIV/AIDS drugs for the first time. Gilead acted quickly to pre-empt the entry of cheap Indian generics by striking a deal with eight Indian generic companies, including Cipla (Pandey 2015). Under the deal, the Indian generic companies have been provided voluntary licenses by Gilead to manufacture the drug, and in return the companies will be restricted by Gilead's strict 'anti-diversion' clause. Under this clause the drug can be exported only to a select list of countries approved by Gilead, thus depriving patients in a range of High and Middle Income Countries (HICs and MICs) such as China, Brazil, Russia, USA, Thailand, Turkey, Mexico, Ukraine, and Georgia. These countries have some of the world's highest Hepatitis C prevalence rates. These, and other HICs and MICs, represent nearly 73 million people with Hepatitis C. Gilead has not included them in their licensing agreements because it sees them as profit-making 'commercial' markets (Hepcoalition 2014).

Precisely at the time when Gilead was negotiating its voluntary licenses, the Indian Patent office was hearing multiple challenges to

Gilead's patent application in India. In other words, Gilead tied up the Indian generic companies even before Gilead was granted a patent. In fact the Indian Patent office rejected Gilead's patent claim in January 2015 (Medecins sans Frontieres 2015). Thus, technically, there is no bar on any Indian generic producer to manufacture the drug and sell and export it at any price it may wish to. But by tying up potential generic manufacturers in India, Gilead has virtually stalled such moves, at least for the time being.

EMERGING CHALLENGES TO GENERIC DRUG PRODUCTION

There are several other IP-related areas, beyond the purview of India's Patent Act, that pose a challenge to generic drug production and access to medicines. These are areas of contestation as a result of pressures from pharmaceutical MNCs and their host countries—the US and the European Union.

Patent Linkage

Bayer, through a writ filed in the Delhi High Court, sought to link the patent status of a drug with the procedures related to the drug's marketing approval. While the court rejected Bayer's original suit in 2009 (Ermert 2009), there are continued pressures to link the patent status of a drug with its marketing approval. This would vitiate the process through which patents are granted as drug control agencies have no competence in adjudicating patent-related issues.

Criminalizing Generic Drugs

Over the past several years, multinational pharmaceutical companies and some developed countries have been pursuing what has come to be known as the 'Intellectual Property (IP) Enforcement Agenda'. The issue became a major international incident in 2009 when generic drugs from India, being exported to Latin America, were confiscated in transit in several European ports (Khor 2009) on the suspicion that they were 'counterfeit'. These drugs were manufactured legally in India and were being exported to countries were these drugs were also legal. The incident served to focus attention on the possible ways in which the IP enforcement agenda could be turned into a ploy to criminalize generic drugs.

Data Exclusivity (DE)

Data exclusivity refers to a practice where, for a fixed period of time (usually five years, but could be more), drug regulatory authorities do not allow data filed by the originator company to obtain marketing approval, to be used to register a generic version of the same medicine. Providing for DE increases costs of generics, delays generic introduction and also provides a 'patent like' protection even when there is no patent on a particular drug. In 2007 a government mandated Committee, called the Satwant Reddy Committee opined that India should not provide for DE in the case of medicines.[6] While the issue should have been laid to rest with the recommendations in the report, the issue of DE continues to be raised by big pharma at various forums (Singh 2009).

Free Trade Agreements

Regional and Bilateral Trade Agreements are an increasingly important part of the governance of global trade, and consequently have large impacts on the health sector across the world. Of particular importance to discussions regarding access to medicines are the ongoing negotiations on the India–EU Free Trade Agreement (FTA). While Indian negotiators appear to have successfully warded off demands by the EU for TRIPS-Plus measures (that is measures requiring stronger IP standards that go beyond the TRIPS agreement) such as data exclusivity, 'patent linkage' and 'patent term extensions', according to leaked texts of the negotiations several areas of concern, especially related to 'IP enforcement', remain (Nagarajan 2013).

Demise of Public Sector-Led Research

The Indian generic 'revolution' was driven by public sector R&D (which quickly and efficiently developed innovative processes for drug manufacture in a 'process patent' regime of IP). However, there has been a shift in public policy and the overall research environment since the 1990s. In synergy with the liberalization of the economy, public R&D centres are increasingly being required to enter into partnerships with private enterprises. Public sector R&D units are also required to generate a portion of their own resources from contract work and partnerships with the private sector. Concurrently, there has been no increase in real terms of public investment in pharma R&D. Overall R&D expenditure is very low and the private sector accounts for approximately two-thirds of gross expenditure on R&D in pharmaceuticals. Further, several Indian companies that had made substantial investments in R&D, have been acquired by foreign companies.

Compounding the problems faced by public sector-led R&D is the almost total demise of public sector manufacturing units—thus denying public R&D with a vital support system for development of new products. There is a need to prioritize investment in areas where research capacity is weak or where 'cutting edge' research is being developed globally. A particularly important area that should be prioritized is the development of capacity in manufacture of and research in biologics (a big proportion of newly introduced products in the global market and those in the pipeline are biologics—a majority of them targeting cancers and auto-immune disorders).

Biosimilar manufacture is a relatively new area as the processes involved are entirely different from those used to produce drugs through the chemical synthesis route. Further, there are regulatory hurdles because the process of getting regulatory approval for biosimilars is more cumbersome than for 'small molecule' drugs. This is because of the nature of biologics—because it is impossible to replicate the original drug and more data is demanded by regulatory agencies to prove that the quality, safety, and efficacy profile of the biosimilar is identical to that of the reference drug (that is, the original biologic). Indian courts and regulatory agencies are yet to work out ways to balance public interest with the necessity for caution while approving biosimilars. This is clearly an area that requires more attention and innovative thinking.

Recent Shifts in Public Policy

The pursuit of neo-liberal reforms has also brought about changes in the industrial climate. Indian generic drug companies are increasingly tying up with foreign MNCs, given their interest in developed country export markets. While domestic demand for medicines has stagnated due to poor public investment in health care, the major source of expansion for large Indian companies is this export market in the EU and US. Against this backdrop, it should come as no surprise that the present government appears to be bent upon decisively abandoning the earlier consensus of adherence to public health goals, which the previous UPA government had nominally retained.

Signalling the clear shift in the Indian government's policy towards IP, the joint communiqué at the end of Prime Minister Modi's visit to the US in 2014, contained the following: 'Agreeing on the need to foster innovation in a manner that promotes economic growth and job creation, the leaders committed to establish an annual high-level Intellectual Property (IP) Working Group with appropriate decision-making and technical-level meetings as part of the Trade Policy Forum'.[7] Indian and US interests will continue to be different with regard to IP protection, because the two countries are very differently placed as regards economic and technological development. By agreeing to a joint IP working group the Indian Government has clearly indicated that it is ready to compromise.

Concurrently, the Indian Government announced the setting up of an 'IP Think Tank' that was, inter alia, tasked to unfold India's new vision on IPRs. The composition of the 'Think Tank' itself has been mired in controversy with several members seen to have conflict of interest as they also, prima facie, appear to represent the interests of pharmaceutical companies (Jishnu 2014).

In January 2015 the Indian Government unveiled its Draft Intellectual Property Policy. The draft policy, significantly, presents a vision of 'intellectual property led growth in creativity and innovation'. The draft has been criticized widely as making ' ... a categorical and critical mistake of promoting intellectual property as an end in itself rather than as a means for achieving social and economic progress through enhanced production of and access to the fruits of creativity and innovation'. (Infojustice 2015)

* * *

While the US and its Northern allies continue to ratchet up pressures on India to change its laws and procedures on intellectual property protection, there has also been a continuous change in the discourse regarding IP protection within India. In a manner, India's relatively 'progressive' patent regime, since its inception, has been out of sync with the consensus between India's two largest political formations—led by the Congress and the BJP, respectively—to aggressively push for neo-liberal reforms. Successive governments have never pushed for a complete realization of the possible benefits of the flexibilities in the Indian Act.

India is now perched on a slippery slope where decades of effort to promote a liberal IP regime that allowed easier access to medical products, stands to be frittered away. It will really be a sad day for millions across the world if India continues to walk the talk and succumbs to the designs of Big Pharma. At stake are poor patients in three continents, who look towards India with hope for medicines that are cheap and effective.

NOTES

1. The application of policies that promote global integration through trade in goods and services and liberalized flow of finances is loosely termed as globalization.

2. Full text of the Order is available at: http://lawmin.nic.in/Patents%20 Amendment%20Ordinance%202004.pdf.

3. For complete text of the Indian Patents Act, see http://ipindia.nic.in/ ipr/patent/patent_Act_1970_28012013_book.pdf.

4. The negotiating history of Section 3(d) of the amended Patent Act is interesting. The Indian Drug Manufacturers Association (IDMA) provided the language for section 3(d). The Left parties in their negotiations with the government had, in fact, asked for an even more stringent definition of patentability by limiting grant of patents for pharmaceutical substances to 'new chemical entities' or to 'new medical entities involving one or more inventive steps'. Section 3(d) was a compromise solution.

5. See *Report of Committee on Price Negotiation of Patented Drugs* here: https://www.pharmamedtechbi.com/~/media/Supporting per cent20Documents/ Pharmasia per cent20News/2012/August/India per cent20Patent per cent20Drug per cent20Pricing per cent20Report.pdf. Accessed on 15 December 2015.

6. The full report is available here: http://chemicals.nic.in/DPBooklet.pdf. Accessed on 7 November 2017.

7. See full text of statement here: http://www.whitehouse.gov/the-press-office/2014/09/30/us-india-joint-statement.

REFERENCES

Arulanantham, David P. 2004. 'The Paradox of the BJP's Stance towards External Economic Liberalization: Why a Hindu Nationalist Party Furthered Globalization in India', *Asia Programme Working Paper*, Chatham House, December 2004.

Basheer, S. 2008. 'Breaking News: Natco Withdraws "Doha" Compulsory Licence Application', Spicy IP. 28 September. Available at: http://spicyip. com/2008/09/breaking-news-natco-withdraws-doha.html. Accessed on 24 April 2014.

Bidwai, P. 1995. 'One Step Forward, Many Steps Back: Dismemberment of India's National Drug Policy', *Development Dialogue* (1): 203–204. Sweden: The Dag Hammarskjöld Centre, Uppsala.

Chandrasekhar, C.P. and J. Ghosh. 2006. *The Market That Failed: A Decade of Neoliberal Reforms in India*. New Delhi: Leftword. Available at: http://cscs. res.in/dataarchive/textfiles/textfile.2008-09-14.6916203095/file.

Chatterjee, P. 2013. 'India's First Compulsory Licence Upheld, But Legal Fights Likely to Continue', *Intellectual Property Watch*, 4 March. Available at: http://www.ip-watch.org/2013/03/04/indias-first-compulsory-licence-upheld-but-legal-fights-likely-to-continue/. Accessed on 24 April 2014.

Chaudhuri, S. 2002. 'TRIPS Agreement and Amendment of Patent Act in India', *Economic and Political Weekly* 37(30): 3354–60.

———. 2013, 'The Larger Implications of the Novartis Glivec Judgment', *Economic and Political Weekly* 48(17): 10–12.

———. 2014. 'Intellectual Property Rights and Innovation, MNCs in Pharmaceutical Industry in India after TRIPS', Working Paper 170, November. New Delhi: Institute for Studies in Industrial Development.

Datta, P.T. Jyothi. 2013. 'Patented Drugs Government Report on Price Negotiation Draws Flak', *Hindu Business Line*, 28 February. Available at: http://www.thehindubusinessline.com/companies/patented-drugs-govt-report-on-price-negotiation-draws-flak/article4459371.ece. Accessed on 15 December 2015.

Ermert, M. 2009. 'Indian High Court Rejects Bayer Complaint for Patent Linkage', *Intellectual Property Watch* 21 August. Available at: http://www. ip-watch.org/2009/08/21/indian-high-court-rejects-bayer-complaint-for-patent-linkage/. Accessed on 24 April 2014.

Hepcoalition. 2014. 'Gilead's License on Hepatitis C drugs, Sofosbuvir and Ledipasvir: A Fool's Bargain'. Available at: http://www.hepcoalition.org/news/article/gilead-s-license-on-hepatitis-c. Accessed on 15 December 2015.

Hill, A., S. Khoo, J. Fortunak, B. Simmons, and N. Ford. 2014. 'Minimum Costs for Producing Hepatitis C Direct Acting Antivirals, for Use in Large-Scale Treatment Access Programs in Developing Countries', *Clinical Infectious Diseases* 58(7): 928–36.

Infojustice. 2015. 'U.S. Law Professors Call for India IP Policy to Promote Balance and Focus on IP's Ends'. Available at: http://infojustice.org/archives/33842. Accessed on 15 December 2015.

Jishnu, L. 2014. 'Rethinking IP Think Tank'. *Down to Earth*, 15 December. Available at: http://www.downtoearth.org.in/content/rethinking-ip-think-tank. Accessed on 15 December 2015.

Khor, M. 2009. 'Row over European Seizures of Low-Cost Drugs', *Third World Resurgence* 228/229: 4–5.

———. 2013. 'Global Trends'. 8 April. Available at: https://www.twn.my/title2/gtrends/2013/gtrends426.htm. Accessed on 7 November 2017.

Marcellin, Sherry S. 2010. *The Political Economy of Pharmaceutical Patents: US Sectional Interests and the African Group at the WTO*. Surrey, England: Ashgate Publishing Ltd.

Medecins sans Frontieres. 2007. 'Examples of the Importance of India as the "Pharmacy for the Developing World"'. Available at: http://www.msfaccess. org/sites/default/files/MSF_assets/Access/Docs/ACCESS_briefing_ PharmacyForDevelopingWorld_India_ENG_2007.pdf. Accessed 25 April 2014.

————. 2011. *Untangling the Web of Antiretroviral Price Reductions* 14th Edition, *Médecins Sans Frontières*, 7 July. Available at: http://apps.who. int/medicinedocs/documents/s18716en/s18716en.pdf. Accessed on 15 December 2015.

————. 2015. 'Gilead Denied Patent for Hepatitis C Drug Sofosbuvir in India'. Available at: http://www.doctorswithoutborders.org/article/gilead-denied-patent-hepatitis-c-drug-sofosbuvir-india. Accessed on 15 December 2015.

Nagarajan, R. 2013. 'European Union-India FTA May Hit Generic Medical Industry', Times News Network, 21 March. Available at: http://timesofindia. indiatimes.com/world/europe/European-Union-India-FTA-may-hit-generic-medical-industry/articleshow/19100738.cms. Accessed on 15 December 2015.

Nair, Gopakumar G., A. Fernandes, and K. Nair. 2014. 'Landmark Pharma Patent Jurisprudence in India', *Journal of Intellectual Property Rights* 19: 79–88.

Padma, T.V. 2007. 'Report on Patent Laws Shames Indian Scientists', *Nature Medicine* 13(4): 392.

Pandey, K. 2015. 'Gilead Expands Hepatitis C Licensing Pacts with Indian Companies', *Down to Earth*, 27 January. Available at: http://www. downtoearth.org.in/content/gilead-expands-hepatitis-c-licensing-pacts-indian-companies. Accessed on 15 December 2015.

Raju, K.D. 2004. 'WTO-TRIPS Obligations and Patent Amendments in India: A Critical Stocktaking', *Journal of Intellectual Property Rights* 9: 226–7. Available at: http://nopr.niscair.res.in/bitstream/123456789/4874/1/JIPR per cent209 per cent283 per cent29 per cent20226-241.pdf. Accessed on 15 December 2015.

Rangnekar, D. 2005. 'No Pills for Poor People? Understanding the Disembowelment of India's Patent Regime', *CSGR Working Paper No. 176/05*, October. University of Warwick. Available at: http://wrap.warwick.ac.uk/ 1926/1/WRAP_Rangnekar_wp17605.pdf. Accessed on 15 December 2015.

Reddy, P. 2010. 'Trends in "Oppositions" against Pharmaceutical Patents', *Spicy IP*, 22 September. Available at: http://spicyip.com/2010/09/trends-in-oppositions-against.html. Accessed 24 April 2014.

Shukla, S.P. 2000. 'From GATT to WTO and Beyond', Working Papers No. 195, World Institute for Development Economics Research, The United Nations University, pp. 14–15, August.

Singh, K. 2009. 'Data Exclusivity Study Draws Flak from Indian Drug Industry', *Economic Times*, 6 December 2009. Available at: http://articles. economictimes.indiatimes.com/2009-12-06/news/27663408_1_data-exclusivity-generic-companies-satwant-reddy-committee. Accessed on 15 December 2015.

Smith, R.D., C. Correa, and C. Oh. 2009. 'Trade, TRIPS, and Pharmaceuticals', *The Lancet* 373(9664): 684–91. Available at: http://www.unc.edu/courses/2010spring/econ/560/002/lancet_trips.pdf. Accessed on 11 June 2014.

Torbett, J. 2001. 'Cipla Sets the Pace on Cut-price AIDS Drugs', *Scrip Magazine* 6: 46–8.

UNAIDS. 2011. 'DOHA+10, TRIPS Flexibilities and Access to Antiretroviral Therapy: Lessons from the Past, Opportunities for the Future', *UNAIDS Technical Brief*. Geneva: UNAIDS. Available at: http://www.unaids.org/sites/default/files/media_asset/JC2260_DOHA per cent2B10TRIPS_en_0.pdf.

Yamey, G. 2009. 'Diving into the Patent Pool', *PLOS Medical Journals* Community *Blog*. Available at: http://blogs.plos.org/speakingofmedicine/2009/11/10/diving-into-the-patent-pool/. Accessed on 25 April 2014.

7

Access to Pharmaceuticals

Role of State, Industry, and Market

S. Srinivasan and Malini Aisola

At the turn of Independence in 1947, India's pharmaceutical production was Rs 10 crore. By 1952, the total turnover of pharmaceutical companies, foreign and Indian, was Rs 35 crore, of which 62 per cent (Rs 21 crore) was of Indian companies. This included Rs 1.16 crore in the public sector. In 1970, the situation was reversed. Multinational companies (MNCs) had 68 per cent of the pharma market. Of the leading 50 pharmaceutical companies in 1971, 33 were foreign. The total formulations market in India in 1972 was Rs 360 crore. There was very little bulk drug (or active pharmaceutical ingredient [API]) production in India by foreign pharma companies despite the government's exhortations on self-reliance and saving foreign exchange. The goal of MNCs in India was minimum risk and maximum profit.[1]

The Patents Act 1970, passed in 1972, replacing the 1911 Patents and Designs Act, changed the entire scenario. The new Act, by excluding product patents for medicines, initiated a dream run for India's local pharmaceutical industry. As a result, several Indian entrepreneurs and business groups started making drug intermediates and bulk drugs. By 1999–2000, most of the bulk drugs that India needed were made in India[2] as also the machinery and the technology that were needed. Scientists at government institutions, the National Chemical Laboratory (NCL), Pune, and the Regional Research Laboratory (RRL, renamed Indian Institute of Chemical Technology, IICT), Hyderabad, played stellar roles in this saga of bulk drug revolution by synthesizing and discovering more efficient ways of making many of the bulk drugs.[3] The domestic formulation industry grew by leaps and bounds to Rs 18,354 crore in 2000–1, which would increase to, by 2017–18, more than Rs 1 lakh crore domestic sales and about an equivalent amount in exports.

India had an enviable spread of public sector enterprises in pharmaceuticals until about 1970. Public sector pharmaceutical plants were set up to control the 'commanding heights' of the Indian economy. The Hindustan Antibiotics Limited (HAL) was set up in 1954, inspired by the experience of the Haffkine Institute, Bombay, and some of its leading scientists. Hindustan Antibiotics Limited and the Indian Drugs and Pharmaceuticals Ltd (IDPL) established in 1961, would do commendable work in laying the foundations of a technological base for making APIs and formulations with the then goals of self-reliance and import substitution in mind. But after the post-Patents Act 1970 boom of the pharmaceutical industry, and the gradual whittling down of public sector undertakings by indifferent governments, IDPL stagnated and was declared a sick industry—a case under the Board of Industrial and Financial Reconstruction (BIFR). A similar fate was shared by other public sector undertakings (PSUs) like HAL, Bengal Chemicals, and others.[4] Many technocrats from IDPL moved on to chart their future in private entrepreneurship.[5]

By the turn of the millennium, India was recognized as the 'pharmacy for the third world'. India started supplying many of the critical medicines for HIV/AIDs to Africa and Brazil. Between 1972 and 2005, any new patented medicine launched in the West, would be manufactured in India within three to four years at a fraction of the price (say, less than 10 per cent of the innovator's price).[6]

By 1995–2000 however, this status of India had eroded for a number of reasons, chiefly because of the predatory moves of global Big Pharma in introducing new definitions, norms, and rules of behaviour for international trade in pharmaceuticals. Consequently, the 'reverse engineering' of Western pharmaceutical innovations being practiced in India took the flavour of a pejorative. With words like 'property' and 'rights' it even acquired connotations of theft, piracy, and violation of inalienable and incontrovertible 'rights' bestowed on the original innovators.[7]

Underlying the World Trade Organization (WTO)/Trade-Related Aspects of Intellectual Property Rights (TRIPS), and the product patent only regime, was/is a politics of extraordinary self-interest of Big Pharma

MNCs and their governments. Big Pharma cartelized but only to have the rug pulled under from their feet in South Africa in 2000 when Cipla cited India-made AIDs drugs prices that were a fraction of those of Western pharma cartels.[8] Under massive worldwide pressure from civil society, the cartel of 39 pharmaceutical companies, was forced to withdraw their case against the South African government over a law to improve access to anti-retrovirals. Big Pharma companies struck back, soon enough, however, riding on the fears and disinformation they had generated and, armed now with overpriced biologicals.

The damage control, post-2005 in the aftermath of disallowing reverse engineering through process patents was initiated by using the flexibilities wrought and won in the final version of TRIPS, and the subsequent reaffirmation in the Doha Declaration of 2001. These flexibilities,[9] enshrined now in the 2005 amendments of the Patents Act, included, famously, Section 3(d) that seeks to prevent ever-greening and patent periods beyond 20 years, by raising the standards of patentability.

Part of global Big Pharma strategy now was to make it difficult for Indian pharmaceutical companies to enter and survive in EU and American markets. However, Indian companies have mostly overcome these entry barriers, defying sceptics, even as the attempts at delegitimizing the quality and efficacy of Indian pharmaceutical products in the post-2005 era continue.

Of late however, many Indian pharma companies, including entities like Cipla and Natco that have been contesting the patent worthiness of several products of Western companies in Indian courts and with some success, have become inclined to partnerships, albeit unequal, with Western pharmaceutical companies. Many have become willing partners in the voluntary licence deal of Gilead for its costly Hepatitis C product Sovaldi (sofosvubir).

Post-1972, as the 'animal spirits' of private entrepreneurship were unleashed in the pharma industry, the scenario especially for the poor in India has become a dismal case of poverty amidst plenty. There has been no consistent grand political vision of health services for all, except for the occasional rhetoric at the time of signing progressive international covenants related to health.

By the turn of the millennium, except for a few states like Tamil Nadu and Kerala, health care of the majority of the populace was left in the hands of the market. The market here meant the poorly regulated private sector consisting of private practitioners and private hospitals who let the bottom line drive the content and quality of their curative practice.

For most state governments and even the central government, health was/is not a political priority. The logic and the brouhaha of expanding horizons of pharmaceutical capital are too much of an alluring narrative for industry as well as the government. Price control of a broad range of medicines that came about in 1979 during the Janata Government has been gradually whittled down over the next 15 years.

Overpriced medicines are a fact of life in India. As we see, a number of historical factors, changing political-economic climate, the state's withdrawal from the social sector, especially health, in the overarching context of the rapacity of global pharmaceutical industry have contributed to whittling down access to affordable medicines in India.

We elaborate in this chapter, three related factors to the above narrative: price regulation and the proliferation of Fixed Dose Combinations (FDCs), pricing of patented drugs, and the interplay of the state, industry, and market therein.

1. PRICE CONTROL, AFFORDABILITY, AVAILABILITY, AND ACCESS

State Intervention and Market Failure

The argument for price regulation/control is the persistence of market failure. The pharmaceutical market is riddled with market failure—the same medicine sells at a wide range of prices, where price has no relation to the cost of production, and the market is distorted by unethical drug promotion. Stiglitz (1989) and Akerlof (1970) have identified the existence of information asymmetries as a cause of market failure.

The doctor–patient–pharmaceutical industry interface is rife with asymmetries. The patient has no power and knowledge to make a decision on what medicine s/he buys as that is decided by the prescriber who, in turn, is influenced by the 'choices' offered by the pharmaceutical industry and its unethical drug promotion. Therefore, the higher priced brands prevail. Each company claims superiority of its brand of the same medicine, promoting the general notion that the higher priced brands are of better quality.[10]

Competition in the classical sense (of many producers entering the field resulting in reduced price of a drug) does not usually occur in the Indian pharmaceutical market. When a generic enters the market for the first time, there is competition and lowering of prices, of the API as well as the formulation, with respect to the price of the innovator.

But after some time when several producers start making the same formulation, the generic formulation is sold at a wide range of prices, positioned as it were to the varying purchasing powers of its buyers. However, because the consumer has little choice, the bulk of the market is skewed towards the higher priced brands. Therefore, the principle that 'many producers will bring down the price of the product' does not work. There is competition of sorts, but it does not work in favour of consumers because they are led to believe, despite actual evidence to the contrary, that the lower the price, the lesser the efficacy of the medicine.

In India, with universal health coverage still a distant dream, electoral compulsions of market failure in medicines has resulted in the pharmaceutical market—at least some parts of it—being brought under price regulation, even if in desultory way.

Contrary Pulls of Price Control

The contentious discourse around price control of medicines in India that began in the 1960s (circa the war with China) has rolled into contemporary neo-liberal times, when the market is considered a better arbiter of prices. Today there is even a semantic hesitation to call it a price control policy—as against price regulation. The former smacks of the 'inefficient' socialist times and the latter is considered tempering wisely unbridled laissez faire in a politically sensitive arena like health care, even as we let the markets play it out.

The policy instruments for price control, the National Pharmaceutical Pricing Policy (NPPP) 2012 and the Drug Price Control Order (DPCO) 2013, have several problems. As we show below, these are at best tokenistic in their attempts at price regulation.

The actual price control, or regulation, always hovers around two factors that see a great deal of lobbying on the part of pharma companies and 'rent collection' on the part of the ruling elite: (i) the range of drugs to be put under price control and therefore, the methodology for selecting these drugs and (ii) the actual formula to determine the ceiling price beyond which the formulation cannot be sold. As a result of successful lobbying over the years, the scope of price control had been successfully restricted to 74 drugs by 1995 from a high of 347 drugs in 1979.[11]

Any 'formula' or 'methodology' based on market considerations (like market share, number of producers and therefore, presence/absence of competition) generally results in an unsatisfactory, if not absurd, list of drugs to be put under price control. Such was the case with the DPCO

1995 and the draft Pharmaceutical Pricing Policy of 2002, the latter being stayed by the Karnataka High Court and the Supreme Court. The DPCO 1995 had only 74 drugs under price control, half of which were drugs rarely in use, an eventuality resulting from the criteria adopted for selecting these drugs.

Likewise, the formula adopted for deciding ceiling prices is important. The usual norm till the onset of DPCO 2013 was cost-based pricing that is, cost of ingredients, plus conversion costs plus margin (in the case of DPCO 1995, the margin called Maximum Allowable Post-manufacturing Expenditure (MAPE) was 100 per cent). The DPCO 2013 relied on the simple average, of price to retailer of brands with 1 per cent market share, plus retailer's commission of 16 per cent, as the ceiling price. The choice of the simple average formula defies logic and has been critiqued by several commentators including the authors (Srinivasan, Srikrishna, and Aisola 2014; Srinivasan, Srikrishna, and Phadke 2013). For instance, among statistical indices that measure spread, why simple average and not mode or median, or weighted average of the lowest three prices?

The current policy, NPPP 2012 and DPCO 2013, were announced hastily after the judicial reprimand in the decade old and still ongoing Public Interest Litigation (AIDAN and Ors vs Union of India and Ors in WP (Civil) 423/2003). The run up to DPCO 2013 saw tremendous lobbying and resulted in modifications amounting to a 'balancing act' in the policy with the following features laden with escape hatches:

1. All 348 drugs in National List of Essential Medicines (NLEM) 2011, in the specified strengths and presentations, were put under price control. (At the time of going to press, a revised NLEM (hereafter NLEM-2015) comprising around 380 medicines has been announced in December 2015.) National List of Essential Medicines-2015 will be the new basket of medicines for price control. In the new list, 70 medicines from the older list have been deleted and replaced with 106 other medicines. (Our comments below and elsewhere in the chapter are applicable to both NLEM lists unless indicated otherwise.)

2. The ceiling price is the simple average price of price to retailer of brands with more than 1 per cent market share plus 16 per cent retailer's trade commission.

3. Only 348 drugs in their *specified* strengths and presentations (totalling about 620) are under price control as specified in the

NLEM-2011. This means the following categories are excluded from price control:

(i)   Strengths, dosage forms and presentations of the 348 essential drugs not mentioned in the NLEM-2011 (for example, paracetamol 650 mg and 1000 mg were excluded from price control as only paracetamol 500 mg tab was specified in the NLEM-2011. Paracetamol 650 mg tab is included in the recently announced NLEM-2015. In a few cases, NLEM-2015 mentions a continuous range of strengths, for example, for migraine, Acetylsalicylic acid, 300 to 500 mg.).

(ii) Chemical analogues of medicines listed in the NLEM-2011 are generally excluded. For example, only Atorvastatin is under price control because it is the only statin mentioned in the NLEM-2011 but all other statins like, Rosuvastatin, Simvastatin, and others are excluded.

(iii) All existing combinations of NLEM plus NLEM, NLEM plus non-NLEM, and non-NLEM plus non-NLEM medicines are excluded.

National List of Essential Medicines-2015 perpetuates, with respect to price control, the problems of NLEM-2011: it leaves out all isomers, derivatives, chemical analogs, limits to specific dosages, and others. This problem arises because the NLEMs, neither 2011 nor 2015, were drafted with price control as the major focus. In fact there needs to be a separate expanded list of essential and life-saving drugs that remedies the problems of relying on an NLEM for price control.

Many useful drugs for asthma—for example, Monteleukast—are excluded from price control. For diabetes only Glibenclamide, Metformin, and Insulin (of a certain kind only) were under price control as only these were mentioned in NLEM-2011. In the NLEM-2015 however Glibenclamide has been replaced by the more useful Glimepiride. But other overpriced and useful diabetics like say Acarbose or Gliptins continue to be excluded. Further, highly expensive drugs like Meropenem, Imipenem, Cilastatin, Tigecycline, Colistin, Abciximab, Tirofiban, and Eptifibatide are out of the NLEM-2015 and hence out of price regulation.

A government affidavit filed in the Supreme Court during November 2013 (Aisola and Zacharias [2015]) declared that only 18 per cent (Rs 13,097 crore) of the then domestic market of Rs 71,246 crore was under price control. This means that a major chunk, of the pharma market, namely, 82 per cent, has slipped out of the DPCO-2013 purview.

A recent estimate (co-author Malini Aisola with Thomas Zacharias, August 2015, unpublished), shows that about 86.6 per cent (Rs 72,730 crore) of the market is out of price control (*PharmaTrac MAT* January 2015 data). The therapeutic category breakdown is as follows: anti-diabetes (93 per cent), anti-malarials (75 per cent), anti-infectives (69 per cent), anti-neoplastics (80 per cent), blood-related (86 per cent), cardiac (80 per cent), derma (95 per cent), gastro intestinal (90 per cent), hormones (65 per cent), neuro/CNS (89 per cent), ophthal/otologicals (95 per cent), pain/analgesics (93 per cent), respiratory (96 per cent), sex stimulants/rejuvenators (100 per cent), stomatologicals (100 per cent), urology (96 per cent), vaccines (71 per cent), vitamins/minerals/nutrients (99 per cent), and others (99 per cent). Of the formulations excluded from price control, combinations account for more than 48 per cent (around Rs 35,413 crore). This corresponds to roughly 42 per cent of the total pharmaceutical market sales (Rs 84,017 crore).

How can a policy that results in more than 86 per cent of the market falling outside price control basket be considered as being aimed at controlling drug prices? Although it apparently meets the directives of the Supreme Court to formulate a price control policy for essential and life-saving drugs, it does not comply with the Supreme Court order[12] stating that the formula for bringing medicines under price control should not be changed. It is a policy that disproportionately reflects prices of brands with a perceived and inflated brand value rather than the actual cost of production. It is a policy which, as we see from Tables 7.1–7.3, legitimizes super profits to the tune of 2,000–4,000 per cent even after price control. These high profits are used in turn to fuel, and are fuelled by, questionable marketing practices in the name of brand promotion.

We present some tabular data below to illustrate some of the averments on overpricing we have made previously. Table 7.1 shows the range of prices used in calculating ceiling prices. The lower prices are closer to the cost of production. If anything, it shows the irrelevance of the cost of the production in calculating the ceiling price. This is quite evident in Table 7.2 when one compares column 7 and column 9.

Table 7.2 shows that in the case of relatively low-priced material, the cost of conversion is almost as much as the cost of the raw material. In the case of amlodipine, the raw material cost is less than the conversion

TABLE 7.1 Range of Prices to Retailer (PTR) Used for Calculating Simple Average Price

Name of drug	Lowest price with 1 per cent market share	Highest price with 1 per cent market share	Simple average price (without 16 per cent retailer markup)*
Acyclovir 200 mg tabs per 10	32.70	148.10	62.90
Atenolol 100 mg tabs per 10	3.00	42.30	32.10
Atorvastatin 5 mg tabs per 10	13.50	52.50	32.90
Azithromycin 500 mg tabs per 10	41.6	393.3	171.2
Losartan 50 mg tabs per 10	9.20	56	37.10

Source: NPPA Working Sheets (2013).

*Ceiling price is the simple average of price to retailer of brands with 1 per cent market share plus retailer's commission of 16 per cent (NPPA Working Sheets 2013).

Note: Prices in INR.

cost. A comparison of the cost price (column 7) and DPCO-2013 ceiling price (column 9), columns shown in bold, shows that the ceiling price methodology legitimizes high margins, making price control an eyewash.

Table 7.3 compares the tender procurement rates of the Rajasthan Medical Services Corporation (RMSC) with the DPCO 2013 ceiling prices. A comparison with that of the Tamil Nadu Medical Services Corporation (TNMSC) reveals similar results of margins of 1,000–3,000 per cent and in the case of Imatinib (Table 7.3, Sr. No 1), generic equivalent of Novartis' Glivec, it is 10,116 per cent! This is not to argue that medicines be sold in the retail market at the prices of the TNMSC/RMSC. Instead, based on the evidence there is room for advocating reasonable cost-based pricing plus sufficient margins so that the prices reflect the cost of production. The tender prices are merely a base and an index of comparative overpricing of the retail market prices of medicines.

To use a minimal list like NLEM for price control is a flawed idea. The basic purpose of minimal lists like NLEM is that Essential Medicines

TABLE 7.2 Conversion or Manufacturing Costs as Per Cent of Cost Price; and Cost Price Compared to DPCO-2013 Ceiling Price

Name (1)	Raw material price per kg (2)	No of tablets per kg of raw material (3)	Cost of API per 10 tabs (4)	Total raw material cost per 10 tabs (5)	Conversion or Mfg costs per 10 tabs (6)	Total cost per 10 tabs (7)	Conv. or Mfg. cost as per cent of total cost (8) [6/7]	DPCO-2013 ceiling price as of Aug 2015, per 10 (9)
Albendazole tabs 400 mg	1,337	2,500	5.35	5.99	2.91	**8.90**	33	**103**
Atorvastatin tabs 10 mg	16,887	89,000	1.90	2.07	1.22	**3.29**	37	**67.40**
Atenolol 50 mg tabs	1,231	20,000	0.62	0.72	0.82	**1.54**	53	**22.80**
Amlodipine 5 mg	3,136	140,000	0.22	0.36	0.59	**0.95**	62	**31.30**
Cetrizine tablets 10 mg	3,499	100,000	0.35	0.45	0.70	**1.15**	61	**19.90**

Source: Authors. Based on data sourced from the in-house records of LOCOST (Low Cost Standard Therapeutics) with which S. Srinivasan is associated.

Note: Costs and Prices in INR.

TABLE 7.3 Comparison of DPCO-2013 and RMSC Rates

1	2	3	4	5	6	7
No.	Name of drug, strength and use	Indication	Simple avg ceiling price as per DPCO-2013 (valid as of August 2015)	RMSC 2015 procurement rates	DPCO-2013 ceiling price/ RMSC rate	DPCO-2013 ceiling price per cent greater than RMSC rate
1.	Imatinib tab - 400 mg, 10 tabs	Anti-cancer	2,962.7	29.0	102.2	10,116
2.	Amlodipine tab - 5 mg, 10 tabs	Antihypertensive	31.3	1.0	32.5	3,150
3.	Enalapril maleate tab - 5 mg, 10 tabs	Antihypertensive	32.7	1.2	28.4	2,739
4.	Atorvastatin tab - 10 mg, 10 tabs	Blood cholesterol lowering agent	67.4	2.5	27.0	2,596
5.	Cetrizine tab - 10 mg, 10 tabs	Antiallergic	19.9	0.8	26.2	2,522
6.	Alprazolam tab - 0.5 mg, 10 tabs	Sedative, sleep inducer	22.2	0.9	25.3	2,428
7.	Domperidone tab - 10 mg, 10 tabs	Antivomiting agent	24.9	1.1	22.7	2,174
8.	Diclofenac Sodium tab - 50 mg, 10 tabs	Painkiller	21.5	1.2	18.3	1,730
9.	Atenolol 50 mg for 14 tabs	Antihypertensive	31.92	1.7	19.2	1,817
10.	Olanzapine tab - 5 mg, 10 tabs	Antipsychotic	32	1.9	16.8	1,580

Source: Prices available at: http://rmsc.health.rajasthan.gov.in/content/raj/medical/rajasthan-medical-services-corporation-ltd-/en/home.html# and http://www.nppaindia.nic.in/. Accessed on November 2017. Data analysis by Aisola and Zacharias (2015).
Note: Prices in INR.

included in it should be available at all times in various public health care facilities. Any essential list is a guide for use mainly for procurement in government health services—if the government restricts its purchases and prescriptions to a limited essential drug list like the NLEM—which are available to about 20 per cent of the population. Even then, as studies and reports have shown, the availability of essential medicines is poor (Kotwani 2013). In rational medical practice, many medicines beyond the NLEM are used. For example, chemical analogues and therapeutic equivalents and life-saving drugs depending on special needs for a patient are also used. If treatment were confined to only the drugs mentioned in the NLEMs 2011/2015, cure and management of chronic life-threatening problems like diabetes and asthma would become impossible for many patients.

The National Pharmaceutical Pricing Policy (NPPP) 2012 is a narrow interpretation of the Supreme Court order to put all essential and life-saving drugs under price control. The DPCO 2013, in turn, has therefore, limited impact. Nevertheless, if justice is to be done to the poorer sections of the population, a separate list of drugs for price control, larger than the NLEMs 2011/2015, needs to be formulated, supported by a free universal public health care system similar, perhaps, to those in the United Kingdom or Canada or the Scandinavian countries.

2. FIXED DOSE COMBINATIONS AND ACCESS TO MEDICINE

The large availability of irrational medicines—mostly in the form of FDCs—comes in the way of patients receiving adequate and appropriate treatment. Initially not many in number, FDCs today are in several thousands, a large proportion having no therapeutic rationale.

What kind of FDCs should be approved? The WHO recommended guidelines for acceptability of FDCs are summarized as follows:

1. Clinical documentation justifies the concomitant use of more than one drug.
2. Therapeutic effect is greater than the sum of the effect of each.
3. The cost of the combination product is less than the sum of individual products.
4. Compliance is improved (that is, when two or more medicines are to be taken separately, as in the case of TB, the user tends to avoid one or two medicines after sometime. This can be avoided if all three medicines are combined into one).

5. Sufficient drug ratios are provided to allow dosage adjustments satisfactory for the majority of the population.

Fixed Dose Combinations that do not satisfy these guidelines should be considered irrational.

Proliferation of Fixed Dose Combinations

Why has India's pharmaceutical industry been manufacturing and marketing FDCs—many of them irrational and harmful—for the last five decades? How, in the first place, did it get licenses for marketing and/or manufacturing these?

Part of the reason for the uncontrolled growth of FDCs is the pressure of competition and new products. Marketing heads of pharmaceutical companies in collaboration with their medical directors, invent combinations of two or more drugs, often launching them without a critical, scientific assessment of their therapeutic benefits and rationale. Moreover, before 1988 the Drugs and Cosmetics Act did not contain the legal provisions relating to FDCs.[13] Between January 1961 and November 2014, the number of FDCs approved by the Central Drugs Standard Control Organization (CDSCO)/Drug Controller Generals (DCGIs) was 1,193,[14] not all of them rational.

Before September 1988, it was a free for all, and manufacturing and marketing of FDCs was not limited to just the list of FDCs approved by the DCGI since 1961. As per these provisions introduced in 1988, FDCs were included in the definition of new drugs (per Rule 122-E), under which they remain new drugs up to four years after the date of its first approval. Notwithstanding the new provisions, there was considerable murkiness with regard to the role of state and central authorities that was clarified only in 2002 when Rule 69(6) and 75(6) were added to the Drugs and Cosmetics Rules. These rules inserted on 1 May 2002 stated that all new drugs including FDCs that qualified as *new drugs* were to have prior approval of the DCGI after which a licence for manufacture may be sought from the state licensing authorities (SLAs). In the absence of this clarificatory rule, a large number of FDCs have been licensed for manufacture by SLAs without being approved for marketing by the DCGI at the centre. Approval by DCGI involved, after 1988, production of proof of safety and efficacy. Part of the problem was also that during the Indian pharma boom during 1998–2002, neither the centre nor the states strictly enforced the laws on that had been passed for FDCs.

Fixed Dose Combinations are, of course, necessary in some select circumstances. These are few in number and cover FDCs for AIDS, TB, malaria, ORS, iron plus folic acid for anaemia, trimethoprim + sulphamethoxazole, and others. In the National List of Essential Medicines 2011, out of 348 medicines, only 18 (5.2 per cent) are FDCs. Estimates of number of FDCs vary between 40 and 60 per cent of the number of formulations in the Indian domestic market; the latter number is estimated around 50,000 (*PharmaTrac* January 2015).

An analysis, done by one of the authors (Aisola with Zacharias 2015) of the 50,000 plus branded medicines in *PharmaTrac* (MAT June 2015), shows about 43 per cent of the market are combinations and more than 50 per cent of which are likely to be irrational. In another study by the authors, in August 2015, of the top selling 300 formulations accounting for Rs 58,452 crore (which is 69.6 per cent of the total domestic market of Rs 84,017 crore [*PharmaTrac*, 12 months ending January 2015]), FDCs assessed to be outright irrational and unscientific accounted for Rs 12,757 crore (21.8 per cent) of Rs 58,452 crore. This comprised 72 items of the top selling 300 drugs. Extrapolating the percentage of the irrational and unscientific FDCs to the then total market of Rs 84,000 crore, irrational FDCs would account for approximately Rs 18,500 crore.

Yet, this is likely to be a gross underestimate. A large proportion of these irrational FDCs contain at least one NLEM medicine. But none of these are under price control. There are numerous similar examples as shown in Table 7.4. In most cases FDCs of an essential drug form 50 to 80 per cent (see column 6) of the total market involving the essential drug. Almost all these FDCs are likely to be irrational.

The pervasive prevalence of unnecessary combinations hits the patient in multiple ways: the patient is burdened with unnecessary extra medication and mostly irrational ones, that cost more (as most of them are out of price control and the patient has to pay for unnecessary extra ingredients) and the patient is put at the risk of avoidable side effects and adverse drug reactions.

Government Response to the Problem of Unscientific Fixed Dose Combinations

The Government of India, through the Central Drugs Standard Control Organization (CDSCO) and its successive Drugs Controller Generals (DCGIs), has been intermittently trying to solve the problem of the

TABLE 7.4 Market for NLEM-2011 Drugs and Combinations

1. Name of NLEM drug	2. Therapeutic category	3. Total annual sales (MAT Jan 2015, Rs cr)	4. Sales of formulations coming under price control (Rs cr)	Sales of formulations excluded from price control (Rs cr)	
				5. Non-NLEM additional strengths and dosage forms	6. Non-NLEM formulations (combinations, isomers, and others)
Ceftriaxone	Anti-Infectives	1,129.9	535	132	462.9
Ofloxacin	Anti-Infectives	1,477.3	151.8	283.3	1,042.2
Domperidone	Gastro Intestinal	1,532.8	33.5	14.9	1,484.4
Pantoprazole	Gastro Intestinal	1,328.8	167.6	460.3	700.9
Paracetamol	Pain/Analgesics	3,285.5	181.6	437.5	2,666.5
Chlorpheniramine	Pain/Analgesics	1,547	0.2	12.5	1,534.2
Amlodipine	Cardiac	1,809.7	299.1	31.5	1,479.1

Source: Data analysis by Aisola and Zacharias (2015).

Note: New formulations involving essential drugs would come under price control on a brand-by-brand basis post-implementation of DPCO 2013. These formulations are not expected to have significant market sales during the time period considered for the analysis.

FDCs, rational, irrational, legal and illegal, and others, over much of the decade of the 2000s.

We will not elaborate here on the chequered history of the relationship and the encounters between the FDC manufacturers and the government since the early 2000s. This includes stay orders by three State High Courts on the attempts by the government to resolve the problem.

The current state of these efforts was initiated with a letter on 15 January 2013, from the DCGI again requesting SLAs to instruct manufacturers to submit to the DCGI within 18 months, data on safety and efficacy of FDCs that were permitted by SLCs but had not been approved by DCGI before 1 October 2012. In response, the DCGI received approximately 6,320 applications. A committee under the Chairmanship of C.K. Kokate was constituted to examine the approximately 6,320 applications in a timely manner. In March 2016, on the basis of the committee's recommendations the Government of India banned 344 FDCs totalling about 1,080 applications as several brands had similar composition of ingredients. Some well-known top-selling brands like Corex, Phensedyl, Vicks Action 500, Saridon, among others, were recommended for ban. Almost immediately, several manufacturers of the banned products approached the Courts, especially the Delhi High Court which issued stay on the ban order even as the court heard the case over the next two months.[15] On 1 December 2016, the Delhi High Court gave an order quashing the ban. The reason given by the Delhi High Court was that the Drug Technical Advisory Board (DTAB) was not consulted in the process leading up to the ban. The order for quashing the ban was appealed in the Supreme Court by the Union of India and the All-India Drug Action Network (AIDAN) in early 2017.

In its final judgment of 15 December 2017, the Supreme Court has set aside the reasoning given by the Delhi High Court in quashing the ban order and ruled that is it is not mandatory for the government to consult the DTAB to ban/regulate/restrict the sale and manufacture of any modern medicine drug. This now gives a leeway to the government to weed out all other irrational FDCs, amounting to at least Rs 25,000 crores of sales by our latest estimates, whereas the current 344 impugned drugs barely affects Rs 2,000 cr of the pharma market. The Supreme Court order makes it clear that as long as the government relies on relevant material it can exercise its powers to ban, restrict or regulate a drug without going through the DTAB. Till such eventuality, all FDCs in the market that contain one or more of essential and life-saving medicines should be brought under price control. This will at the least minimize the economic burden on patients.

A footnote is in order: In view of the 'peculiar circumstances' of the case the ban on 344 drugs was stayed nevertheless with a direction by the Supreme Court to the DTAB, or a committee appointed by it, for re-scrutiny of the 344 impugned drugs within a time frame of 6 months, and then recommend a ban or otherwise (see judgment available at the Supreme Court website in the matter of Civil Appeal No. 22972 Of 2017.

ACCESS TO PATENTED MEDICINES

Pricing of Patented Drugs: Price Negotiations

Notwithstanding the many provisions in the amended Indian Patents Act of 2005 that protect Indian generic manufacturers, several medicine-related product patents that have been granted to foreign companies in India between 2005 and 2015. These medicines are often life-saving, but unfortunately, high priced. So how may these be made more affordable and accessible? If the government brings them under price control, how is the ceiling price to be decided? Are price negotiations the answer? If so, how is a negotiable price to be determined in the absence of transparent data on the cost of discovery of the drug? The experience of other developing countries has shown that price negotiations do not yield low enough prices to be affordable for the majority of the population and constitute a strategy far inferior to generic competition in lowering prices. For example, in Brazil, the lack of transparency, the lengthy time frame for negotiations, frequent re-negotiations in the background of public health emergencies, and others proved futile and local industry suffered even as patients lost out on much needed treatment.

It may be recalled that Novartis was selling at a high of Rs 1.2 lakh per month per patient (Rs 40,000 per 10 tablets) during the days when the company was arguing before the Indian courts on the patent worthiness of its anti-cancer drug Glivec (Imatinib mesylate). The patent was denied. In Table 7.3, we showed the same Imatinib 400 mg tabs had now a DPCO 2013 ceiling price of Rs 2,962.70 for 10 tablets and the Rajasthan Medical Services Corporation's procurement price is

100 times less at Rs 29.00 per 10 tablets. Likewise, as mentioned earlier, even when Bayer was arguing the case against Natco, Bayer's price for Nexavar (Sorafenibtosylate) in India was Rs 2,88,425 per person per month while Natco's was Rs 8,800 per person per month (and the Cipla costs as of April 2015 were Rs 6,840 for a month's treatment). These are price reductions that no amount of price negotiation could have achieved.

Nor are the current prices of these patented drugs in India a cause for cheer: Sunitinib caps, anticancer, at Rs 8,715 per 50 mg cap; Dasatinib, anticancer, Rs 2,761 per 50 mg tab; Posaconazole, antifungal, Rs 14,443 for a 40 mg/105 ml suspension; Eltrombopag, anticancer, Rs 8,715 per 50 mg cap; and so on. Given the lack of public financing for provision of medicines, the government will de facto end up as the 'price taker'. Therefore, alternative strategies are needed.

Efforts at setting a formula for price control of patented medicines factoring in per capita GDP adjusted for PPP, and others do not seem to have found agreement across the board. Nor do they give acceptable results all the time. There is no agreed way to 'discover' the real cost of patented drugs. It is not possible to discover prices without the cooperation of the innovator/first formulator and the patent holder has not been transparent in this regard anywhere in the world. Estimates of cost of R&D, for discovery of a new medicine, vary widely—the highly disputed figure of USD 2.6 billion has been put forth by the Tufts Center for the Study of Drug Development while Drugs for Neglected Diseases (DNDI)'s estimate is around USD 112–69 million for full development of a new chemical entity.

Yet, efforts have been made by a team of researchers led by Andrew Hill at the Liverpool University, UK. Hill and his colleagues have published estimates of mass producing oral direct acting medicines for the treatment of hepatitis (for example, sofosbuvir) and more recently several tyrosine kinase inhibitors (TKIs) for cancer (Imatinib, Erlotinib, Sorafenib, Lapatinib, Dasatinib) which demonstrate that generic production has the potential to drastically reduce prices to increase access globally to patients who can benefit from these treatments (van de Ven et al. 2015). While efforts to discover the production costs are yielding results and may present an opportunity to impose price control on patented medicines using a cost-based mechanism (with adequate margins), implementing these measures in India given the current fixation on market-based approaches, is unlikely to happen soon.

The only workable strategy to make patented drugs affordable is to let them be made by Indian drug manufacturers under compulsory licence (CL) or government use provisions of the Patents Act (Sections 84, 92, and 100). These are TRIPS-sanctioned flexibilities and therefore do not violate TRIPS obligations. Further, this approach laid down by the law makers also ensures strategic manufacturing capacity in the pharmaceutical sector.

What is Voluntary Licence?

A recent trend is to enter into voluntary licenses with pharma companies to make the product cheaper. Recently in India, Gilead entered into voluntary licences with seven major Indian companies over Sovaldi (sofosvubir), for treatment in hepatitis C. Gilead's price was USD 1,000 per 400 mg pill in the USA working out to USD 84,000 for the full 12-week course of treatment. As a result, in the first six months after Sofosbuvir (brand Sovaldi) entered the market, Gilead made nearly USD 6 billion on sofosbuvir. There was uproar at the high prices from consumers and civil society. The voluntary licence was partly to ward off the criticism. The Indian price would be USD 335 for a 12-week course. Research from Liverpool University shows however that Sofosbuvir could be produced for roughly USD 1 per pill, or USD 101 per treatment course.[16]

Gilead's voluntary licence deal with the Indian companies purchased the silence of these Indian companies that had filed patent oppositions in India.[17] In fact, Natco withdrew its patent opposition after accepting the voluntary license from Gilead. These are thecompanies that could have worked the compulsory licence in India. Allowing Gilead (and other MNCs) to issue a voluntary licence to Indian companies makes the legal case for CL weaker in India as the likes of Gilead will argue in the Courts how it has reduced the prices compared to the American price—although still unaffordable in India. It also closes the gate for the Indian voluntary licensees by buying the silence of the few companies capable of working the compulsory licence in India.

As an editorial in the *Economic and Political Weekly* in 2015 pointed out:

> [L]et us state it clearly. Going by this trend, no patented medicine in India on cancer, HIV/AIDS, infectious/chronic diseases, et al., can be sold at affordable prices or their access made easy. Nor can price

control on these high-priced patented medicines be an option as these companies will simply not sell in India arguing that the prices are too low. And if the prices are set high, issuing a CL would be difficult as these companies will argue that they are selling at government-approved prices ... If we need patented medicines at affordable prices, they have to be made in India by Indian pharma companies for Indian patients, and for those in developing countries without restrictions or conditions. Compulsory licensing of high-priced patentable/patented medicines is the only option—an option exercised by even smaller countries like Thailand which has a relatively smaller pharma industry. (Anonymous 2015)

* * *

India's pharmaceutical industry has made long strides since 1947, and from 1972. Access issues, however, remain along with the challenges of affordability, availability, and rationality of products. Allowing the market to regulate itself will not work. Proactive state intervention is necessary in pricing and provision of medicines and health care services to deal with the extraordinary crisis of public health in India. But for a couple of state governments like that of Tamil Nadu, Rajasthan and Kerala, the availability of medicines in the public health system is erratic and uncertain.[18]

The dilution of key flexibilities in India's patent laws, at the behest of Big Pharma lobbies, will put the clock back. Nor is such dilution necessary as India is fully TRIPS compliant. Efforts at opening up India to international trade must build on, not undo, the enormous strides made in the domestic pharma sector over the last 40 years.

ACKNOWLEDGEMENTS

The authors, along with Anant Phadke, Mira Shiva, Anurag Bhargava, and T. Srikrishna contributed to a Representation, on the issues discussed herein inter alia, to the Union of India in compliance with an order dated 15 July 2015 of the Supreme Court in *AIDAN and Ors. v. UOI and Ors. in WP* (Civil) 423/2003. This chapter reflects formulations in the Representation, especially on issues related to essential drugs and FDCs, credit for which is due to the above named friends. Errors of omission and interpretation are that of the authors alone. The authors are grateful to Thomas Zacharias for his assistance in the data analyses related to the DPCO 2013.

NOTES

1. For a more detailed history, see Chapter 2 in Chaudhuri (2005).

2. As of writing, India is dependent for 60 per cent of its APIs on imports, mostly from China. The Government of India appointed Katoch Committee whose recommendations are available at: http://pharmaceuticals.gov.in/document/salient-features-recommendations-katoch-committee-report-apis-0 (accessed on 3 March 2016), has targeted API self-sufficiency of India on par with India's formulations industry.

3. Interview with Yusuf Hamied by Tarun Khanna, Bombay, India, 29 April 2013, 'Creating Emerging Markets Oral History Collection', Baker Library Historical Collections, Harvard Business School. Available at: http://www.hbs.edu/businesshistory/Documents/emerging-markets-transcripts/Hamied_Yusuf_Web per cent20Transcript.pdf. Accessed on 27 September 2015. Also see Rao (2014), and 'Indian Pharma Industry: Decades of Struggle and Achievements' by Y.K. Hamied on the occasion of A.V. Rama Rao's 70th birthday, 2 April 2005 (available at: http://www.arvindguptatoys.com/arvindgupta/avra-hamied.pdf. accessed on 26 September 2015).

4. For details, see http://pharmaceuticals.gov.in/cpses. Accessed on 30 September 2015.

5. For a first person account of these transitions, see Reddy (2015).

6. See Table 6.1 in Chapter 6 of this book, "Globalization, Intellectual Property Rights and Pharmaceuticals" by Amit Sengupta.

7. For the politics in the run up to WTO/TRIPS, see Bhagwati (2004) pp.182ff. The author, a leading economist and international trade theorist, has been adviser to the WTO and GATT.

8. See Chapter 3 of Lofgren (2013).

9. These flexibilities include the following:

- Section 3(d) of the Patents Act was amended to exclude patentability of new forms (including derivatives of old drugs or combinations of old drugs) of known substances unless there is significant enhancement of efficacy;
- New use of an old drug, is not to be considered an invention and hence not patentable;
- Pre-grant opposition to patents applications was retained; and
- Post-grant opposition to granted patents was introduced.

In addition, definitions related to patentability criteria were modified by the 2005 amendments, especially definitions of 'invention', 'inventive step'. Other safeguards against patent abuse were introduced/modified through the 2005 amendments as well as earlier amendments of the 1970s law: Compulsory license, Bolar exception (preparation for generic launch, that is production for marketing approval, and marketing approval) and parallel importation. Also see Chapter 6 in this volume on IPR.

10. On Pharmaceutical Market Failure, see Bennett, Jonathan, and Velásquez (1997).
Public-Private Roles in the Pharmaceutical Sector—Implications for Equitable Access and Rational Drug Use. Health Economics and Drugs Series, No. 005, (WHO, 1997; 115 pages).

11. For a more complete history of price control since 1962, see Chapter 8 in Chaudhuri (2005) and LOCOST/JSS (2004).

12. In the order passed on 3 October 2012, in WP(Civil) No. 423 of 2003, AIDAN and Ors. Versus UOI and Ors., the Supreme Court ruled: 'While adjourning the case, we make it clear that the Government should not alter the price structure of the drugs as notified vide Notification dated 13 July 1999 and similar notifications which may have been issued thereafter.' This order was completely ignored in the formulation of DPCO 2013.

13. Specifically, Rules 122 A, B, D, and E and Schedule Y in Part X-A related to requirements and guidelines for import and manufacture of new drugs including FDCs. Appendix VI of Schedule Y gives requirements for approval of various categories of FDCs.

14. Available at: http://www.cdsco.nic.in/writereaddata/Aprroved per cent20FDC per cent20list per cent20till per cent20november per cent202014. pdf. Accessed on 18 January 2015.

15. For a background in the context of a case filed by pharma companies regarding the ban of the 344 FDCs, see Srinivasan, Shiva, and Aisola (2016).

16. Dr Andrew Hill quoted at http://www.ip-watch.org/2015/01/14/key-hepatitis-c-patent-rejected-in-india-for-lack-of-novelty-inventive-step/. Accessed on 29 September 2015.

17. For patent oppositions filed, see http://patentoppositions.org/en/drugs/51dfee9097961f0002000020#patent-oppositions (accessed on 3 March 2016). Among these the opposition filed by the Initiative for Medicines, Access & Knowledge (I-MAK) in November 2013 together with the Delhi Network of Positive People (DNP+) were heard in February 2016. Its lawyers argued that sofosbuvir was 'old science,' and 'did not meet the standard needed for patenting in India ... Patents for sofosbuvir have been rejected in Egypt, China and Ukraine, and further patent oppositions have been filed in Argentina, Brazil, Russia, Thailand, and the EU'. Available at: https://donttradeourlivesaway.wordpress.com/2016/02/29/patent-challenge-hearing-on-gilead-hepatitis-c-drug-sofosbuvir-starts-in-india/. Accessed on 3 March 2016.

18. At the time of going to the press, a free drugs initiative (http://nrhm.gov.in/images/pdf/in-focus/Shimla/Guidelines/Free_Drugs_Service_Intitiative.pdf) has been initiated to provide support to the states to initiate delivery mechanisms like the Tamil Nadu and Rajasthan Medical Service Corporations. The details of financial support to the states are not clear. The Jan Aushadhi scheme (http://janaushadhi.gov.in/) for availability of

affordable essential drugs at the retail level has also been streamlined and 3,000 outlets are to be opened.

REFERENCES

Aisola, Malini and Thomas Zacharias. 2015. 'Analysis for the Representation to the Union of India in Compliance with the Hon'rble Supreme Court order of July 15, 2015'. AIDAN and Ors. *v* UOI and Ors. In WP(Civil) 423/2003 (Unpublished report).

Akerlof, George A. 1970. 'The Market for "Lemons": Quality Uncertainty and the Market Mechanism', *Quarterly Journal of Economics* 84(3): 488–500.

Anonymous. 2015. 'Pharma Patents after 10 Years', *Economic and Political Weekly* 50(18): 7–8.

Bennett, Sara, Jonathan D. Quick, and Germán Velásquez. 1997. 'Public-Private Roles in the Pharmaceutical Sector - Implications for Equitable Access and Rational Drug Use', *Health Economics and Drugs Series* 005. Geneva: WHO.

Bhagwati, Jagdish. 2004. *In Defense of Globalization*. New Delhi: Oxford University Press.

Chaudhuri, Sudip. 2005. *The WTO and India's Pharmaceutical Industry*. New Delhi: Oxford University Press.

Kotwani, Anita. 2013. 'Where Are We Now: Assessing the Price, Availability and Affordability of Essential Medicines in Delhi as India Plans Free Medicine for All', *BMC Health Services Research* 13: 285.

LOCOST/JSS. 2004. *Impoverishing the Poor: Pharmaceuticals and Drug Pricing in India*. Vadodara/Bilaspur: LOCOST/JSS.

Lofgren, Hans. 2013. *The Politics of the Pharmaceutical Industry and Access to Medicines: World Pharmacy and India*. New Delhi: Social Science Press.

NPPA Working Sheets. 2013. June. Available at http://www.nppaindia.nic.in/. Accessed on 15 December 2017.

PharmaTrac. 2015. MAT. January. AIOCD/AWACS.

PharmaTrac. 2015. June. AIOCD-AWACS Pharma Data Platform. Available at: http://www.aiocdawacs.com/ProductDetail.aspx.

Rao, Rama A.V. 2014. 'Indian Organic Chemical Industry: Decades of Struggle and Achievements', *Indian Journal of History of Science* 49(2): 399–412.

Reddy, Anji K. 2015. An *Unfinished Agenda: My Life in the Indian Pharmaceutical Industry*. Gurgaon: Portfolio/Penguin Books India.

Srinivasan, S., T. Srikrishna and Anant Phadke. 2013. 'Drug Price Control Order 2013: As Good as a Leaky Bucket'. *Economic and Political Weekly* 48 (26–27): 10–12.

Srinivasan, S., T. Srikrishna, and Malini Aisola. 2014. 'Pharma Price Control Policy: Unrealistic and Unfair', *Economic and Political Weekly* 49 (23): 13–15.

Srinivasan, S., Mira Shiva, and Malini Aisola. 2016. 'Cleaning Up the Pharma Industry. A Landmark Ban on Irrational Drugs', *Economic and Political Weekly* 51(14): 21–3.

Stiglitz, Joseph E. 1989. 'Markets, Market Failures, and Development', *The American Economic Review* 79(2): 197–203.

Van de Ven, N., J. Fortunak, B. Simmons, N. Ford, G.S. Cooke, S. Khoo, and A. Hill. 2015. 'Minimum Target Prices for Production of Direct-Acting Antivirals and Associated Diagnostics to Combat Hepatitis C Virus', *Hepatology* 61: 1174–82.

COURT CASE

Pfizer Limited and Another *v.* Union of India and Another in WP (C) No. 2212 of 2016, order dated 1 December 2016.

8

Structure, Organization, and Knowledge Production of Clinical Trial Industry

Roger Jeffery, Gerard Porter, Salla Sariola, Amar Jesani, and Deapica Ravindran

In India, the number of clinical trials (CTs) has been radically transformed in two directions since 2005. In that year, legislation was changed to make it easier for 'Big Pharma' to carry out multisited trials in India and at the same time as elsewhere in the world. After a period of rapid growth up to 2010, numbers of new trials registered with the 'Clinical Trials Register-India' dropped from 500 in 2010 to 321 in 2011 and 262 in 2012 (Chawan, Gawand, and Phatak 2015). Following a series of adverse reports, the number of approvals in 2013 dropped further to 107 in 2013, 150 in 2014, 121 in 2015, and 85 in 2016, and then rose to 172 in 2017. It remains to be seen if it will be possible to maintain the current rate of growth.

This chapter reviews the evidence about the scale and significance of these trials, using a theoretical approach derived from the theories of 'global assemblages'. We set out some of the new social forms that have arisen to service these trials, before assessing the growth in CTs in India since 2005. The chapter also analyses the ethical implications of CTs for India and its 'public health'. We conclude by considering the implications of the reforms that have been introduced since 2013 as a result of several highly publicized scandals that highlighted problems in the management of CTs.

Our main arguments are that *firstly*, the claims of the Indian CTs industry and its supporters have been massively exaggerated; and *secondly*, that the Indian generics pharmaceutical industry, and the nascent contract research organizations, were well prepared for the changes introduced by India signing up to the Trade-Related Aspects of Intellectual Property Rights (TRIPS) element when joining the World Trade Organization in 1995. India's regulators have been much slower to come to terms with the ethical, political, and public health implications of this change (Yee 2012). We draw on research funded by the UK's Economic and Social Research Council (ESRC) and its Department for International Development (DfID), carried out between 2009 and 2012.[1] We also draw on the detailed understanding of the pharmaceutical sector and the growth of CTs from previous research and engagement with issues of medical ethics.

DEFINITIONS OF 'CLINICAL TRIAL' AND THEORETICAL APPROACH

Clinical trials take a variety of forms. They range from computer simulations and testing of drugs on animals, through initial testing of pharmaceuticals, appliances, biologicals, or surgical techniques on healthy patients, to applying them to patients and finally reviewing their costs and benefits in 'real-world' use. The most common and popular image is of the international, multisited trial of new chemical molecules run by a contract research organization, sponsored by large pharmaceutical companies with the aim of establishing a patented drug that will win them large profits. But publicly funded trials, or indeed trials funded by a combination of public and private sponsors also take place. Some trials are community-based, some are conducted by and for particular hospitals or medical colleges, and some within the confines of pharmaceutical companies. The existing classification of CTs—by 'phase'—is not entirely satisfactory, since the boundaries between phase can be unclear and, occasionally, subject to fierce disputes (Sarojini et al. 2010). Nonetheless, for heuristic reasons we focus, in this chapter, mostly on Phase III trials—trials carried out on large numbers of patients who are ill with the target disease, in order to compare new medicines or treatment protocols with an existing treatment or a placebo, to see if it is better in practice, and if it has important side effects. Most are carried out by commercial sponsors (many, but not all, based outwith India), for which the most common focus is on drugs and biologicals.

Until the late 1980s, most multi-sited Phase III clinical research trials were carried out in relatively wealthy countries in North America, Western Europe, and Oceania (Theirs, Sinskey, and Berndt 2008). Since the early 1990s, however, there has been a rise in the numbers of foreign and locally sponsored CTs conducted in the so-called 'pharmerging' regions of Africa, Asia, South America, and Eastern Europe (Theirs, Sinskey, and Berndt 2008). This shift has been linked to several factors, including the rapid growth in these markets (IMS Institute for Healthcare Informatics 2011) and the possibility of using CTs to create a presence for the company or the drug in the regions. Other reasons cited include the increasing problems and costs of carrying out trials in relatively wealthy countries, and difficulties in accessing patients who are 'treatment naïve'. Nonetheless, even as late as 2012 the USA, Canada, and Europe remained the dominant locations of CT sites. Low- and middle-income countries hosted only 21 per cent of clinical research sites (Drain et al. 2014).

Even for those trials that take place entirely within India, the form they take is heavily influenced by a global industry, one that has come to prominence in India since 2005. In the outsourcing of CTs to developing and transitional countries, complex mediations occur at a series of levels between sponsors and the populations that become CT subjects. The flows generated by such biomedical research involve bilateral transfers within and between the Global North and South; the mediations produce transnational networks. In joining the global assemblages (Collier and Ong 2005; Sassen 2008) that constitute international CTs, actors based in India look to capture the economic benefits of scientific innovation. The promise of these partnerships is of internationally transferable knowledge and commodities that generate other benefits along the way—employment, career development, infrastructure, medical, and public health as well as entrepreneurial possibilities.

Global assemblages are constructed from institutions, roles, and relationships that are global in origin and yet are locally specific in the particular forms of combinations that emerge. They involve expectations of and aspirations to universal standards of design, method, reliability, validity, ethics, and reporting of results. Although the sponsors—often but not always from 'Big Pharma' (Sariola et al. 2015)—take a leading role and attempt to control the whole process, they inevitably lose a degree of oversight as they negotiate with local partners for trial approval, recruitment of patients, and others. The local teams co-construct—from very unequal starting points—the practicalities of any particular research project, always within externally dictated protocols, rules, and guidelines. They are also responsible for communicating the risks and hazards that feature prominently as part of these processes. Thus, clinical trial assemblages are the 'cutting edge' in a process of de-territorialization (Deleuze and Guattari 1980, 1988) which bring global procedures into everyday settings (hospitals, laboratories, and others) and render them coeval and continuous with others around the globe (Timmermans and Berg 1997). Further, they manage trial subjects and induct them into the global laboratory that such procedures represent. They are gatekeepers to a global modernity for members of these assemblages, who regulate access to different regimes of care but also to new temporalities (via the research process), new spaces (in the clinic/hospital as laboratory), and most importantly, futures (as biological citizens [Rose and Novas 2005], biomedical citizens [Petryna 2005], therapeutic citizens [Nguyen 2005], pharmaceutical citizens [Ecks 2005], or bioethical citizens [Simpson et al. 2015]).

Entry into such global assemblages, however, presents challenges as well as opportunities for Contract Research Organizations (CROs), Principal Investigators (PIs), and regulators in India (see for example, Cassese 2004; Held and Koenig-Archibugi 2003; Slaughter 2004). The opportunities are largely financial—access to a world market-place for the skills and patient population available in the country—the advantages of the place they know well. The challenges arise from the mismatch between the interests of the various stakeholders, and because India's democracy ensures some voice to the patient population, to try to ensure that the industry works to their benefit as well. Foreign-sponsored CTs being conducted in India have to orient towards weak regulatory systems (Sama 2012; see also Ana et al. 2013; Glickman et al. 2009; Jesus and Higgs 2002). With little experience of structured medical research and plagued by poverty, inadequate public medical facilities, excessively expensive private medical care options, and stark social inequalities, Indian regulatory institutions struggle to achieve their stated goals in the face of mounting public, legal, and parliamentary criticism. These standards are not uniformly reached elsewhere in the world, including in developed countries, and a case can be made that such standards should be adapted to take account of local conditions in resource-poor settings. For most Indian commentators, however, the aspirational norms of Western science remain unchallenged. While commercial interests quickly took note of the new opportunities that outsourced CTs might offer them in India, the procedures to regulate these activities in the interests of wider societal goals were much slower to become established (Yee 2012). After describing the legal framework for regulating CTs in India, in the following section we turn to evidence about the growth and form that CT activity in India has taken since 2005.

REGULATION OF CLINICAL TRIALS

The regulation of clinical trials in India consists of both a legislative framework and an active role 'on the ground' for research ethics committees (RECs). The Drugs and Cosmetics Act, 1940 (as amended) entrusts the approval of CTs to the Drugs Controller General of India (DCGI). The Drugs Controller General of India is part of the Central Drugs Standard Control Organization (CDSCO), India's main regulatory body for pharmaceuticals and medical devices, situated within the Ministry of Health and Family Welfare. The Drugs and Cosmetics Act also gives the central government the power to draft secondary legislation for the regulation of CTs, mainly through Schedule Y of the Drugs and Cosmetics Rules 1945 (as amended). Criticism has been less addressed to the rules themselves, and more to their patchy implementation (see Parliament of India 2012, 2013a, and 2013b).

India signed the World Trade Organization's (WTO) Agreement on TRIPS in 1995. It then introduced three amendments to the Patents Act (in 1999, 2002, and an ordinance in December 2004 which was converted in to an Act in 2005) to implement TRIPS (Sengupta 2013). The Patents (Amendment) Act 2005 encouraged CTs to move to India by removing the fear that Indian firms would copy a test drug by 'reverse-engineering' and produce a generic competitor. A further boost to the Indian CTs industry was given in 2005, when Schedule Y of the Drugs and Cosmetics Rules 1945 was amended to remove the 'phase lag' requirement. This allowed companies to 'conduct trials of new drugs in India at the same time that trials of the same phase are being conducted in other countries' (Nundy and Gulhati 2005: 1633; Sariola et al. 2015). Simultaneous Phase II and III CTs of molecules were thenceforth permitted, but not Phase I. An exception allows drugs developed abroad that relate to a pressing health need to be marketed without undergoing trials in India. This exception also permitted simultaneous Phase I trials of the AIDS vaccine (whose patent was held by a US firm) by the International AIDS Vaccine Initiative (IAVI) in collaboration with the Indian Council of Medical Research (ICMR).

The 2005 amendments to Schedule Y also require an application to conduct a clinical trial to first receive, inter alia, the approval of a properly constituted REC before it can then be authorised by the DCGI. The Research Ethics Committees evaluate clinical trial protocols in light of the ICMR's 'Ethical Guidelines for Biomedical Research on Human Participants', as well as India's 'Good Clinical Practice' guidelines[2] and the Declaration of Helsinki. In 2000 and 2006, the ICMR updated its guidelines to bring them into line with the Declaration of Helsinki (Indian Council of Medical Research 2006). Nevertheless, the ICMR guidelines diverge from the Declaration of Helsinki as they are more flexible on controversial issues in international research, including the use of placebo controls and post-trial access to medicines.[3]

The Clinical Trials Registry-India (CTR-I), launched in 2007, is maintained by the ICMR's National Institute of Medical Statistics. Since 2009, the online registration of CTs in the CTR-I is mandatory. There are, nevertheless, recurrent concerns that the submitted data are often incomplete and fail to provide sufficient information, for example, on sponsors, CROs and sites, and several amendments have been made to the form (Pandey et al. 2013; Pandey et al. 2009; Pandey et al. 2008). The editors of eleven major Indian biomedical journals declared that only articles emerging from registered trials would be considered for publication (Pandey et al. 2009; Pandey et al. 2008).

The changes after 2005 made it possible for Indian CROs to bid for work in multisited global trials, and gave the Government of India (and to some extent, the wider interested public) much useful information. However, identifying the scale and form that clinical trial activity has taken in India has been hard to extract from the registration system, and many of the 'facts' that enter into public debate turn out to have been provided by interested parties for their own purposes. Separating facts from claims is the focus of the following section.

SCALE AND NATURE OF CLINICAL TRIALS ACTIVITY

The earlier attitude was that we should block [clinical trials development] because as I told you it was a nation of traders at that time and now because our own people are innovating, we want the innovation to be there, we want to be landscaped for the innovation, so the trials are to be permitted … you don't feel threatened; not at all. But the only thing, I feel heavy as a person.

(Author interview with a senior Government of India official 2008;
emphasis added)

India apparently offered great cost-cutting opportunities to pharmaceutical companies and other research sponsors (van Huijstee and Schipper 2011: 49–54). Compared to competitor countries, India seems to be very attractive for inclusion amongst the new countries considered for multi-sited trials. According to industry sources, costs for recruiting patients and managing data collection are as little as half of those in North America; India's large pool of doctors, nurses, and trial assistants usually have good English; and a huge number of patients, many of whom are treatment-naïve, provides a large pool of potential easily-recruitable trial participants (Gupta and Padchy 2011). Carrying out trials also offers sponsors opportunities to build market access for patented drugs, by creating networks of key physicians who are well-disposed to prescribing their products, old and new (Glickman et al. 2009). Regulatory structures in India are simpler (and in English) compared to many other competing countries, and more likely to accommodate the demands of sponsors and Contract Research Organizations (CROs), allowing for quicker recruitment. But weaker regulatory structures are vulnerable to accusations of unethical practice and poor quality observance of international standards in data collection and management. There is a risk that data from one country or research site might become suspect and unusable in the pivotal trials that are submitted to the US Food and Drug Administration (FDA) or to European or Japanese drug regulatory bodies (Ana et al. 2013; MacMahon, Perkovic, and Patel 2013).[4]

Managing trials in India—in some cases more so than elsewhere in LMICs—can be a frustrating process. In India, multiple regulatory agencies have to be satisfied—not only the CDSCO but also the New Drugs Advisory Committee (NDAC), Drug.Technical Advisory Board (DTAB), ICMR, and Directorate General of Foreign Trade (DGFT)—several of which are under-staffed, with time taken to seek approvals ranging from five to eight months (Saini et al. 2013). Table 8.1 suggests that difficulties continue after the trial has received approval, with perhaps around 50 per cent of trial participants initially identified failing to continue through to the end of the trial.

How successful have Indian firms been in attracting trials to India? The main sources of evidence are the CTR-I and the US FDA register at clinicaltrials.gov. These sources do not include those 'trials' that do not register; there is anecdotal evidence that off-register 'trial-like' activity is common practice, for example, in experimental treatment of autistic children or in the use of stem cells (Editorial 2014; Sleeboom-Faulkner and Patra 2011). Furthermore, data entry into the CTR-I is not

TABLE 8.1   Start-up Times, Screening Failure, and Median Drop-out
Rates for Phase III Oncology Studies

Indicator	Brazil	Russia	India	China
Protocol approval to first site initiated— weeks of delay	55.0	31.5	40.2	35.6
Percentage of patients who, through the screening process, were disqualified from participating in the study	20 per cent	20.5 per cent	32.3 per cent	10.2 per cent
Median drop-out rate	8.3 per cent	18.1 per cent	18.2 per cent	10.6 per cent

Source: Authors. Tabulated from Saini et al. (2013: 47).

complete: for example, the trial design is not always recorded, with no real indication of why this is the case. The BA/BE (Bio-availability and Bio-equivalence) trials carried out on healthy subjects for testing generic drugs to satisfy regulators in developed countries for exports are also not listed in the CTR-I. They probably number as many as the other CTs listed in the CTR-I. Large public health experiments are also often not listed unless they are using 'new drugs'.

Until 2008–09, clinicaltrials.gov was the main source of evidence about trial activity globally, but this covered only those trials for which a US registration was required or desired: in June 2009, the US FDA registered 1,040 CTs with a site in India: 618 were active in some form; 422 were completed. The data kept on the CTR-I showed little information until after the registration of trials was made mandatory in 2009. The number of trials approved by the DCGI increased from a few per year until 2009 with 500 registered in 2010. As on 30 June 2010 CTR-I listed 1,078 trials, out of which 757 were reported to be trials sponsored by pharmaceutical companies. Of these, 442 had multinational pharmaceutical sponsors (for more details, see Tables 8.2 and 8.3).

TABLE 8.2   Clinical Trials Registered in the CTR-I by Sponsor,
as of 30 June 2010

Sponsor category	No. of trials	Percentages
Public/Govt. funded	128	12 per cent
Private funded	789	73 per cent
Other sources	112	9 per cent
No information on sponsors	49	5 per cent
Total Trials	1068	99 per cent

Source: Database created by Centre for Studies in Ethics and Rights, Mumbai,
from CTR-I on-line website. Available at: http://ctri.nic.in/Clinicaltrials/login.
php.

TABLE 8.3   Clinical Trials Registered with the CTR-I by Country
of Origin of Sponsors of 30 June 2010

Origin of sponsor	No. of trials	Percentages
Indian	486	45 per cent
Foreign	515	48 per cent
Collaborative	22	2 per cent
No information	55	5 per cent
Total	1078	100 per cent

Source: Database created by Centre for Studies in Ethics and Rights (CSER),
Mumbai, from CTR-I online website. Available at: http://ctri.nic.in/Clinicaltrials/
login.php.

Our preliminary analysis of CTR-I registered trials at 30 June 2010
showed that substantial minorities of the trials registered do not involve
pharmaceutical products. Table 8.4 shows the pattern for India's five
largest medicines trial sites, and demonstrates that while trials of drugs
are the largest category, other types are also carried on. For the purposes
of this chapter, we restrict ourselves to the pharmaceutical trials, which
constitute the vast majority of the field.

The total number of trials being conducted in India has indeed risen
sharply since the early 2000s, but different sources give different estimates
of the actual total number of trials, and trial participants, depending
on methodologies and definitions. One study gives a figure of 1,156
trials active in 2012. This represents a growth rate from 2005–12 of over

TABLE 8.4   Distribution of Trials by Type at Five Leading Institutions, 2011

Trial type	AIIMS	Tata Memorial	KEM	Ramaiah	CMC Vellore	All selected institutions
Behavioural	2					2
Biologicals	43	18	14	18	18	111
Devices	4		3		4	11
Dietary Supplements	5				2	7
Drug	88	46	36	56	58	284
Other	8		2		2	12
Procedure	7	2			6	15
Radiation		3			2	5
All trials	*157*	*69*	*55*	*74*	*92*	*447*

Source: CTR-I data, analysed by CSER, Mumbai. For further detail, see Ravindran and Nikarge (2010).
Note: Not all data have been entered into the CTR-I, and the classification by type of trial is according to the categories selected by the trial registrant.

30 per cent per annum (Drain et al. 2014). Although this growth was faster than for Brazil, it was less than in China, South Korea, Egypt, and Japan and well below industry projections. According to the same study, India was involved in 3.7 per cent of all registered trials in the world in 2012 (Drain et al. 2014: 166 and S2). Another study for 2012 found 2,091 of the 129,099 trials listed on the clinicaltrials.gov registry involved India. Of 4,823 breast cancer trials, 70 had sites in India.[5] So India, with about 17 per cent of the world's population, was involved in between 1.5 per cent and 3.7 per cent of all CTs, depending on the indicator and the data source chosen (Saini et al. 2013).

The global significance of Indian clinical trial sites depends on whether the indicator chosen is the number of trials with an Indian site, the number of Indian sites, or the number of patients recruited. In addition, not all trials have the same significance to the sponsor. 'Pivotal' trials are the ones over which most care is taken, since these are the ones to be submitted to the US FDA or the European Medicines Agency (EMA) and are the trials used to make specific claims about efficacy and safety. While Indian trial sites may appear significant according to some indicators, they seem to be less important if pivotal trials are considered.

One estimate, based on a sample of 650 completed industry-sponsored trials listed on clinicaltrials.gov on January 2011, and for which a publication could be identified, 53 (8.1 per cent) included a site in India (Hoekman et al. 2012: 4), making India 28th in a list of countries involved in such trials. For the EMA over 80 per cent of patients who participated in pivotal trials submitted to them in 2005–10 were recruited in North America, Europe, or Australasia, and only 1.6 per cent in India (EMA 2012: 7). Of a sample of 15 PhRMA companies surveyed in 2010, eight had allocated pivotal registration trials to India over the preceding 10 years, but in only three cases was this for more than 5 per cent of their trials (Scott et al. 2011: 610).

The research and development offshore outsourcing amongst larger companies (so-called Big Pharma, who account for between 60 and 80 per cent of global pharmaceutical R&D) remains predominantly within low value, low risk parts of the R&D value chain (Haakonsson, Jensen, and Mudambi 2013: 686–7). In 2013, for example, Roche—one of the largest of the Big Pharma companies, with nearly 340,000 participants in CTs across the globe—recruited only 0.3 per cent of the total from low-income countries, and 1.2 per cent from middle-income countries.[6] An analysis of data from clinicaltrials.gov suggests that in the period 2008–12 there was little change in the percentage of Phase III trial sites outwith Western Europe and North America. Over that period, however, the share of India declined, while that of China increased (Glass, Glass, and DiFrancesco 2015). This shift was recognized by some of our interviewees:

> India has participated in global research longer than China has. But we're also seeing a significant amount of turnover in our staff in India, but also wage inflation in the country, which leads to workforce migration, instability, which is a challenge for any company operating there, not just ours. And there are also concerns about the quality of the data at times that comes out of India, so we have to do a lot of additional work to make sure the quality is there, and that human subjects are protected. Literacy is kind of low for some areas. We have to make sure that people aren't coerced.
>
> (Author interview with a senior executive with a Contract Research Organization 2008)

While India was 15th in a listing in terms of the total number of trials in the period 2005–12, and 11th in terms of trials as at 2012, its trial density, at 0.97 per million population, was well below that for high-income countries, where rates of 20 or more are common (Drain et al. 2014: S5). Achieving even this limited success, however, has required the creation of a wide range of organizational forms, and transformations in others. In the next section, we consider the most important of the new actors, the CROs.

ROLES PLAYED BY CONTRACT RESEARCH ORGANIZATIONS IN CLINICAL TRIALS

The Contract Research Organizations commonly perform one or more of the sponsor's trial-related duties and functions on their behalf. The functions include, for example, regulatory submission, clinical operations, data management, biostatistics, medical writing, quality assurance, IT, human resources, training and development. Since January 2010, clinical researchers have started a journal, *Perspectives in Clinical Research*[7] with financial support originally from Pfizer.[8] Commonly repeated estimates of the number of CROs in India are around 120, and they are probably involved in most trials reported in India. We analysed data on 101 CROs, using their websites as the source. There were 72 Indian companies (in some cases subsidiaries of Indian generics producers such as Zydus-Cadila or Ranbaxy), while 29 were branches of international CROs such as Quintiles or Pharmaceutical Product Development (PPD). Some foreign multinational pharmaceutical companies established branches in India to run their own trials: GlaxoSmithKline (hereafter GSK), Roche, Pfizer, and Sanofi-Aventis manage some or all functions for their CTs in-house, from Mumbai offices. Foreign-based CROs account for the majority of trials, whether conducted by Indian or foreign sponsors. The Contract Research Organizations have a variety of relationships with trial sponsors (Sariola et al. 2015). Some independent Indian companies provide capital to drug discovery enterprises. Contract Research Organizations usually manage trial design, trial management, data analysis, medical writing, and assist with navigating regulatory requirements. Local Principal Investigators (PIs) are responsible for patient recruitment, and host teams of clinical research assistants who manage the day-to-day relationships with patients, CROs, and sponsors.

The number of full-time workers in the CRO sector has been estimated to have grown from 4,000 in 2008 to 20,000 in 2010, with site-workers expanding from 6,000 to 30,000. Such individuals occupy a plethora of specialist roles which are needed to accomplish internationally credible trials: Clinical Research Associates, Clinical Research Investigators, Clinical Project Managers, Study Coordinators, Clinical Research Managers as well as various managers, auditors, statisticians, and safety

officers. One estimate claimed that about 150 CROs registered with
the US Food and Drug Administration (US FDA) operate in India
(Srinivasan 2009).

Indian CROs and their advisers have a vested interest in exaggerating
the scale and opportunities of the income and other benefits to be gained
from hosting CTs. Indian CROs and PIs have worked hard to attract
business within this growing market since 2005, helped by international
accountancy firms such as KPMG. Optimistic estimates of the current
and future size of the 'industry' have been used to leverage assistance
from the Government of India, which views CTs as an economic
and developmental opportunity. Industry analysts estimate that the
burgeoning Indian clinical trial service industry was worth USD 450
million (£282 million) in 2010–11 and would pass the USD 1 billion
(£594 million) mark by 2016. The Indian CTs lobby has claimed that
their businesses strengthen indigenous medical research capacity, as well
as being a source of foreign exchange and increasing employment. While
the predicted financial benefits have been heavily overestimated (and
not just because of the crisis in trial registration that developed in 2013,
discussed in the following sections), other aspects of the benefits of CTs
to India have also been exaggerated. In the next section, 'Knowledge
Production', we look in particular at the role of knowledge production,
and the possibilities for indigenous innovation in the field.

KNOWLEDGE PRODUCTION

> The academics have started to shape themselves based on clinical trials,
> which is really pre-cooked research. It is not research, it is operations,
> and I think it is a dreadful thing that has happened to India. India is
> becoming a service centre economy for the middle class, extending to
> academics and research.
>
> (Author interview with retired dean of medicine in a prestigious
> medical faculty in India, 2009)

Commercial CTs in India produce particular forms of 'research culture'
which may not neatly fit familiar conceptual frameworks (Simpson and
Sariola 2012). Within these settings, the requirements of protecting their
intellectual property from the scrutiny of competitors means that those
on the periphery—including the PIs at Indian field-sites—have little
access to the fundamental knowledge behind decision-making about
research protocols and are unable to challenge key decisions. Scientific
leadership roles within these trials—trial design and authorship of

results, in particular—remain very firmly within the countries where the trials are initiated, that is, overwhelmingly in North America, Europe, and Japan. '[A]lthough clinical trial activities are now executed across the globe, scientific leadership in these trials is disproportionally concentrated in traditional research locations. This geographical decoupling of patient enrolment and clinical trial management is most pronounced in industry funded research' (Hoekman et al. 2012: 4).

As peripheral participants in a global science network, Indian PIs and managers of CROs in India carry out the less crucial tasks—following the rules laid down elsewhere, being concerned mostly with learning discipline in carrying out tasks that are complex, but which have been defined elsewhere. With respect to India, in the 53 trials in the Hoekman et al database, only 16 (30 per cent) of the linked publications listed someone based in India as a co-author, compared to 98 per cent in the case of the USA-based authors, 68 per cent for Germany, 65 per cent for the UK, and 60 per cent for Canada (Hoekman et al. 2012: 6). Indeed, one analysis of the impact of this opening up of India to CTs concludes that it has had little impact on indigenous R&D:

> … a large number of R&D investment projects are focused on developing facilities for phase III clinical trials and other such modules that only integrate Indian talent and facilities into foreign pharmaceutical firms' global objectives (Abrol, Prajapati, and Singh, 2011: 342) … liberalisation of foreign investment has opened the door for outsourcing of clinical trials to India [rather] than to new investment on R&D from basic stages for the development of new drugs.
>
> (Joseph 2011: 43–4, citation and emphasis as in the original quote)

The US Food and Drug Administration and the EMA determine key elements in global approvals and resultant access to the markets where most profits are made. Therefore, key decisions are made outside India, in light of the superior knowledge held by sponsors about how to convince the USFDA and the EMA that they have robust evidence that their new product is safe and effective. Benefits and value flow to the active, managerial participants rather than to those whose involvement is more passive. Collaborations between sponsors, CROs, and PIs rarely translate into equalizing or equal benefits but rather serve to reproduce inequality in knowledge production. Nonetheless, involvement in CTs is attractive for some doctors who have the time and energy to spare. Outside government hospitals, PIs may be paid per participant recruited, but for others we interviewed, the possibility of acquiring more up-to-date equipment and improvements to laboratory facilities may play a larger role.

In this context of feverish competition to join a global scientific research community, allied to undershooting their claims so far, it is not surprising that most of the reported trials are managed by CROs, most of which are either foreign-owned or have a close relationship with a foreign-based CRO, and that the research model used closely follows international standards. According to data supplied to the CTR-I, RCTs constitute 431 out of 644 trials in 2011, and 475 out of 787 trials in 2012 (see Table 8.5). Use of a placebo in study design is remarkably common, with 134 trials in 2011 and 149 trials in 2012, and also multiple arm trials might employ both active control and placebo controls (Ravindran 2013: 73).

In order to achieve their goals, sponsors have to engage in research capacity building and to deliver transferable methodological skills, enhanced employment opportunities, foreign exchange earnings, and profits. Innovation, creativity, and shifts in global economic and political

TABLE 8.5 Trials Registered with the Clinical Trials Register of India, by Study Type, 2011 and 2012

Study type	Number of trials	
	2011	2012
Non-randomised, placebo-controlled trial	2	2
Single arm trial	90	152
Non-randomised, active-controlled trial	10	11
Non-randomised, multiple arm trial	14	10
Randomised parallel group trial	79	125
Randomised, parallel group, placebo-controlled trial	134	147
Randomised, parallel group, active-controlled trial	151	124
Randomised, parallel group, multiple arm trial	41	45
Randomised, crossover trial	23	29
Cluster randomised trial	5	8
Randomised factorial trial	3	5
Other	92	129
Total	644	787

Source: Ravindran (2013: 73).

power in favour of Indian participants over the next 10 years cannot, therefore, be ruled out. Activist groups within India, along with the championship of relevant Parliamentary Committee, have highlighted ethical problems in research and have been an important driver towards changes in how research is conducted. The international perception that India's CTs are not run on an ethical basis has led to a dramatic loss of confidence in the industry. In the next section, 'Ethical Concerns', we look at the ethical issues, and finally the impact this has had in generating reform processes.

ETHICAL CONCERNS

Given the bad press that the Indian CTs industry has received on ethical issues, it is important to state that most trials in India are probably run in accordance with national and international ethical standards. Given also that if ethical concerns are raised about a trial, its chances of acceptance by regulatory authorities are reduced, most CROs and sponsors have a strong incentive to follow the rules in spirit as well as letter. Nevertheless many 'outlier' cases have been reported in the Indian media. Controversies have exposed improper informed consent procedures, dysfunctional ethics committees, and failures to pay compensation for clinical trial-related injuries or death.[9]

To illustrate, survivors of the 1984 Bhopal gas explosion being treated at the Bhopal Memorial Hospital and Research Centre were enrolled in CTs without their knowledge or consent. Adverse events were not properly reported, deaths were not investigated and compensation was not paid to the families of patients who died during the trials (Lakhani 2011). Concerns over informed consent were also highlighted in a mass vaccination demonstration project (or a Phase IV trial—accounts differ) against Human Papilloma Virus. Tribal girls in Andhra Pradesh and Gujarat, many living in hostels, were enrolled when their wardens gave mass consent (PATH 2013; Sarojini et al. 2010; Talwar 2013). Seven girls who participated in the trial died. Their deaths were not promptly investigated by an independent body. Even though a later Parliamentary committee concluded that the deaths were unrelated to the vaccine, the image of CTs remained badly affected (Terwindt 2014).

These examples highlight several weaknesses in the regulatory framework. The Drugs Controller General of India was understaffed even in 2005, and has remained unable to cope with the surge in clinical trial activity that it is supposed to regulate (Nundy and Gulhati 2005).

Furthermore, after the DCGI grants approval to commence a clinical trial, it plays little further role in monitoring trial activity. With respect to ethical review in India, it is claimed that members of RECs do not apply the relevant rules consistently; that their members are inadequately trained, have too little time to understand the implications of complex trials and often include people with conflicts of interest; that they do not inspect clinical trial sites to check that the promised procedures are being followed; and that they do not (or cannot) take decisive action when violations have been alleged (Desai 2012). Grassroots activism, working through Parliament as well as the Supreme Court, has been an important driver for reform.

In February 2012, a Public Interest Litigation (PIL) petition was filed by the NGO Swasthya Adhikar Manch (SAM), which sought to halt the conduct of CTs in India for new products. Swasthya Adhikar Manch alleged that weak regulatory controls on the conduct of CTs, combined with their poor enforcement, have contributed to an unacceptable number of deaths and adverse events. It also sought to halt trials for drugs and devices that will not be sold or marketed in India, and will thus not advance Indian healthcare. Swasthya Adhikar Manch submitted documents claiming that over 2,262 clinical trial participants in India had died in 2006–11. In an internationally unprecedented interim ruling of 30 September 2013, the Supreme Court of India halted the approval by DGCI of new CTs, pending a more effective review and monitoring system.

The Supreme Court ruling prompted a raft of reform measures aimed at strengthening protections for Indian clinical trial participants. These include: (*i*) a more rigorous 'three tier' committee system for screening clinical trial protocols at the DCGI; (*ii*) three new criteria for evaluating CTs, namely, (*a*) assessment of risk versus benefit to the patients, (*b*) innovation vis-à-vis existing therapeutic options, and (*c*) unmet medical need in the country; (*iii*) audio-visual recordings of the informed consent process; and (*iv*) the mandatory registration of Indian RECs.

The most controversial of the recent reforms, however, have been those relating to compensation for clinical trial-related injuries or death. Some measures, which aim to strengthen procedural oversight so that incidents are investigated properly and compensation paid if appropriate, are in line with international approaches. Yet, some of the new criteria for compensation depart radically from the regimes in other countries. For example, one provision states that 'In the case of an injury occurring to the clinical trial subject, he or she shall be given free medical management as long as required' (Ghooi 2013). This would seem to apply regardless

TABLE 8.6 Approvals of Trials by DCGI by Year and Type, January 2013–December 2017

Type of trial	2013	2014	2015	2016	2017	Total	Percentage
Global Clinical Trial	17	87	54	37	97	292	46.7 per cent
New Drug	17	28	25	28	43	141	22.6 per cent
Subsequent New Drug	6	4	21	10	15	56	9.0 per cent
Fixed dose combination	9	11	12	9	17	58	9.3 per cent
Biological (recombinant)	17	1	0	0	0	18	2.9 per cent
Biological (vaccine)	22	0	0	0	0	22	3.5 per cent
Institutional	18	10	9	0	0	37	5.9 per cent
Medical device	1	0	0	0	0	1	– per cent
Total	*107*	*141*	*121*	*84*	*172*	*625*	*100.00 per cent*

Source: http://www.cdsco.nic.in/forms/SearchMore.aspx?Id=11. Accessed on 19 January 2018.

of whether the trial itself had caused a medical problem. Another rule states simply that subjects shall be eligible for compensation for 'use of placebo in a placebo-controlled trial'. Entitlement to compensation was also established for failure of an investigational product to provide the intended therapeutic effect.

These changes caused serious concerns about legal risks and led to an exodus of CTs from India. The numbers of CTs approved by CDSCO fell from 500 in 2010 to just 107 in 2013 (see Table 8.6). It is reported that sponsors and CROs shifted their activities to 'rival' countries with more favourable regulatory systems. Alarmed by the impact on its clinical trial industry, the Indian government is currently watering down some of the reform measures for compensation. Furthermore, in January 2015, and in line with the Modi government's pro-business strategy, the Ministry of Health proposed 'pre-submission meetings' between drug regulators and stakeholders so as to increase efficiency and speed up approval times (Nair 2015). It remains to be seen whether the efforts to entice business back to India can be made compatible with the enhanced protections for Indian trial participants that is, rightly, demanded by advocacy groups in civil society.

* * *

The scandals that have highlighted problems in the management of CTs have been widely publicized, and may have encouraged the managers of global trials to look elsewhere—particularly China—for a setting that is less likely to generate controversy. But the CTs industry in India has always massively exaggerated the potential for growth, whether in terms of total numbers of trials, of foreign exchange earnings, or of benefits to India's public health. Clinical trials are still taking place in large numbers—not of new drugs, but of generics that need to be assessed for bio-equivalence or bio-availability. Now that these are also coming under threat, the industry has a considerable job to do in reassuring external and internal regulators that their results can be trusted. For example, in September 2015, the Gujarat FDA called in some German and French media for 'assuaging the fear and confusion emanating from the European nations over the quality of the drugs that are manufactured in the country after the GVK fiasco' (Anon. 2015).

Although the Indian generics industry, and CROs seemed well prepared for joining the WTO in 2005, they underestimated the cultural and regulatory shifts needed if Indian firms were to establish their position in the complex global assemblage that is the contemporary CTs industry. On the positive side, a necessary debate has begun about how this assemblage can be reshaped to maximise its benefits to India as a whole, and not just the pharmaceutical industry, whether CROs, 'Big Pharma' or generics producers. In many respects, India is leading the way, by taking seriously issues of whether so-called 'new' drugs really offer advantages over existing ones, and trying to ensure that public health issues take precedence over profits. But this struggle has only started: we cannot be sanguine about the outcome.

NOTES

1. For more details about this project, see http://www.bhesa.org/. Accessed on 14 November 2017.

2. Central Drugs Standard Control Organization's Good Clinical Practice guidelines were based on a synthesis of the ICMR guidelines and international Good Clinical Practice documents (Central Drugs Standard Control Organization 2001).

3. See generally, Nuffield Council on Bioethics (2002).

4. For example, in May 2015 'The European Medicines Agency (EMA) has confirmed its recommendation to suspend a number of medicines for which

authorisation in the European Union (EU) was primarily based on clinical studies conducted at GVK Biosciences in Hyderabad, India'. Available at: http://www.ema.europa.eu/ema/index.jsp?curl=pages/medicines/human/referrals/GVK_Biosciences/human_referral_000382.jsp&mid=WC0b01ac05805c516f. Accessed on: 15 August 2016.

5. At the same time, the CTR-I listed 77 breast cancer studies.

6. http://www.roche.com/research_and_development/who_we_are_how_we_work/clinical_trials.htm. Accessed on 5 January 2015.

7. Available at: http://www.picronline.org/.

8. This is mentioned neither in the print issue nor on the website.

9. For more details on the issues covered by this section, see Porter (2017).

REFERENCES

Abrol, Dinesh, Pramod Prajapati, and Nidhi Singh. 2011. 'Globalization of the Indian Pharmaceutical Industry: Implications for Innovation', *International Journal of Institutions and Economics* 3(2): 327–65.

Ana, Joseph, Tracey Koehlmoos, Richard Smith, and Lijing L. Yan. 2013. 'Research Misconduct in Low- and Middle-Income Countries', *PLoS medicine* 10(3): e1001315.

Anon. 2015. 'Gujarat FDCA Clarifies Misconceptions over Quality Issues at a Meet with Western Media', *Pharmabiz*. 12 September. Mumbai.

Cassese, Sabino. 2004. 'The Globalization of Law', *New York University Journal of International Law and Politics* 37(4): 973–93.

Central Drugs Standard Control Organization. 2001. *Good Clinical Practices: Guidelines for Clinical Trials on Pharmaceutical Products in India*. New Delhi: Directorate-General of Health Services, Ministry of Health and Family Welfare, Government of India.

Chawan, Vihang S., Kalpesh V. Gawand, and Abhishek M. Phatak. 2015. 'Impact of New Regulations on Clinical Trials in India', *International Journal of Clinical Trials* 2(3): 56–8.

Collier, Stephen J. and Aihwa Ong. 2005. 'Global Assemblages, Anthropological Problems'. In *Global Assemblages: Technology, Politics, and Ethics as Anthropological Problems*, Stephen J Collier and Aihwa Ong (eds), pp. 3–21. London & New York: Blackwell.

Deleuze, Gilles and Felix Guattari. 1980. *Capitalisme et schizophrénie Vol. 2: Mille plateaux*. Paris: Éditions de Minuit.

———. 1988. *A Thousand Plateaus: Capitalism and Schizophrenia*. London: Athlone Press.

Desai, Mira. 2012. 'Ethics Committees: Critical Issues and Challenges', *Indian Journal of Pharmacology* 44(6): 663–4.

Drain, Paul K., Marion Robine, King K. Holmes, and Ingrid V. Bassett. 2014. 'Trial Watch: Global Migration of Clinical Trials', *Nature Reviews Drug Discovery* 13(3): 166–7.

Ecks, Stefan. 2005. 'Pharmaceutical Citizenship: Antidepressant Marketing and the Promise of Demarginalization in India', *Anthropology and Medicine* 12(3): 239–54.

Editorial. 2014. 'Regulating Stem Cell Therapy'. *The Hindu*, Chennai, 12 March.

EMA. 2012. 'Reflection Paper on Ethical and GCP Aspects of Clinical Trials of Medicinal Products for Human Use Conducted Outside of the EU/EEA and Submitted in Marketing Authorization Applications to The EU Regulatory Authorities'. London: European Medicines Authority.

Ghooi, Ravindra B. 2013. 'Injury and Death in Clinical Trials and Compensation: Rule 122 DAB,' *Perspectives in Clinical Research* 4(4): 199–203.

Glass, Harold E., Lucas M. Glass, and Jeffrey J. DiFrancesco. 2015. 'ClinicalTrials.gov: An Underutilized Source of Research Data About the Design and Conduct of Commercial Clinical Trials', *Therapeutic Innovation & Regulatory Science* 49(2): 218–24.

Glickman, Seth W., John G. McHutchison, Eric D. Peterson, Charles B. Cairns, Robert A. Harrington, Robert M. Califf, and Kevin A. Schulman. 2009. 'Ethical and Scientific Implications of the Globalization of Clinical Research', *New England Journal of Medicine* 360(8): 816–23.

Gupta, Y.K. and B.M. Padchy. 2011. 'India's Growing Participation in Global Clinical Trials', *Trends in Pharmacological Sciences* 32(6): 327–9.

Haakonsson, Stine Jessen, Peter D. Orberg Jensen, and Susan M. Mudambi. 2013. 'A Co-Evolutionary Perspective on the Drivers of International Sourcing of Pharmaceutical R&D to India', *Journal of Economic Geography* 13(4): 677–700.

Held, David, and Mathias Koenig-Archibugi (eds). 2003. *Taming Globalization: Frontiers of Governance*. London: Polity Press.

Hoekman, Jarno, Koen Frenken, Dick de Zeeuw, and Hiddo Lambers Heerspink. 2012. 'The Geographical Distribution of Leadership in Globalized Clinical Trials'. *PloS one* 7(10): e45984.

IMS Institute for Healthcare Informatics. 2011. 'The Global Use of Medicines: Outlook through 2015'. New Jersey NJ: IMS Health Incorporated.

Indian Council of Medical Research. 2006. *Ethical Guidelines for Biomedical Research on Human Participants*. New Delhi: ICMR.

Jesus, J.E. and E.S. Higgs. 2002. 'International Research Ethics: Progress, but not Perfection', *Trends in Molecular Medicine* 8(2): 93–5.

Joseph, Reji K. 2011. 'The R&D Scenario in Indian Pharmaceutical Industry', *RIS Discussion Papers*. New Delhi: Research and Information System for Developing Countries.

Lakhani, N. 2011. 'From Tragedy to Travesty: Drugs Tested on Survivors of Bhopal'. *The Independent*, London. 15 November.

MacMahon, Stephen, Vlado Perkovic, and Anushka Patel. 2013. 'Industry-Sponsored Clinical Trials in Emerging Markets: Time to Review the Terms of Engagement', JAMA 310(9): 907–8.

Metzger-Filho, Otto, Evandro De Azambuja, Ian Bradbury, Kamal S. Saini, José Bines, Sergio D. Simon, Veerle Van Dooren, Gursel Aktan, Kathleen I. Pritchard, and Antonio C. Wolff. 2013. 'Analysis of Regional Timelines to Set Up a Global Phase III Clinical Trial in Breast Cancer: The Adjuvant Lapatinib and/or Trastuzumab Treatment Optimization Experience', *The Oncologist* 18(2): 134–40.

Nair, A. 2015. 'Clinical research: Regulatory uncertainty hits drug trials in India', *The Pharmaceutical Journal* 294(7853). DOI: 10.1211/PJ.2015.20068063.

Nguyen, Vinh-kim. 2005. 'Antiretroviral Globalism, Biopolitics, and Therapeutic Citizenship'. In *Global Assemblages: Technology, Politics, and Ethics as Anthropological Problems*, Aihwa Ong and Stephen J. Collier (eds), pp. 125–44. London: Blackwell.

Nuffield Council on Bioethics. 2002. 'The Ethics of Research Related to Healthcare in Developing Countries'. London: Nuffield Council on Bioethics.

Nundy, Samiran, and Chandra M. Gulhati. 2005. 'A New Colonialism? Conducting Clinical Trials in India', *New England Journal of Medicine* 352(16): 1633–6.

Pandey, Arvind, Abha Aggarwal, Mohua Maulik, Jyotsna Gupta, and Atul Juneja. 2013. 'Challenges in Administering a Clinical Trials Registry: Lessons from the Clinical Trials Registry-India'. *Pharmaceutical Medicine* 27(2): 83–93.

Pandey, Arvind, Abha Rani Aggarwal, Mohua Maulik, and S.D. Seth. 2009. 'Clinical Trial Registration Gains Momentum in India [Letter to Editor]'. *Indian Journal of Medical Research* 130(1): 85–6.

Pandey, Arvind, Abha Rani Aggarwal, S.D. Seth, Mohua Maulik, R. Bano, and Atul Juneja. 2008, 'Clinical Trials Registry-India: Redefining the Conduct of Clinical Trials', *Indian Journal of Cancer* 45(3): 79–82.

Parliament of India (Rajya Sabha). 2012. *Department-related Parliamentary Standing Committee on Health and Family Welfare. 59th Report on the Functioning of the Central Drugs Standard Control Organisation (CDSCO).* New Delhi: Rajya Sabha Secretariat.

———. 2013a. *Department Related Parliamentary Standing Committee on Health and Family Welfare. Seventy-Second Report on Alleged Irregularity in the Conduct of Studies Using Human Papilloma Virus (HPV) Vaccine by PATH in India.* New Delhi: Rajya Sabha Secretariat.

———. 2013b. *Department Related Parliamentary Standing Committee on Health and Family Welfare. Sixty Sixth Report on Action Taken by the Government on the Recommendations/ Observations Contained in the 59th Report of the Functioning of Central Drugs Standards Control Organisation (CDSCO).* New Delhi: Rajya Sabha Secretariat.

PATH. 2013. 'Statement from PATH: Cervical Cancer Demonstration Project in India'. Seattle, WA: PATH.

Petryna, Adriana. 2005. 'Ethical Variability: Drug Development and Globalizing Clinical Trials', *American Ethnologist* 32(2): 183–97.

Porter, Gerard. 2017. 'Regulating Clinical Trials in India: The Economics of Ethics', *Developing World Bioethics*. DOI: 10.1111/dewb.12156, electronic version prior to print version, 9 July 2017.

Ravindran, Deapica. 2013. 'Clinical Trials Watch', *Indian Journal of Medical Ethics* 10(1): 73.

Ravindran, Deapica and Sachin Nikarge. 2010. 'Clinical trials watch', *Indian Journal of Medical Ethics* 7(4): 259–62.

Rose, Nikolas and Carlos Novas. 2005. 'Biological Citizenship'. In *Global Assemblages. Technology, Politics, and Ethics as Anthropological Problems*, Aihwa Ong and Stephen J. Collier (eds), pp. 439–81. London: Blackwell.

Saini, Kamal S., Gaurav Agarwal, Ramesh Jagannathan, Otto Metzger-Filho, Monika L. Saini, Khurshid Mistry, Raghib Ali, and Sudeep Gupta. 2013. 'Challenges in Launching Multinational Oncology Clinical Trials in India', *South Asian Journal of Cancer* 2(1): 44–9.

Sama: Resource Group for Women and Health (ed.). 2012. *National Consultation on Regulation of Drug Trials*. New Delhi: SAMA.

Sariola, Salla, Deapica Ravindran, Anand Kumar, and Roger Jeffery. 2015. 'Big-Pharmaceuticalisation: Clinical Trials and Contract Research Organisations in India', *Social Science and Medicine* 131: 239–46.

Sarojini, N.B., Sandhya Srinivasan, Y. Madhavi, S. Srinivasan, and Anjali Shenoi. 2010. 'The HPV Vaccine: Science, Ethics and Regulation', *Economic and Political Weekly* 45(48): 27–34.

Sassen, Saskia. 2008, 'Neither Global nor National: Novel Assemblages of Territory, Authority and Rights'. *Ethics and Global Politics* 1(1–2): 1–8.

Scott, Nick, Bruce Binkowitz, Ekopimo Okon Ibia, Tonya Houck, Belinda Field, Steven D. Talerico, Yoko Tanaka, and Andy Lee. 2011. 'Results of a Survey of PhRMA Member Companies on Practices Associated with Multiregional Clinical Trials', *Drug Information Journal* 45(5): 609–17.

Sengupta, Amit. 2013. 'Two Decades of Struggle', *Economic and Political Weekly* 48(32): 43–5.

Simpson, Bob and Salla Sariola. 2012. 'Blinding Authority Randomized Clinical Trials and the Production of Global Scientific Knowledge in Contemporary Sri Lanka', *Science, Technology & Human Values* 37(5): 555–75.

Simpson, Robert, Rekha Khatri, Tharindi Udalagama, and Deapica Ravindran. 2015. 'Pharmaceuticalisation and Ethical Review in South Asia: Issues of Scope and Authority for Practitioners and Policy Makers', *Social Science & Medicine* 131: 247–54.

Slaughter, Anne-Marie. 2004. *A New World Order*. Princeton: Princeton University Press.

Sleeboom-Faulkner, Margaret, and Prasanna Kumar Patra. 2011. 'Experimental Stem Cell Therapy: Biohierarchies and Bionetworking in Japan and India', *Social Studies of Science* 41(5): 645–66.

Srinivasan, Sandhya. 2009. 'The Clinical Trials Scenario in India', *Economic and Political Weekly* 44(35): 29–33.

Talwar, Pankaj. 2013. Editorial. *Indian MIMS*, September.

Terwindt, Carolijn. 2014. 'Health Rights Litigation Pushes for Accountability in Clinical Trials in India', *Health and Human Rights* 16(2): 84–95.

Theirs, F.A., A.J. Sinskey, and E.R. Berndt. 2008. 'Trends in the Globalization of Clinical Research', *Nature Rev Drug Discovery* 7: 13–14.

Timmermans, Stefan and Marc Berg. 1997. 'Standardization in Action: Achieving Local Universality through Medical Protocols', *Social Studies of Science* 27(2): 273–305.

Van Huijstee, Mariëtte, and Irene Schipper (eds). 2011. *Putting Contract Research Organisations on the Radar*. Amsterdam: Stichting Onderzoek Multinationale Ondernemingen, Salud y Fármacos & Centre for Studies in Ethics and Rights.

Yee, Amy. 2012. 'Regulation Failing to Keep Up with India's Trials Boom', *The Lancet* 379(9814): 397–8.

9

Body as 'Resource' in Surrogacy and Bio-Medical Research

New Frontiers and Dilemmas

Sarojini Nadimpally and Vrinda Marwah

Advances in the life sciences have created new markets for body parts and bodily labour today. The economic climate of the post-liberalization era in India has given new direction and intensity to the ways in which poor people's bodies become a resource. In the current context of deepening inequalities, worsening access to essential services, and the marginalization of the poor, technology and commerce have combined to create new markets in biomedicine; this has resulted in an unprecedented traffic in body parts, and their renting and selling.

Scholars of science have called our attention to the co-production of the social and the scientific (Martin 1998); in particular, they have understood the life sciences as representing a new face and phase of capitalism (Rajan 2006). Even the criteria we have traditionally employed to understand categories like labour, body, kinship, and property are in flux today. In such a situation, the phenomenal growth of industries of assisted reproduction and clinical trials (CTs) in India raises many pressing questions.

This chapter is based on two different studies conducted by Sama-Resource Group for Women and Health,[1] which tries to explore and understand the commonalities in the experiences of commercial surrogates and bioavailability and bioequivalence (henceforth BA/BE)[2] trial participants. While acknowledging fundamental differences between commercial surrogacy, egg donation, clinical trials, and BA/BE clinical trials, this chapter is a preliminary attempt to draw out ethical, regulatory, and political–structural concerns, and to explore ways that these may be addressed.

BRIEF DESCRIPTION OF STUDIES

Commercial Surrogacy

India has become a global hub for assisted reproductive technologies (ARTs)—a group of procedures designed to circumvent infertility by assisting in conception, or the carrying of pregnancy to term. Surrogacy, enabled through the use of ARTs, is an arrangement in which a woman agrees to carry another individual's or couple's baby to term, usually in exchange for money. In commercial surrogacy, the more invasive in vitro fertilization (IVF) is preferred over intrauterine insemination (IUI). In IVF many embryos are fertilized, of which the healthiest ones—with the greatest chances of success—are implanted into the woman. It is common to find multiple—three to four—embryos being implanted, which often results in twins and triplets being born.

While official statistics on the number of surrogacies being arranged in India are not available, anecdotal evidence and media reports suggest that ARTs are a multimillion dollar industry (Smerdon 2008: 24). The following factors create a conducive environment for the ART industry in India: lack of regulation; comparatively lower costs; shorter waiting time; close monitoring of surrogates; quality medical services; and large numbers of women willing to be surrogates. More recently, the government appears to be moving to close down surrogacy services for foreigners and non-resident Indians (NRIs), but this has not been finalized into law yet and regardless, the domestic markets continue to function and flourish as before.

Several complex, contemporary contestations are contained within the issues of surrogacy and ARTs. During 2011–12, Sama conducted a multisited qualitative study in Delhi and Punjab, with the aim of understanding the experiences of surrogates, as well as uncovering the processes followed in surrogacy arrangements. The research report *Birthing a Market: A Study on Commercial Surrogacy* (2012) analyses data from interviews with 12 surrogates, two agents, five doctors, and one commissioning parent. Most women interviewed and their spouses were employed in low-paying, insecure, informal sector jobs. Women were mostly engaged in informal garment work, factory work, and domestic work or were not employed outside their household. Their spouses were engaged in work such as driving, cooking, and garment factory work. The motivation for doing surrogacy was mainly monetary.

The research revealed that the current operation of the surrogacy industry is unfavourable to surrogates, who occupy the lowest rung of the industry. The potential surrogate must be married, with biological children ('proven fertility'), and must have her husband's consent, to be a surrogate. For surrogacy, the more invasive IVF-ET (Embryo Transfer) is preferred over IUI, in the interest of severing all genetic links between the surrogate and the child (imagined as the possible source of a claim by the surrogate over the child in future). Surrogates have little to no information about multiple ET cycles, multiple embryo implantation (and possible foetal reduction), or the likelihood and implications of a Caesarean section delivery.

The surrogate relies entirely on the agent or the doctor for information regarding the surrogacy arrangement, including the payment process, drugs, procedures, and others. Her ability to negotiate is severely constrained. She signs a contract that is drawn up by the intended parents in English, and is usually not explained to her well enough. She is not provided with any legal counsel, or any counselling for her emotional and psychological needs. The amount and pattern of payment varies. The surrogacy agent's commission may come out of the surrogate's fees, and this is not always clarified in advance. The health risks to mother and child from the drugs and procedures in ARTs are both under-researched, and in the case of surrogacy, under-communicated. Post-delivery, the surrogate must relinquish the child but has no control over the terms of relinquishment; for instance, she usually cannot breastfeed the child. Surrogacy arrangements currently regulate the lifestyle of the surrogate—her sexual and physical activity, mobility, diet, and so on, but not other important areas like the maximum number of surrogacies and the interval between surrogacies.

Bioavailability/Bioequivalence Trials

India's pharmaceutical industry is globally renowned for its traditional strengths in manufacturing, including contract manufacturing of drugs. India's domestic drugs market is the fourteenth largest globally, and is seen by the global pharmaceutical market as having huge potential for further growth (Reuters 2013). This recognition of India's pharmaceutical industry is in the context of substantive global shifts currently. As a preferred manufacturing location with a wide range of outsourcing arrangements, partnership initiatives, and other contractual arrangements that enable the creation of vast networks, India is expected to be an important player.

The rising cost of medicines and overall cost of health care received considerable attention and during the last few years, there is a significant increase in new drug discoveries as well as generic drug production to reduce those costs. Generic equivalents of branded drugs have captured more than 65 per cent of the global market (Shah 2013). Because of the importance of generic drugs in health care, it became imperative that the pharmaceutical quality and in vivo performance of generic drugs be reliably assessed.

A large number of BA/BE trials are specific to those countries that are exporting generic drugs to other countries and are carried out to satisfy regulatory requirements. The offer of compensation is a good inducement to enrol to participate in BA/BE studies. In India, currently BA/BE studies are being carried out by pharmaceutical and contract research organizations (CROs) for generic submission.

Sama conducted a multisited qualitative exploratory study during 2012–13 with the objective of understanding the motivations and perceptions of BA/BE trial participants in Gujarat and Andhra Pradesh. The study examined the perspectives of 15 participants about recruitment, reasons for participation, informed consent, adverse events, and payments. Most participants came from the marginalized sections of the society such as Dalit, Muslim, and economically backward communities, and were usually employed in low-paying and informal jobs such as construction workers, agricultural labourers, working in lime quarries and factories, domestic workers, and auto rickshaw drivers.

The study reported two pathways of recruitment. One, through local area recruitment agents in contact with the local families. Interestingly, these agents were also engaged in recruiting egg donors and surrogates, particularly in Gujarat. Two, through word of mouth, the families who were recruited informed other family members and friends about these trials. The major motivation for participation was monetary gain that served to supplement participants' incomes. There were many issues regarding informed consent, the most important of which was that the complex biotechnical language did not translate to clearly set out information leading to an ambiguous understanding of the process, and other details. The study's probes on adverse events threw up a number of findings. While participants from Andhra Pradesh mentioned that they were sent back home without care for possible side effects once the blood was drawn; in Gujarat, participants had been provided a contact person with the CRO for health issues, deemed to be side effects within a month of initial participation. However, the majority of the participants said that CROs were apathetic towards side effects once the study had been completed, with treatment costs mostly borne by the participants themselves.

THE POLITICAL ECONOMY CONTEXT TODAY

> I am planning to go to Lambda for a study on an arthritis drug the day after tomorrow. It's a 10-day study in two parts and they will pay me Rs. 10,000. Schools are going to re-open in 15 days. I have to get my second son admitted [to school]. So I have to earn some money for his admission, new books, commuting, monthly fees, etc. If livelihood options were made stronger and if today I was to get a good, steady income then why would I need to take risks like these? If everyone had a well-paying job, then people would think twice. —Mahesh
>
> My children are studying in an English medium school, the house rent has increased, expenses have increased, and I am not able to handle this. So when someone told me about this (surrogacy), I thought I can do something to better my children's lives. That's what I thought. I am not doing this for myself. I have this dream, since I couldn't study, I want my children to be educated. Whatever I couldn't get, my children should have, that is why I came here. I just thought one thing that my children should not suffer as I have There's nothing else, sisterji. I was not keen to do surrogacy. I'm scared even now. I have taken a big risk. But you have to bear some pain in life to gain something, how else will you get anything in life. Even this money is not enough, but we will help them at least a little bit in our lifetime. —Manjit
>
> If a house was rich, would any lady do surrogacy? —Hasina
> (Excerpts from interviews conducted with surrogates and clinical trial participants for the research report by Sama [2012])

The phenomenal growth of industries such as ARTs and clinical trials in India has been enabled by the economic climate of the post-liberalization era. We are living in a time when the priorities of the Indian state have shifted away from strengthening the public health system, to promoting the private health sector, and public–private partnerships. The bioavailability and bioequivalence trials and surrogacy create medical indication within market logic, rather than respond to a medical indication in the best interests of collective health.

Drawing from the concept of 'bio capital', Cooper and Waldby (2014) introduce the concept of 'clinical labour'. They contend that post-Fordist economies have moved away from mass manufacture models, and are instead dominated by the service sector, knowledge creation and culture industries, financial markets and information capitalism, and biomedical production. Cooper and Waldby (2014) argue that surrogacy, participation in clinical trials, and gamete donation represent new forms of embodied labour that have proliferated at the lower ends of this post-Fordist biomedical economy. They use the term 'clinical labour' to refer to this extensive yet unacknowledged labour force that the life science industries rely on, and whose service consists in visceral experiences like experimental drug consumption, more or less invasive biomedical procedures, tissue extraction, and gestation.

Clinical labour sustains the biomedical economy, and yet most of its workforce 'intersects with the lowest echelons of informal service labour, recruiting from the same classes marginalised by the transition from Fordist mass manufacture to post-Fordist informatics production' (Cooper and Waldby 2014). So, 'far from representing an exceptional or extreme manifestation of the underground economy, [it] is emblematic of the conditions of twenty-first-century labour' (Cooper and Waldby 2014).

When we consider the class of women from which surrogates are being drawn, the troubling issues in commercial surrogacy stand out as not just of rights for surrogates in the arrangement (though that is also urgent and needs intervention), but of the larger issue of reproductive justice and autonomy. Surrogates have little autonomy over their own pregnancies; they are from a class that has traditionally been targeted for population control, coercive or incentivized tubectomies, has high maternal mortality and morbidity, and little access to the health care that should be their entitlement. A longer term, life cycle view of the reproductive health of these women, and its linkages with interrelated questions of livelihoods, nutrition, education, and others, helps us understand surrogacy not only in individual terms but also in the context of its political economy, particularly state responsibility and communal rights, and the conditions of women's labour under globalization.

There is a relationship between the restructuring of the global economy since the 1980s and the restructuring of reproduction.

As public funding is rolled back, women are finding employment as maids, nannies, cleaners, and others, jobs that recast their traditional capacities for nurturance, maternity, and sexuality as negotiable assets for the consumption of households where these services are no longer performed by educated, professional women (Ehrenreich and Hochschild 2003; Sassen 2002). In India particularly, there has been a move towards flexibilization of labour and informalization of economic activity since the 1990s. As Cooper and Waldby (2014) note, there are continuities between surrogacy and other kinds of feminized work: 'They are recruited through brokerage; the work may be undertaken at home, although many move to a clinic-endorsed hostel for part of their pregnancy; and they service a component of a production chain while nevertheless falling outside the formal labour sector.'

These continuities are also visible in BA/BE trial participation. A Dalit participant from Gujarat, who works as a part-time driver with a monthly income of Rs 4,000–5,000 explained how he came to participate in these trials:

> You probably know that Gujarat is famous for its diamond industry. I was working in Surat. Large number of us used to work in this industry. We were mainly doing cutting, polishing, and shaping of diamonds. We were all wageworkers but we got good wages for the work. We could afford to live with basic facilities and buy our vegetables and other things. Before the crisis, life was very different. About four-five years ago, the diamond industry crashed. Many warehouses were shut down. After the crash we became unemployed. Most of us shifted to other cities for work. Houses were locked down. Owners left and the workers had to move on. It was the worst time. Women were pushed into embroidery work or some other piece meal work. But for men there was no regular work and income. Jignesh

Another instance of the relationship between lack of livelihoods and the decision to participate in BA/BE trials is demonstrated in the quote:

> We are landless labourers. We came and settled here because of the work at the limekilns. Since the work begins at early hours, we stay close by. We don't have the money to rent a place in the town. As you have already seen, we live in this small hut, closer to these big limekilns in the lime dust. We don't have ration cards or Arogyasri cards. We don't exist for the govt. There is no proper infrastructure, like a pucca house, electricity, water, toilet facility, etc. We work in the limekilns half the day and in the remaining time, we are involved in agricultural work/'coolie' work

(as wage labour) and work in the chilli and cotton fields. At the kilns we are paid Rs 100 per day.

(Excerpt from a personal interview conducted by Sama [2012] with Dhanamma)

In addition, intersections with other circuits of vulnerability also came up in Sama's BA/BE study. In Gujarat, some of the trial participants interviewed were from the Muslim community and had been victims of the 2002 communal violence. One of them said,

Juhapura swelled in numbers after 2002. Many families came from violence-affected areas in Ahmedabad, and even outside. The majority here are still struggling for employment. Whatever we had, we lost during the riots. There is not much work, no jobs. Many families in Juhapura are struggling for survival. Men generally drive auto rickshaws, or go for wage labour work. They cannot go and work in big shops in the city. After 2002, there is a lot of fear and insecurity. Many Hindus don't even employ us nowadays. Everything is expensive here. Juhapura is in between Sarkhej and Bejalpur (both Hindu majority areas). Facilities are distributed between these two areas and Juhapura ends up with nothing. Take the example of land itself. After the riots we have all come here, but the area is small and the people are many. So now, you cannot buy land in Juhapura and build a place unless you are very, very rich. In Bejalpur, one square foot of land may be Rs 500 but in Juhapura it would be Rs 5,000.

(Excerpt from an interview conducted for the research report by Sama [2013])

These experiences do not represent a causal story. They are presented here not to argue that 'events' such as communal violence or the collapse of a livelihood become the reason that individuals get pushed into surrogacy or BA/BE participation. Certainly enough cases exist where we cannot make such linear linkages. However, these narratives should remind us of the precariousness of life for a large section of India's population. This precariousness that is part of the fabric of life for a class of people in India is what makes options like surrogacy and BA/BE participation attractive.

ETHICAL DILEMMAS: EXPLICIT AND IMPLICIT QUESTIONS ABOUT BIOETHICS AND REGULATION

The field of bioethics grapples with the ethical dilemmas that arise from advances in medical science and technology. Towards this, it lays out the principles of non-malfeasance, beneficence, autonomy, and justice.

It is clear from interviews with BA/BE trial participants and surrogates that their arrangements with CROs, clinics, and agents leave much to be desired from a bioethics perspective. One of the BA/BE study participants recounted her experience of giving informed consent as follows:

> They gave us a form of around 5–6 pages but they did not give us enough time to read it or ask questions. Moreover, the papers were in English. They asked us to sign it. We were in a big hall with about 40–50 other women but were not allowed to interact much. They gave us a pill to swallow and later took our blood samples. I asked the person who gave me the pill what it was for. She said it was for abortion. I asked if anything would happen to me. They said that nobody had any problem. They get very irritated if anyone asks too many questions ... I was very scared throughout the time I was there.
>
> (Excerpt from an interview with Satyavati, conducted for the research report by Sama [2012])

Similarly, another BA/BE study participant reported the following experience:

> We don't usually know what medicine it is. We only know how much blood is taken and how much money it will fetch. Yes, you have to sign documents. I did. But anyway that is written in English and not Gujarati, and they keep it. They don't give it to us after we sign it. Kamleshben

A surrogate mother from Punjab elaborated on her recruitment process:

> Before the embryo transfer, they took all my signatures stating that I am willing to have their child for them and I will finish my entire responsibility. The documents said that I have no problems in giving away the child. They, I and my husband, signed. Everything was through their lawyer. (Did the doctor offer to provide you with a lawyer if you needed one?) No, nothing like that. Their lawyer read out the document in Hindi since it was in English. There was no mention of money. About money, we had a general conversation, a verbal discussion. Nothing was written. They didn't tell me anything about medicines or injections. Whatever was needed for my treatment—medicines, injections, Horlicks, etc.—was provided to me completely by them. The day the embryo had to be put in, they informed me. They would tell me that today we will perform an ultrasound; today we will check the baby's heartbeat, etc. The doctor madam gave me some information

in the beginning. She informed me that she would put two embryos first and if the result comes negative, then four can also be put.

(Excerpt from an interview with Rekha, conducted for the research report by Sama [2012])

These narratives reveal that the process of obtaining informed consent did not follow the required norms, that is, a delineation of risks and side effects of drugs and procedures in the language of the surrogate or BA/BE trial participant, ensuring that the person understands what is being communicated, can freely ask questions, and upon satisfaction, signs the informed consent form, and retains a copy of it. When this protocol is not followed, it constitutes an explicit violation of informed consent.

However, this was not always the case. Sama's studies also found a few cases where the process was duly followed. A BA/BE participant recalled:

When you first enter the complex after getting selected, they explain everything about the study. We all sat in one big hall and the scientists and doctors explained the drug, what it is used for, its dosage, and its side effects. They gave us a document to read as well but also explained everything on the board. They explained why this study was being undertaken. They said that as we know, we get medicines from the market; sometimes there is a need to manufacture new drugs. To make a new drug similar to the one we buy from the market, they have to study whether this new medicine works like the drug in the market. They gave us a form to read of about 4–5 pages in Gujarati that we signed. However, some things in the form I could not understand. I feel it is important to keep these forms with you because if something happens to us, our family members should know what happened and why.

(Excerpt from an interview conducted with Paresh, for the research report by Sama [2013])

The stigma associated with clinical labour makes trial participants and surrogates secretive about their work. Many go to various lengths to conceal what they are doing from family members, friends, and neighbours. This process of concealment also generates its own anxieties. More worryingly, the concealment compounds vulnerability, and individualizes the burden of risk from participation in drug trials and surrogacy arrangements.

In our village they will say that we sold our child. That we earn from selling babies. People say such things. It's not good here (in Delhi) either, people say things here as well that you are selling sex. So it's not appropriate to tell everyone about these things. Once the belly becomes big, I will shift to some other place.

(Excerpt from an interview with Lata, conducted for the
research report by Sama [2012])

Other concerns from a bioethics perspective include the inadequate nature of care given to the surrogate mothers. The surrogacy arrangement entails subjecting the surrogate's body to long-drawn-out and significant medical interventions. While aspects such as the benevolence of surrogacy and financial gain for the surrogate are repeatedly highlighted, the medical procedures and their implications are completely invisibilized.

They had transferred four eggs (embryos) inside me and I was not told about it. One day, I got a call asking me to visit the hospital. They told me that the heartbeat of one of the foetus was not there and that one has to be taken out by surgery. I was very scared. I didn't understand how you could take one out. What if something happens to me? I called my husband, but before he could reach, they had taken me inside for the surgery. That night there was too much pain in my stomach and I could not walk or mover.[3]

(Excerpt from an interview with Radha, conducted for the
research report by Sama [2012])

These are important gaps that need attention from many quarters, including the government, public health and bioethics, civil society, and the biomedical industry. The present conjuncture is particularly critical because regulatory frameworks for these new industries are being debated, drafted, and amended. This is an exercise in deciding which practices are to be codified in law as legitimate and ethical, and which are not, as well as what the rights and duties of various parties in these arrangements will be.

It becomes important then to ask in this moment, what kind of ethics and regulation do we want? What constitutes an ethical surrogacy or an ethical study, and how are these regulatory regimes to be enforced?

Currently, the surrogacy industry in India operates with little regulation. A set of non-binding guidelines by the ICMR was drafted in 2005. A Draft Assisted Reproductive Technology (Regulation) Bill and Rules (2014) has been tabled in Parliament but is yet to be passed into a law. Most recently, directives regarding surrogacies commissioned by foreign couples were issued by the Ministry of Home Affairs.[4] Given the complex nature of the ethical issues in surrogacy, the proposed regulatory frameworks merit greater debate among multiple stakeholders than has ensued. For instance, while the 2014 draft lays out the mandatory nature of informed consent, and a mandatory waiting period between repeat egg donation and surrogacy arrangements, it uncompromisingly permits only gestational and not genetic surrogacy (in the interest of severing all genetic links—and thus potential parenthood claims—of the surrogate to the child). However, where feasible, genetic surrogacy is both the less invasive and less expensive option and should be allowed. Further, the 2012 MHA guidelines discriminate against single persons, gay couples, and unmarried couples. These are some examples of ethical issues arising within the framework of regulation.

Similarly, all bioavailability and bioequivalence studies should be conducted according to the Guidelines for Bioavailability and Bioequivalence studies as prescribed. The guidelines do not address the issues related to recruitment and informed consent. However, according to the ICMR guidelines (2006) on biomedical research on human participants,

> BA/BE studies are also clinical studies conducted most often in normal volunteers. Hence, all safeguards to protect participants must be in place, including ethical review of protocol, recruitment methods, compensation for participation, evidence of non-coercion and consent procedures. It is in such studies that volunteers often participate at short intervals and may participate at different centres within less than the prescribed period of three months between two studies. Mechanisms to prevent this must be developed at the study site.

BEYOND ETHICS: MORE QUESTIONS THAN ANSWERS

In addition to the issues raised in the previous section, biomedical economies are throwing up challenges that fall outside narrow regulatory frameworks. These challenges tend to be largely absent from industry and policy-level discourse, but they are nonetheless critically important. In this concluding section, we will consider some of these larger concerns.

In the surrogacy contract, for instance, there is no space to negotiate the relinquishment of the baby-to-be by the surrogate. The surrogate cannot abort, but the commissioning parents can demand 'foetal reduction' in the event of a multiple pregnancy. In fact, the requirement that the surrogate must give up the child is a strict non-negotiable and an overarching concern, one that is reiterated at every stage and in every way. Further, the terms of relinquishment are decided by the commissioning parent/s, such as the decision to stay in touch with the surrogate or not. Can we imagine an arrangement that respects the surrogate's relationship with the child as not being necessarily as alienable as other commodities produced or services rendered in the market? Arlie Hochschild (2012) highlights the unaccounted emotional labour of surrogacy, the 'backstage work' that surrogates do of separating themselves from the babies they carry and from the part of their bodies that carry the babies. A surrogate mother from Delhi described to us her feelings about this:

> We will give the child as soon as it is born, what else. They (commissioning parents) will not talk to us. We are poor people, we would talk, but they won't. These rich people won't. Once you've done the work, they pay and that's it. This I also understand. I am not very educated but I understand. She (commissioning mother) becomes the mother because she has spent the money when she is not even the mother. I am the mother, it's in my womb. But when I give them the child, they will take her and go away, so what relationship can we build? The more we try to build relations, the child would get to know (about the surrogacy) and would have to be told that this is how it happened, your mother is there. These people do not enable a relation. They forget, and try to forget as well.
>
> (Excerpt from an interview conducted with Sonia, for the research report by Sama [2012])

Perhaps there is a larger question here. Biomedical economies depend literally on the bodies of the poor and the vulnerable. While all work is embodied, in that, it is 'of the body'; in biomedical economies, like BA/BE study and surrogacy, the biology of the body 'is the work'. In such a scenario, how are terms of an arrangement to be decided? What is 'fair' when what is at stake is the body itself?

> Everything else is fine with me but I feel that since we are taking more risk, we should be paid more money. The sahebs who orient us get Rs 80,000–1 lakh and all they do is monitor on the computer. I think more money is important. Rajesh
> This is any day better than begging for alms.
>
> (Excerpts from personal interview conducted with Bhanu by Sama [2012] for an exploratory study on participants perspectives in Clinical Trials)

Medical ethics must answer to social justice concerns. It cannot confine itself to the four walls of a clinic setting; it must address the world outside the clinic that bears down on the world inside it. Clearly, money, even a relatively small amount, is the primary reason most people participate in BA/BE studies. For clinical labour to be undertaken in more equitable ways, Cooper and Waldby (2014) argue that the current terms of exchange must change, such as through a just wage and social insurance. They are careful to clarify that the category of labour cannot account for all instances in which patients donate tissues, participate in clinical trials, and so on. Rather, they suggest that these services should be regarded as labour when the activity is intrinsic to the valorization of a particular bio-economic sector, when therapeutic benefits to participants and their communities are absent or incidental or when experimental effects may be actively harmful, and when clinical labour is performed in exchange for health care.

As bodies become resources in new ways, we are confronted with a range of implications, and possible responses to these implications. It is important to understand which of these responses are being enabled by the structures and politics of the present moment, and which are being disabled. Finally, to take a life cycle view of the clinical labour participant would mean to ask deeper political questions about social justice. Why are surrogates drawn from a class of women otherwise targeted for population control and subject to high maternal risks? Why are livelihood options so poor that BA/BE study participation has become as popular as it has? Why should the people who most depend on the physical labour of their bodies have to risk those very bodies to live? A neo-liberal paradigm that rolls back social securities like universal health and education, generates scant and insecure employment, and individualizes risk, robs people of robust alternatives and creates the conditions for clinical labour to flourish. Ultimately, it is this paradigm that must be challenged at all levels.

NOTES

1.   Sama is a Delhi-based resource group on gender and public health that works through research, policy advocacy, and movement building. For more information check, samawomenshealth.org.

2.   According to *ICMR Guidelines on Biomedical Research on Human Participants* (2006), Bio Availability Studies—For all new drug substances and for new dosage forms administered for systemic absorption, which are approved elsewhere in the world, bioequivalence studies with the available formulation should be carried out wherever applicable. Data on the extent of systemic absorption may be required for formulations not meant for

systemic absorption. Evaluation of the effect of food on absorption following oral administration should be carried out if the food absorption data is not submitted. Bio Equivalent Studies are also clinical studies conducted most often in normal volunteers. Hence, all safeguards to protect participants must be in place, including ethical review of protocol, recruitment methods, compensation for participation, evidence of non-coercion, and consent procedures. It is in such studies that volunteers often participate at short intervals and may participate at different centres within less than the prescribed period of three months between two studies. Mechanisms to prevent this must be developed at the study site.

3.   According to the *ICMR National Guidelines Accreditation, Supervision and Regulation of ART Clinics in India Guidelines 2005*: No more than three oocytes or embryos may be placed in a woman in any one cycle, regardless of the procedure/s used, excepting under exceptional circumstances (such as elderly women, poor implantation or poor embryo quality), which should be recorded.

4.   Ministry of Home Affairs (2012). Available at http://www.icmr.nic.in/ icmrnews/art/MHA_circular_July%209.pdf. Accessed on 8 July 2015.

REFERENCES

Cooper, Melinda and Catherine Waldby. 2014. *Clinical Labor: Tissue Donors and Research Subjects in the Global Bioeconomy*. Durham and London: Duke University Press.

Ehrenreich, Barbara and A.R. Hochschild (eds). 2003. *Global Woman: Nannies, Maids, and Sex Workers in the New Economy*. New York: Henry Holt and Company.

Hochschild, A.R. 2012. *The Managed Heart: Commercialization of Human Feeling* (3rd edition). Berkeley: University of California Press.

Indian Council of Medical Research (ICMR). 2006. *Ethical Guidelines for Biomedical Research on Human Participants*. New Delhi: Director General-Indian Council of Medical Research.

Martin, E. 1998. 'Anthropology and the Cultural Study of Science', *Science Technology and Human Values* 23: 24–44.

Rajan, K.S. 2006. *Biocapital: The Constitution of Postgenomic Life*. Durham and London: Duke University Press.

Reuters. 2013. 'Novartis Loses Landmark India Patent Case on Glivec by Kaustubh Kulkarni and Suchitra Mohanty', 2 April. Available at: http:// in.reuters.com/article/2013/04/01/india-drugs-patent-novartis-glivec-idINDEE93000920130401. Accessed on 31 August 2015.

Sama—Resource Group for Women and Health. 2012. *Birthing a Market: A Study on Commercial Surrogacy*. New Delhi: Sama—Resource Group for Women and Health.

————. 2013. *Trials and Travails: Perceptions and experiences of Clinical Trial Participants in India*. New Delhi: Sama—Resource Group for Women and Health.

Sassen, S. 2002. 'Global Cities and Survival Circuits'. In *Global Woman: Nannies, Maids and Sex Workers in the New Economy*, Barbara Ehrenreich and Arlie Hochschild (eds), pp. 54–74. New York: Metropolitan Books.

Shah, Kalpesh S.K. 2013. 'Bridging the Gap of Indian regulations and Major Global Regulations for Bioequivalence Studies with Emphasis on Adaptive Sequential Design and Two-Stage Bioequivalnce Studies', *Journal of Pharmaceutical and Scientific Innovation* 2(2): 14–19.

Smerdon, U.R. 2008, 'Crossing Bodies, Crossing Borders: International Surrogacy between the United States and India', *Cumberland Law Review* 39(1): 15–85.

III

EQUITY ISSUES IN HEALTH CARE—GENDER, CASTE, DISABILITY, AND VIOLENCE

10

Health, Disability, and Equity
Conversations among Bodies, Discourses, and Law[1]

Renu Addlakha

One billion people, or 15 per cent of the world's population, experience some form of disability.[2] One-fifth of this population group experiences significant disabilities. Persons with disabilities (PWDs) as a group are more likely to experience adverse socio-economic outcomes than persons without disabilities, such as worse health outcomes, less education, less employment, and higher poverty rates. It may reasonably be argued that disability[3] is the latest entrant to the identity politics-driven social movements that spawned in the 1960s and 1970s in the West—women's movement, civil rights movement, gay and lesbian movements were the most prominent revolts against a social order that marginalized specific groups on a presumption of inferiority embedded in biology.

In India, the caste system provides another context for operationalization of the human rights paradigm. With the opening up of the Indian economy to global forces in the 1990s, accompanied by a diminution of state activity in the social sector, many so-called 'social welfare' activities have become the critical sites of civil society activism which engage the state as an advocate both on behalf of the general population and more specifically on behalf of marginalized groups such as PWDs. Non-government organizations (NGOs) become the medium for this advocacy and the tool for intervention in the areas of health, education, livelihoods, and social security. This work generates an army of professionals like women's activists, health activists, disability activists, and others. A substantial amount of this activity is made possible through the transfer of resources in the form of funds and expertise from the Global North to the Global South. Another approach to empowerment is through garnering resources in the form of corporate social responsibility (CSR) where private companies are given tax breaks to invest in social arenas like health and education. State–NGO partnership has also become standard practice in the formulation and implementation of social welfare programmes and schemes. It is within this broad framework that the disability sector operates.

This chapter seeks to engage with the contemporary debates around health and equity from the perspective of disability focusing on the contemporary interface between health disability, and law that is panning out in public policy in India. The first section of the chapter maps the multidimensional nature of the disability concept as it is deployed in the medico-bureaucratic state paradigms and the human rights and identity politics activist discourses of civil society, with a particular focus on its linkages with health. The second section discusses the attempt to balance the demands of health and equity and social justice in the disability sector through the Mental Health Act 2013 passed by the Parliament in August 2016, and the proposed disability legislation, namely the Rights of Persons with Disabilities Bill 2014 which is awaiting approval in the Parliament.[4]

DISABILITY, HEALTH, AND EQUITY: DISENTANGLING THE INTERCONNECTIONS

Till the 1990s, disability in India was largely viewed as a lifelong medical problem for which there was no cure. The individual (and by extension his/her family) had to adjust to the physical, mental, sensory, or communication limitations; education and employment were secondary considerations. The primary concern was basic survival and improvement in the impairment condition(s) through medical intervention. Of course, other variables like caste, class, gender, and place of residence, as also family disposition and support, modified the experience of disability, but the discursive framework was one of deficit, dependency, pity, and compassion. Welfare and charity paradigms configured the state response as well. Medical rehabilitation was given primacy; the disabled had to be provided services free of cost, given concessions in education, and employment wherever possible. The disabled person was still very much visualized as a subject requiring assistance rather than an individual agent with rights.

Given this perspective, it is not surprising that the issue of disability (and consequently disabled individuals) remained at the margins of the social system where they would have continued to remain were it not for the convergence of two factors. Firstly, individuals with disabilities who had managed to navigate the system to achieve a level of personal and professional status, that is, intelligent, determined articulate PWDs with access to resources and information beyond their own society. For instance, some writers like Meenu Bhambani (2005) argue that the disability rights movement in India began with the pioneering work of the Disability Rights Group that came into existence in the early 1990s in Delhi, and canvassed for the passage of the Persons with Disabilities Act (1995) through a coalition of different disability groups constituting a cross disability platform.[5] And secondly, social reforms, which not only opened up the Indian economy to global influences but also brought in new ideas, aspirations, and inspirations. Economic globalization brought in its wake pressures on the state to institute necessary socio-economic changes in compliance with global standards and international law. After its passage by the United National General Assembly in 2006, India's signing of the United Nations Convention on Rights of Persons with Disabilities (UNCRPD) in 2007 articulated a commitment to change laws, policies, and programmes making disability a human rights and not only a medical and social welfare issue.

These developments sought to eject disability from the thraldom of bodily inferiority and illness into the domain of social exclusion and marginalization through a new vocabulary of oppressions and rights. It was argued that the physical, economic, legislative, and social environments, and not bodily deficits, create and/or maintain barriers to the participation of people with disabilities in economic, civic, and social life. Barriers include inaccessible buildings, transport, information, and communication technology; inadequate services, and funding for those services; and too little basic data on disability and its analysis for effective policies. Poverty may increase the risk of disability through malnutrition, inadequate access to education and health care, unsafe working conditions, polluted environment, and lack of access to safe water and sanitation. Disability may increase the risk of poverty, through lack of employment, lower wages, and increased cost of living with a disability.

The fundamental change in thinking on disability has been moving it out of the configuration of medical definitions and control to the social domain wherein it intersects with other variables, such as caste, class ethnicity, socio-economic status (SES), gender, and others, to emerge as a particular kind of oppression which can be addressed more through social and infrastructural engineering than medical technology. Hence one of the aims of the disability rights movement all over the world has been to break the stranglehold of the medical model, and by extension, the location of disability from the health-related sectors to other domains of social, economic, political, and cultural life. This line of argument is in keeping with the power of the medical model in practically all walks of life in the West. Western medicine has not had that kind of influence in other parts of the world including India. Our appraisal of the medical model has to be tempered by this historical backdrop. This chapter contends that the analysis of disability and medicine are inextricably intertwined in distinctive ways when it comes to applying the social model to the Indian reality. And law emerges as a critical site for this analysis.

Without going into the nitty-gritty of the evolution of the disability category, it suffices to say that the concept has evolved over the past few decades from referring to sensory, mental, and communication conditions like blindness, deafness, mental retardation, and different kinds of mobility limitations ranging from muscular dystrophies to paralysis to the functional limitations and societal prejudices linked to these and many other somato-psychic conditions. The underlying premise is that every physical condition occurs, or is experienced or managed, within a multilayered context incorporating the social, cultural, economic, and political factors at a given place and time. This viewpoint sits well with the holistic definition of health of the World Health Organization (WHO) as the state of complete physical, mental, and social well-being and not merely the absence of disease or infirmity.[6]

The trajectory of the disability concept in the United Nations system over the past half a century shows its transition from a purely health issue to one of social exclusion and marginalization (Sundaresan 2013). For instance, the International Classification of Impairments, Disabilities and Handicaps (ICIDH) propounded the tri-dimensional experiential nature of any disease, illness, or injury at the levels of the body, person, and society, respectively (World Health Organization 1980). Impairment is defined as any loss or abnormality of anatomical or psychological structure or function. Impairment may lead to a restriction or lack of ability to perform an activity in the manner and within the range considered normal for a person resulting in disability or disabilities.

Handicap, on the other hand, is a social disadvantage resulting from an impairment or disability hindering the person from performing a social role. In 2001 WHO put forward the International Classification of Functioning, Disability and Health (ICF). While ICIDH focused on the consequences of diseases or disorders at the levels of the body, the person and society in a causal fashion, ICF is based on a components approach to human functioning, which connotes holistically the range of bodily functions, restrictions, and social participation. In this framework, disability is an umbrella term that covers impairments, activity limitations, and participation restrictions. Consequently, the ICF presents a well-rounded definition of disability that encompasses the bodily differences, activity levels, and social dimensions embedded in the tripartite classification of ICIDH.

Concomitant with these medically based conceptual changes led by the WHO were two other developments that shaped the contours of the disability rights movement across the world with its roots within and outside the United Nations system: one was the deployment of a legal machinery to make visible and guarantee fundamental human rights to persons with disabilities including persons with mental illness and intellectual disabilities through a range of declarations, recommendations, guidelines, and action plans beginning in the 1970s and culminating in the United Nations Convention on Rights of Persons with Disabilities passed by the General Assembly in 2006. The other was a vibrant social movement championing a rights discourse for PWDs in which self-advocacy was a pivotal modality. This civil society initiative derived its ideological inspiration from identity politics and human rights discourses configuring disability as a form of social oppression embedded in a minority identity (Barnes 1998, 1991; Barnes and Mercer 1996; Barnes, Oliver, and Barton 2002; Davis 1995; Driedger 1989; Finkelstein 1980; Linton 1998; Oliver 1996, 1990; UPIAS 1976). In fact, disability law, disability rights movement, and disability studies as an academic speciality took shape in these emerging crosscurrents.

The United Nations Convention on Rights of Persons with Disabilities proposes a definition of disability that is strongly embedded within the social model while not discounting its biological reality. Convention places disability firmly within a sociopolitical and economic framework. Article 1 states that: 'Persons with disabilities include those who have long-term physical, mental, intellectual or sensory impairments which in interaction with various barriers may hinder their full and effective participation in society on an equal basis with others'.[7]

This definition addresses both the biomedical concerns with types of disabilities and the historically embedded reality of social exclusion in the form of social, economic, and cultural barriers to social participation and inclusion. In fact, Article 2 of the Convention specifically defines disability-based discrimination which:

> means any distinction, exclusion or restriction on the basis of disability which has the purpose or effect of impairing or nullifying the recognition, enjoyment or exercise, on an equal basis with others, of all human rights and fundamental freedoms in the political, economic, social, cultural, civil or any other field. It includes all forms of discrimination, including denial of reasonable accommodation.[8,9]

Widening the frame of the medical discourse to issues of human rights and fundamental freedoms is as much a part of the disability paradigm as it is of the health paradigm. Health is also as much a biological as a social economic, political, and cultural issue. The two intersect and overlap in different ways, and it is the purpose of this paper to highlight some of these patterns of conflation. While the UNCRPD does not explicitly define health, Article 25 addresses some of the disability-associated discriminatory practices in the health sector such as inaccessible health care and rehabilitation services at the community level, neglect of sexual and reproductive health of women and girls with disabilities, lack of sensitization of health care providers to the concrete needs and concerns of disabled persons in an ethical and sensitive manner, denial of health insurance in the public and private sectors, and so on. United Nations Convention on Rights of Persons with Disabilities not only explicitly recognizes the sociomedical dimensions of disability, but also acknowledges its intersectional connections with other social variables such as gender and age, For instance, it has dedicated articles on women and children with disabilities.

However, even within highly socialized frameworks and definitions that place disability within social construction perspectives of the social model and minority identity, the originary dialectical relationship between health and disability cannot be obscured. This is illustrated in disability legislation worldwide; for instance. in the Disability Discrimination Act (2005) of the United Kingdom, people with HIV, cancer, and multiple sclerosis are deemed disabled. Similarly, the proposed Rights of Persons with Disabilities Bill (2014) in India has expanded the number of conditions deemed as disabling from seven (low vision, hearing impairment, speech impairment, locomotor disability, mental retardation, mental illness, and leprosy-cured contained in the Persons with Disabilities Act 1995) to 19 (autism, low vision and blindness, cerebral palsy, deaf blindness, haemophilia, hearing impairment, leprosy, intellectual disability, mental illness, muscular dystrophy, multiple sclerosis, learning disability, speech and language disability, sickle cell disease, thalassemia, chronic neurological conditions, and multiple disability). But other chronic and acute infectious conditions with major disabling consequences like heart disease, asthma, cancer, and communicable diseases like TB, HIV, hepatitis, are not regarded as disabilities in the proposed Indian legislation.[10]

The above discussion shows that disability is a multidimensional, heterogeneous, and cross-cutting concept not only in terms of the intersecting socio-demographic variables but also in terms of the type of disabilities (sensory, physical, mental, and communication). This heterogeneity extends to its temporal status as well, that is, whether it is congenital or acquired, whether it is static, episodic or degenerative. Impairments may be visible or invisible, may generate disability or may entail no functional limitations. Examined from the perspective of the lifecycle, such ideas as the temporarily able bodied person (TAB) or the contingently able bodied (CAB) underscore the possibility of anyone and everyone being/becoming disabled at some point or other in their lifetime.

Nuancing Medical Model in Disability Legislation

As discussed in an earlier publication on the interface between women, health, and law in India (Addlakha 2011), law is one of the sites of cultural engagement and is very much embedded in and the product of prevailing values, norms, and practices; it is not outside culture. Although separate in terms of their form, applicability, social status, law and culture are inextricably linked. For instance, customs, religion, and traditions are sources of laws. Given the number of statutes enacted to protect the interests of different marginalized groups in India like the minorities, scheduled castes and scheduled tribes, women, the disabled, and others, law is viewed as a powerful agent of social change to make social justice a reality. However, the contestations between formal and substantive equality highlight how the legal regime is operationalized. According importance, for instance, to corporeal differences gives rise to disability-specific legislation like the PWD and Mental Health Acts. However, the difference in treatment espousing formal equality is based on the notion of the neutral human subject, but factoring in the unique experiences of PWDs flies in the face of formal equality. In the difference approach, discrimination is allowed by highlighting the difference(s) and hence thwarting their claims to formal equality. This perspective has given rise to protectionist legislation. The substantive equality model moves from treatment by the law to its impact and combines both the sameness and difference approaches. Aiming to compensate for past injustices and take account of disability-specific differences, the substantive approach endorses both affirmative action and protectionist legislative regimes in the pursuit of social justice. This is the rationale for disability-specific legislation.

Earlier legislations like the Mental Health Act of 1987 and the Persons with Disabilities Act 1995 primarily focused on criteria for identification, assessment, and prevention of disabilities, training of manpower in the mental health and disability sectors, maintenance of standards, licensing of facilities, and expanding infrastructure. One of the major criticisms of these existing laws is the use of an overtly medical approach to definitions and management of disabilities. For instance, Chapter IV of the Persons with Disabilities Act (PWD Act) 1995 is devoted to early detection and prevention of disabilities. The Mental Health Act of 1987 at no point defines mental illness apart from using tautological expressions like unsoundness of mind to refer to the same. There is an assumption of the psychiatric diagnosis constituting the undisputed subtext of the issue.

With the signing of the UNCRPD and a more deeply embedded human rights perspective that emphasises the social dimensions of disability being adopted by the state within a larger framework of social inclusion and empowerment, India is obliged to modify its legislative regime to harmonize with the Convention. Initially, the route of amendment was adopted but consultations with different stakeholders in the disability sector revealed that to make the PWD Act compliant with the UNCRPD would require over 100 amendments. Consequently, the government decided to overhaul existing disability laws. Between 2010 and 2014 different committees[11] were constituted comprising a wide range of stakeholders, including medical professionals, caregivers, activists, and persons with disabilities by the ministries of Social Justice and Empowerment and Health and Family Welfare to draft new mental health and disability laws respectively. The frenzy of discussions resulted in many substantive and procedural controversies arising out of the fractiousness among different disability activists and groups as also the government taking final unilateral decisions, thus aborting the very process of wide consultation it had earlier initiated. For instance, there were significant differences between the versions of the Persons with Disabilities Bill arrived at through nationwide consultations and the one approved by the cabinet for enactment. This move divided disability activists, with some in favour of enacting the Cabinet-approved legislation because it included impairments like autism; and others rejecting the bill on grounds of omission of the right to legal capacity and an explicit prohibition on discrimination on grounds of disability, which are the heart and soul of the UNCRPD. Such rumours that government was thinking of the ordinance route to push through the new law further added to the chaos and confusion. Drafts of the Mental Health Care Act (Government of India 2010) were severely criticized by mental health advocates, particularly persons with psychosocial disability; they decried the overweening authority vested with psychiatrists, no right to refuse treatment in emergency situations, and the continuing approval for Electro-Convulsive Therapy (ECT) as a treatment modality. While a historical analysis of the debates around the drafting of these Bills is worthy of a separate study beyond the scope of this chapter, it is suffice to say that the outcome of this process is that the Mental Health Care Bill 2013 (as introduced in the Rajya Sabha) and Draft Rights of Persons with Disabilities Bill 2014 (as introduced in the Rajya Sabha) went to Parliamentary Standing Committees. While the former awaits approval from the Lok Sabha or Lower House to become a law, the latter has been enacted.

This section will focus on how the equity issue is articulated in the proposed bills drafted to make the local legislative regime compliant with the mandate of the UNCRPD, with a specific focus on the disability-health dynamic. A perfect match between the Convention and the proposed legislation is the ideal which can only be approximated. While critiquing this attempt, a weighted analysis factoring in both positive and negative aspects is adopted. The proposed bills are brought in conversation through a comparative approach focusing on a few common features connected with the issue of health like medicalization definition of disability, conditions identified as disabling, early detection, treatment refusal, right to live with the family and in the community, health insurance, disabled-friendly health centres, sport, and others. It may be noted that there are really not many departures between the proposed bills and the enacted laws on these specific themes.

The proposed legislations, in contrast to their predecessors, namely, the Mental Health Act of 1987 and the Persons with Disabilities Act 1995, attempt a more holistic view, moving beyond infrastructural and institutional issues, to the experiential dimensions of marginalization, exclusion, and inequities experienced by different categories of individuals with disabilities in the diverse areas of health education, employment, leisure and recreation, and others. The proposed bills also impose a new section on penalties (in the form of fines and imprisonment) for violations of the rights of PWDs, whose absence is a major weakness of existing disability legislation.

Both legislations begin with the UNCRPD's unequivocal commitment to principles of equality, dignity, autonomy, and non-discrimination. Core concepts of the social model of disability such as barriers,[12] reasonable accommodation,[13] inclusive education,[14] universal design,[15] and others, constitute the language of the draft laws highlighting a strong rights-based approach. While the conceptual and linguistic scaffolding of the UNCRPD constitute the rationale and the body of the two laws, a medicalized protectionist regime continues to subsist being expressed through a range of caveats and reservations, which cast doubt on the move from a social welfare to an anti-discrimination legislation to disability. The legislations appear to be struggling to balance the often competing demands of individual choice and family autonomy on the one hand, and a medico-legal paternalism, on the other.

Secondly, while universal access to health care, identification, treatment/rehabilitation, and prevention of disabilities are unquestionably important, they also lead to the configuration of disability as something to be feared, avoided, and eradicated. How valid is this in the face of a social model of disability that regards it as a form of social oppression expressed through physical capital, and the ICF of the WHO, which regards it as form of human variation?

So, while beginning with the UNCRPD definition of disability, the Rights of Persons with Disabilities (RPD) Bill presents a tripartite model of the same as contained in the following definitions in Chapter 1:

(p) "person with benchmark disability" means a person with not less than forty per cent of a specified disability where specified disability has not been defined in measurable terms and includes a person with disability where specified disability has been defined in measurable terms, as certified by the certifying authority;

(q) "person with disability" means a person with long term physical, mental, intellectual or sensory impairment which hinder his full and effective participation in society equally with others, and;

(r) "person with disability having high support needs" means a person
with benchmark disability certified under clause (*a*) of sub-section
(*2*) of section 57 who needs high support;
(As given in Chapter 1 of the Rights of Persons with Disabilities
Act 2016, titled 'Preliminary'. Available at: http://lawmin.nic.in/ld/
P-ACT/2016/A2016-49.pdf. Accessed on 1 June 2017)

The Mental Health Care Bill (2013) gives an explicit medical definition
of its core concept.

(i) 'Mental illness' for the purpose of this Act, means a disorder of mood,
thought, perception, orientation or memory which causes significant
distress to a person or impairs a person's behavior, judgment
and ability to recognize reality or impairs the person's ability to
meet the demands of normal life and includes mental conditions
associated with the abuse of alcohol and drugs, but excludes mental
retardation.
(ii) Mental illness shall be determined in accordance with nationally and
internationally accepted medical standards such as the latest edition
of the International Classification of Disease of the World Health
Organization.

The rationale for juxtaposing the UNCRPD's socially embedded
definition with the medical criteria for disability assessment is not
explained. What it ultimately indicates is that medicalization is the *sine
non quo* of the disability category. Is this in keeping with the avowed
spirit of the UNCRPD?

Section 10 on Right to Equality and Non-discrimination of the
Mental Health Care Bill attempts to challenge the historically embedded
stigma to mental illness by unequivocally equating it with physical
illness. While the medical model has been highlighted as a source of
social injustice for PWDs because of its neglect of the sociocultural
dimensions of impairment, in the case of mental illness medicalization
has sometimes helped in removing some of the stigma associated with
mental illness by reconfiguring it as a disease that can be treated rather
than a lifelong curse (due to bad 'karma') that has to be endured.
The Bill states:

Persons with mental illness shall be treated equal to persons with physical
illness in the provision of all health care:

(i) No discrimination on any basis including gender, sex, sexual
orientation, religion, culture, caste, social or political beliefs, class or
disability.

(ii) Public and private insurance providers shall make provisions for medical insurance for treatment of mental illness on the same basis as is available for treatment of physical illness.

(iii) Emergency facilities and emergency services for mental illness shall be of the same quantity and quality as those provided to persons with physical illness, including ambulance services in the same manner, extent and quality as provided to persons with physical illness.

(iv) Living conditions in health facilities shall be of the same manner, extent and quality as provided to persons with physical illness;

(v) Any other health services provided to persons with physical illness shall be provided in same manner, extent and quality to persons with mental illness.

How much does medicalization reduce the stigma of mental affliction? It takes the issue out of the religious-magical domain into the arena of secular science diminishing the element of blame and evil attributed to the afflicted; and opens up the possibility of reduction in suffering and the hope of a cure through medication. As far back as 1982 the National Mental Health Programme sought to integrate mental health services with general health services through inter-sectoral collaboration from primary to tertiary levels. This underlying institutional philosophy is also the backdrop of the proposed mental health legislation.

Nowhere in this Bill is the term psychosocial disability (or even disability, for that matter) even mentioned once, even though the current trend in the mental health field is to deploy it to highlight the social, economic, political, and cultural concomitants of mental illness. While the RPD Bill numerates 19 disability conditions, the MHC relies on a psychiatric diagnosis for a condition to be recognized as mental illness. It does not specify when a mental illness becomes a disability.

Chapter V of the RPD Bill puts forth state policies and programmes for ensuring the social security, health, rehabilitation, and recreation of PWDs like ensuring affordable aids and appliances, medicine and diagnostic services, and corrective surgery. From the health perspective, the chapter also talks about guaranteeing a basic standard of living to all PWDs, which includes access to safe drinking water and appropriate and accessible sanitation facilities especially in urban slums and rural areas; and, community centres offering an environment that guarantees safety, sanitation, health care, and counselling.

In addition, the RPD Bill makes provisions for:

(a) Free health care in the vicinity especially in rural area subject to such family income as may be notified.

(b) Barrier-free access in all parts of the hospitals and other healthcare institutions and centres run or aided by them.

(c) Priority in attendance and treatment.

The concern with prevention and early identification of disabilities, particularly in children, is a health matter that is central to the legislation.

(2) The appropriate Government and the local authorities shall take measures and make schemes or programmes to promote health care and prevent the occurrence of disabilities and for the said purpose shall.

(a) Undertake or cause to be undertaken surveys, investigations and research concerning the cause of occurrence of disabilities;

(b) Promote various methods for preventing disabilities;

(c) Screen all the children at least once in a year for the purpose of identifying "at-risk" cases;

(d) Provide facilities for training to the staff at the primary health centres;

(e) Sponsor or cause to be sponsored awareness campaigns and disseminate or cause to be disseminated information for general hygiene, health and sanitation;

(f) Take measures for pre-natal, perinatal and post-natal care of mother and child;

(g) Educate the public through the pre-schools, schools, primary health centres, village level workers and anganwadi workers;

(h) Create awareness amongst the masses through television, radio and other mass media on the causes of disabilities and the preventive measures to be adopted;

(i) Health care during the time of natural disasters and other situations of risk;

(j) Essential medical facilities for life saving emergency treatment and procedures;

and

(k) Sexual and reproductive health care especially for women with disability.

25. The appropriate Government shall, by notification, make insurance schemes for their employees with disabilities.

26. (1) The appropriate Government and the local authorities shall within their economic capacity and development, undertake or cause to be undertaken services and programmes of rehabilitation, particularly in the areas of health, education and employment for all persons with disabilities.

(2) For the purposes of sub-section (*1*), the appropriate Government and the local authorities may grant financial assistance to non-Government Organisations.

(*The Rights of Persons with Disabilities Bill* 2014, Bill No. 1 of 2014)

In this comprehensive listing of health-related provisions for PWDs, the critical rider is 'The appropriate Government and the local authorities shall within their economic capacity and development ...' effectively putting breaks on the extent to which resources may be deployed to accommodate the health concerns of PWDs. This application of the principle of reasonable accommodation to the provision of health is ethically problematic. Many disabilities are accompanied by health complications, for example, post-polio syndrome,[16] kidney problems in the absence of disabled-friendly toilets, arthritis symptoms due to long term use of a wheelchair, and others. Consequently, to make health services conditional goes against a basic human right to a minimum standard of health.

Then, clubbing together identification and prevention of disabilities communicates the problematic message that disability is and should be eradicable. While we know that the effects of most disabilities can be moderated through early identification and possible intervention (particularly in the case of nutritional and infection-induced disabilities), a large segment of disabilities are acquired during the life course arising out of various contingencies like automobile and industrial accidents, environmental pollutants, and ageing-associated degeneration. Consequently management of disability becomes another element of the larger package of comprehensive health care going beyond standard medication and surgery. Indeed, a very small number of disabilities (less than 5 per cent) are congenital, which appears to be the stereotypical mode of representation of disability both in lay and legal discourses.

Physical culture is a critical component of health particularly as a part of the education system. People with disabilities have always been excluded from sports under the false assumption that disability is a barrier to sporting capacity. This assumption has been contested by the world-wide Paralympics and Abilympic movements. The connections between physical fitness, sports culture, and health are too well known to be elaborated. Section 29 of RPD bill pitches for developing the sporting potential of PWDs.

While many clauses of the RPD Bill apply to persons diagnosed with a mental illness, the reverse is not true. The disability paradigm is trying to disengage itself from the biological impairment model while the mental health legislation is trying to marshal it to empower persons with mental illness. This underscores the legitimate power of the psychiatric profession to define and regulate the domain in which persons with psychosocial disability have limited negotiating power.

Although underplayed in its text, even the RPD Bill exclusively relies on medically certified criteria, given the importance accorded to the disability certificate in accessing the benefits that it confers upon PWDs.

EQUITY ENHANCING MEASURES

In addition to facilities for the education and employment of PWDs— taking into account their needs, talents, and aspirations through inclusive education policies (free education till 18 years of age), affirmative action, reasonable accommodation actualized through such concrete measures as reservation (enhancing from 3 to 5 per cent),[17] establishment of special employment exchanges, finance corporations for providing loans to start self-employment ventures, job identification in government departments, incentives to the private sector to employment persons with disabilities, and others—the proposed bills outline other modalities to create an enabling environment for PWDs to lead fulfilling lives

Historically, PWDs (and not just mental illness) have been deprived of the basic right to living at home with their families and right to decision-making including the right to refuse treatment. Institutionalization has been a method to manage the disabled in society. Both the RPD and the MHC Bills guarantee the right to live in the community for PWDs.[18] Section 7 on right to access to mental health care clearly states:

> (iv) Mental health services shall provide treatment in a manner which supports persons with mental illness to live in the community and with their families. Long term hospital based mental health treatment shall be used only in exceptional circumstances, for as short a duration as possible, and only as a last resort when appropriate community based treatment has been tried and shown to have failed.

Section 8 on the Right to Community Living clarifies:

> All persons with mental illness have a right to live in, be part of and not be segregated from society. No person with mental illness shall continue to remain in a mental health facility merely because he or she does not have a family or is not accepted by his or her family or is homeless or because of the absence of community based facilities. The Government shall therefore provide for and/or support the establishment of less restrictive community based facilities including halfway homes, group homes and like, for persons who no longer require treatment in a more restrictive mental health facility.

The RPD Bill states that no child with disability shall be separated from his or her parents on the ground of disability except on an order of a competent court, if required, in the best interest of the child. Where the parents are unable to take care of a child with disability, the competent court shall place such child with his or her near relations, and failing that within the community in a family setting or in exceptional cases in a shelter home run by the appropriate government or non-governmental organization. The relevance of this section is intriguing because in India we have more instances of the opposite problem, namely, children with disabilities in need of care and protection because of being abandoned by their families.

While the widespread use of anti-psychotic drugs from the 1960s made it possible for many severely ill mental patients to live in the community resulting in what has now come to be called the de-institutionalization movement, the situation in India is more complicated. While the deplorable, almost inhumane living conditions in many mental hospitals have been well documented and no new mental hospitals have been built since Independence, there is at the same time a burgeoning private industry of institutions. So, in addition to talking about the right to family and community living, it would have been more appropriate to put in place measures to regulate the privatization of the institutional management of PWDs.

But some attempts (perhaps cosmetic) have been made to attenuate the experience of institutionalization. Earlier mental health legislation focussed on guaranteeing human rights of persons in mental health intuitions from the perspective of health care providers and administrators with the focus being on maintaining basic standards of living and care of inmates. The proposed legislation directs attention to such issues as patients' right to information (Section 11); confidentiality (Section 12); access to their medical records (Section 13); right to personal contacts and communication including personal visitors, email, and mobile communication (Section 14); right to free legal aid (Section 15); and make complaints about deficiencies in services (Section 16). Recognizing the new realities of persons self-identifying as mentally ill and the incidence of mental illness in children, there are sections on Independent (without Support) Admission and Treatment (Section 42) and Admission of a Minor (Section 43).[19]

Support arrangements are a critical element in disability legislation. While plenary or total guardianship has been the dominant mode of support, the UNCRPD put forward the idea of supported guardianship, and the proposed Indian legislation seem to be incorporating all these modes According to the RPD bill,

(i) 'plenary guardianship' means a guardianship whereby subsequent to a finding of incapacity, a guardian substitutes for the person with disability as the person before the law and takes all legally binding decisions for him and the decisions of the person with disability have no binding force in law during the subsistence of the guardianship and the guardian is under no legal obligation to consult with the person with disability or determine his or her will or preference whilst taking decisions for him;[20]

(ii) 'limited guardianship' means a system of joint decision which operates on mutual understanding and trust between the guardian and the person with disability.

Why has the proposed legislation taken a compromise position by adopting both plenary and limited guardianship? Who exercises the option between the two, especially in a sociocultural context where most important decisions are outcomes of a family-based process? To what extent do such guardianship provisions limit the avowed commitment to independent decision-making of the person with a disability? While independent decision-making is an issue in connection with all types of disabilities because of a presumed innocence or incapacity of a PWD to exercise autonomy, it has historically been overwhelmingly discussed with regard to mental illness.

The MHC Bill states that a person having a mental illness shall not by itself be taken to mean that he or she is not competent to make decisions That is why the proposal of an advance directive[21] to counter the deep-rooted legally sanctioned prohibitions limiting the functioning of persons regarded as mentally ill. An Advance Directive may be made irrespective of a person's mental health status in the past or present. It is a kind of living will, which is ratified by a medical practitioner certifying that the person is competent at the time of writing the Advance Directive. Of course, it may be revoked, amended, or cancelled at any time. But there are three caveats to the validity of a valid advance directive since, which dilutes the competence and free will of the person with a mental illness in treatment, which are as follows:

(v) If a person makes an Advance Directive which contains a refusal of all future medical treatment for mental illness, then such an Advance Directive shall not be valid unless it has been submitted to the District Panel of the Mental Health Review Commission.

(vii) If a mental health professional or a relative or a care-giver of the person desires to over-rule a valid Advance Directive when treating a person with mental illness, the mental health professional or the relative or the care-giver of the person, may apply to the District Panel of the Mental Health Review Commission for review and cancellation of the Advance Directive.

(viii) Notwithstanding any provision in this section, it shall not apply to any emergency treatment given under Section 50.

(x) A medical practitioner or a psychiatrist shall not be held liable for any unforeseen consequences on following a valid Advance Directive.

Is an advance directive practicable (or even relevant) in a context like India? Is there not a class bias in its introduction? Is it another way of ensuring more control to the medical practitioner and/or family in the guise of an autonomy granting measure? This is indeed what the accompanying caveats seem to suggest.

One of the central features of stigma is that it taints the entire life course once a person has been labelled with a particular attribute. The label becomes a lifelong liability even if and when the stigma-inducing features ceases to exist. Thus once a person enters a psychiatric facility, s/he gets saddled with a new identity that has social, cultural, political, economic, and most importantly, legal consequences going beyond the phases of diagnosis, treatment, and rehabilitation. It is this legal burden that the MHC Bill seeks to remove by:

(v) A background of past treatment or hospitalization to a mental health facility though relevant, shall not by itself justify any present or future determination of mental illness.

This section has attempted to point to some features of the draft disability legislation that attempt to de-medicalize it by focusing on issues that impact the total well-being of a person like participation in community life, exerting choice in treatment, having access to humane institutional arrangements, and others. The medical model in locating the problem within the individual seeks individual remedies; whereas the social model recognizing that the problems of disability arise due to the manner in which the physical and normative world is structured looks for structural solutions. Disability rights activists are attempting to move public discourse from the medical to the social but only with partial success. The law is attempting a compromise position that appears fraught with inconsistencies. So, is it the case that the purity of analytical models cannot be replicated by life?

An analysis of the texts of the MMC and RPD Bills shows the definite imprint of the majority voice authoring them. While the former is largely the product of mental health professionals, predominantly psychiatrists, the latter are more the product of the thinking and experiences of caregivers and PWDs themselves. Perhaps that is why the law text in the one reads more like a laundry list of demands to the state on behalf of PWDs and the other, a set of concessions accorded to persons with mental illness by medico-administrative authorities. The sum and substance of this overriding caveat is contained Section 64 of the MHC Bill on protection of action taken in good faith, which unequivocally states:

(i) No suit, prosecution or other legal proceeding shall lie against any person for anything which is in good faith done or intended to be done in pursuance of this Act or any rules, regulations or orders made thereunder.

(ii) No suit or other legal proceeding shall lie against the Government for any damage caused or likely to be caused for anything which is in good faith done or intended to be done in pursuance of this Act or any rules, regulations or orders made thereunder.

Disability is the term marshalled to break the umbilical link with health by shifting the focus from impairment (the purely physiological/anatomical anomalous condition) to the experiences of discrimination, segregation, and deprivation due to social attitudes and practices that systematically marginalize persons with such impairments in society. But much of the debate in the development sector on disability focuses on poverty, malnutrition, absence of medical services, and re-establishing (and at times reinforcing) the primordial connection between the two. While the move from the medical to the social model is largely uncontested, it is neither epistemically nor empirically possible to completely abandon biology. The umbilical cord between medicine and disability lies in a set of definitional parameters that set up biological norms against the backdrop of which disability takes shape. And yet the tension between the two is the conceptual reality that current legislation and policy have to constantly grapple with. The proposed legislative regime discussed here is but one instance of this ongoing contestation.

* * *

This chapter has attempted to examine conceptual linkages between disability, health, and law at a critical moment in the history of disability legislation in India by examining two landmark bills in the last stages of their journey to becoming laws. The health-disability dialectic that configures the disability category emerges just as strongly in the proposed legislation as it does in the disability rights movement and disability studies not only in India but across the world. The legislation only reflects this ubiquitous reality.

While pioneering proponents of the social model of disability (many of who were themselves persons with disabilities) persuasively questioned the power of the medical model in defining disability by invoking the role of social, economic, political, and cultural factors in creating and sustaining the problems faced by PWDs, the limitations of the social model in the face of the reality of embodied pain and suffering cannot be denied. While de-medicalization of the disability category may be theoretically viable under the overwhelming weight of social constructionism and identity politics, the pragmatic lens of collective well-being militates against a total separation. Indeed, health becomes the bridge connecting disability as a form of social oppression to disability as a form of bodily and personal difference.

So, when the state machinery tries to operationalize a scheme of laws and policies to address the needs and aspirations of the disability community in a social climate in which human rights and medicalization are almost competing for supremacy, it is likely to lead to some quandaries and contradictions which are reflected in the proposed legislation. It is the contention in this chapter that although the final legislation may depart in some ways from the proposed bills, this underlying conceptual tension discussed here is unlikely to be touched because it lies at the very heart of the disability category.

ACKNOWLEDGEMENTS

My gratitude to Purendra Prasad and Amar Jesani for inviting me to contribute to this volume. Their suggestions and the incisive comments of the anonymous reviewers have been instrumental in bringing this chapter to completion.

NOTES

1. This chapter was completed before the passage of both the Rights of Persons with Disabilities Act and the Mental Health Care Act by Parliament in 2016. Consequently the chapter is based on the analysis of different drafts of the above bills that were in the public domain for an extended period of time like Mental Health Care Bill 2010 and 2013 and Rights of Persons with Disabilities Bill 2014.

2. Available at: http://www.un.org/disabilities/default.asp/default.asp?id=18. Accessed on 15 January 2015.

3. This chapter will not dwell on the multiple connotations of the disability category, which is discussed in detail in other writings (Addlakha 2010a, 2010b, 2013 and Addlakha et al. 2009).

4. It may be noted that the Rights of Persons with Disabilities Bill was passed by Parliament on 16 December 2016 with some amendments after the completion of this chapter. This chapter will not take up the enacted legislation but the 2014 version of the Bill which was introduced in Parliament in 2016.

5. This is one attempt to situate the origin of disability rights activism in India. For a detailed discussion of different perspectives, see Mehrotra (2011).

6. Available at: http://who.int/about/definition/en/print.html. Accessed on 15 January 2015.

7. Available at http://www.un.org/disabilities/default.asp?id=26. Accessed on 19 November 2016.

8. It 'means necessary and appropriate modification and adjustments not imposing a disproportionate or undue burden, where needed in a particular case, to ensure to persons with disabilities the enjoyment or exercise on an equal basis with others of all human rights and fundamental freedoms' (UNCRPD Article b, 2).

9. Available at: http://www.un.org/disabilities/default.asp?id=26. Accessed on 19 November 2014.

10. In the Rights of Persons with Disabilities Act 2016 the number of disabilities has been increased from 19 to 21. In addition to the aforementioned disabilities, acid attack and Parkinsonism have been added to the list of conditions identified as disabling.

11. The task of drafting the new legislation was given to Centre for Mental Health Law and Policy of I.L.S. (Pune) under the chairmanship of Dr Soumitro Pathare in 2011 by the Ministry of Health, Government of India. The RPD Bill went through several drafts after initially be worked through by a Committee appointed by the Ministry of Social Justice and Empowerment with Dr Sudha Kaul (Director, Spastic Society of Easter India, Kolkata) as the chair.

12. The first chapter of the RPD states: 'barrier' means any factor including communicational, cultural, economic, environmental, institutional, political, social, or structural factors which hampers the full and effective participation of persons with disabilities in society.

13. The first chapter of the RPD states(t) 'reasonable accommodation' means necessary and appropriate modification and adjustments, without imposing a disproportionate or undue burden in a particular case, to ensure to persons with disabilities the enjoyment or exercise of rights equally with others;

14. The first chapter of the RPD states(k) 'inclusive education' means a system of education wherein students with and without disability learn together

and the system of teaching and learning is suitably adapted to meet the learning needs of different types of students with disabilities;

15.   The first chapter of the RPD states(z) 'universal design' means the design of products, environments, programmes and services to be usable by all people to the greatest extent possible, without the need for adaptation or specialised design and shall apply to assistive devices including advanced technologies for particular group of persons with disabilities.

16.   Typically it may appear 15–30 years after recovery from the original paralytic attack, at an age of 35 to 60. Symptoms include muscular weakness, pain, and fatigue.

17.   The RPD Bill 2016 has capped reservation to higher educational institutions at 5 per cent for persons with benchmark disabilities and in employment at 4 per cent in public institutions based on cadre strength.

18.   Right to home and family is guaranteed by the RPD when it states, '4. (1) The persons with disabilities shall have the right to live in the community; (2) The appropriate government shall endeavour that the persons with disabilities are: (a) not obliged to live in any particular living arrangement and (b) given access to a range of in-house, residential and other community support services, including personal assistance necessary to support living with due regard to age and gender'.

19.   Mental Health Care Bill (2010) states, 'Any person under the age of eighteen years (minor) may be admitted to a mental health facility only in exceptional circumstances through a nominated representative. (c) the mental health care needs of the minor cannot be met unless he or she is admitted as proposed and in particular, all community based alternatives to admission have been shown to have failed or are demonstrably unsuitable for the needs of the minor.

The nominated representative or an attendant appointed by the nominated representative shall under all circumstances stay with the minor in the mental health facility for the entire duration of the admission of the minor to the mental health facility. In the case of minor girls, where the nominated representative is male, a female attendant shall be appointed by the nominated representative and shall under all circumstances stay with the minor girl in the mental health facility for the entire duration of her admission'.

20.   The RPD Bill 2016 has done away with the notion of plenary guardianship opting for the provision of limited guardianship.

21.   As the MHC explains the right to an advanced directive is a declaration in writing how a person wishes to be treated in the event of a mental illness in the future: in terms of the following options: (i) the way the person wishes to be cared for and treated for a mental illness and/or; (ii) the way the person wishes not to be so cared for and treated for a mental illness and/or; (iii) the individual or individuals, in order of precedence, the person wants appointed as their nominated representative under Section 6 below in the event of his or her having a mental illness in the future.

REFERENCES

Addlakha, R. 2010a. 'Engendering Disability in the Developmental Agenda in India: A Policy Perspective'. In *Interrogating Social Development: Global Perspectives and Local Initiatives*, Debal K. Singharoy (ed.), pp. 269–300. New Delhi: Manohar.

———. 2010b. 'From Invalidation and Segregation to Recognition and Integration: Contemporary State, responses to Disability in India', *Occasional Paper Series* No. 55. Centre for Women's Development Studies.

———. 2011. 'Women's Health, Law and Culture in India: A Contemporary Perspective', *Stance: The Thai Feminist Review* 4(2553): 27–65.

———. 2013. *Disability Studies in India: Global Discourses, Local Realities*. New Delhi: Routledge.

Addlakha, R., Stuart Blume, Patrick J. Devlieger, Osamu Ngase, and MyriamWinance (eds). 2009. *Disability and Society: A Reader*. New Delhi: Orient Blackswan.

Barnes, Colin. 1991. *Disabled People in Britain and Discrimination: A Case for Anti-Discrimination Legislation*. London: C. Hurst & Co.

———. 1998. 'The Social Model of Disability: A Sociological Phenomenon Ignored by Sociologists?'. In *The Disability Reader: Social Science Perspectives*, Tom Shakespeare (ed.), pp. 65–78. London: Cassell.

Barnes, Colin and Geoff Mercer (eds). 1996. *Exploring the Divide: Illness and Disability*. Leeds: Disability Press.

Barnes, Colin, Mike Oliver, and Len Barton (eds). 2002. *Disability Studies Today*. Cambridge: Polity Press.

Bhambani, Meenu. 2005. 'The Politics of Disability Rights Movement in India', *International Journal of Disability Studies* 1(1): 3–28.

Davis, Lennard J. 1995. *Enforcing Normalcy: Disability, Deafness and the Body*. London: Verso.

Driedger, Diane. 1989. *The Last Civil Rights Movement*. London: C. Hurst & Co.

Finkelstein, Victor. 1980. *Attitudes and Disabled People: Issues for Discussion*. New York: World Rehabilitation Fund.

Government of India. 1982. National Mental Health Programme.

———. 1995. *Persons with Disabilities (Equal Opportunities, Protection of Rights and Full Participation) Act 1995*. Extraordinary Gazette of India Part II, Section I. New Delhi: Ministry of Law, Justice and Company Affairs. Available at: http://www.disabilityaffairs.gov.in/upload/uploadfiles/files/RPWD%20ACT%202016.pdf.

———. 2010. *Mental Health Care Act (Draft Document)*. New Delhi: Ministry of Women and Child Development. Available at: http://www.prsindia.org/uploads/media/draft/Draft%20Mental%20Health%20Care%20Act,%202010.pdf.

———. 2013. *The Mental Health Care Bill, 2013*. Bill No. LIV of 2013.

————. 2014. *The Rights of Persons with Disabilities Bill, 2014.* Bill No. 1 of 2014.

————. 2016. *The Rights of Persons with Disabilities.* Extraordinary Gazette of India Part II, Section 3 (i). New Delhi: Ministry of Law, Justice and Company Affairs. Available at http://lawmin.nic.in/ld/P-ACT/2016/A2016-49.pdf.

Linton, Simi. 1998. *Claiming Disability: Knowledge and Identity.* New York: New York University Press.

Mehrotra, N. 2011.'Disability Rights Movememnts in India: Politics and Practice', *Economic and Political Weekly* 46(6): 64–73.

Mental Health Act 1987. Available at: https://www.legalcrystal.com/act/51111/men. Accessed on 1 December 2016.

Oliver, Michael. 1990. *The Politics of Disablement: Critical Texts in Social Work and the Welfare State.* London: Macmillan Press.

————. 1996. *Understanding Disability: From Theory to Practice.* New York: St. Martin's Press.

Sundaresan, N. 2013. 'Tracking Disability through the United Nations'. In *Disability Studies in India: Global Discourses, Local Realities,* R. Addlakha (ed.), pp. 78–93. New Delhi: Routledge.

Union of the Physically Impaired Against Segregation (UPIAS). 1976. *Fundamental Principles of Disability.* London: UPIAS.

United Kingdom. Disability Discrimination Act 2005. Available at: https://www.legislation.gov.uk/ukpga/2005/13/contents., Accessed on: 1 December 2016.

United Nations. 2006. *United Nations Convention on the Rights of Persons with Disabilities.* Available at: http://www.un.org/disabilities/documents/convention/convoptprot-e.pdf. Accessed on 19 November 2014.

World Health Organization. 1980. *International Classification of Impairments, Disabilities and Handicaps* (ICIDH). Geneva: WHO Press. Available at http://whqlibdoc.who.int/publications/1980/9241541261_eng.pdf. Accessed on 15 January 2015.

————. 2001. *International Classification of Functioning, Disability and Health* (ICF). Geneva: WHO Press. Also available at: http://www.who.int/classifications/icf/zh/index.html. Accessed on 15 January 2015.

11

Caste, Class, and Gender on the Margins of the State

An Ethnographic Study among Community Health Workers

Madhumita Biswal

Ethnographic studies on the working of the state have gained considerable attention in the recent times (see for instance, Das and Poole 2004; Ferguson and Gupta 2002; Scott 1998; Sharma and Gupta 2006). One of the concerns of such ethnographic investigations is to critically engage with the interface between the bureaucratic apparatus of the state and local communities. This chapter attempts to focus on the activities at the points of intersection of the state and local community through an enquiry into the state-health interventions. Drawing on an ethnographic study[1] carried out in Boudh district of Odisha, the chapter engages with the working of the state at two levels. In the first part it tries to map how the Indian state-health discourse intervenes in the lives of women from marginalized communities through the routinized practices of its bureaucratic machinery. The second part examines questions of the identity of the institutional agents of the state, and how the embodiment of their identity intersects with their modern professionalism in everyday negotiations.

Partha Chatterjee (1997: 279) has observed that the postcolonial Indian state conceives its bureaucracy to be a 'universal class', 'working for the universal goals of the nation', and thereby claiming to be working on a single rational consciousness or will of the state. However, it may also be argued, as we do here, that the embodiment of the caste and gender identities of the institutional agents of the state seem to be playing an active role in giving expression to the practices of the state.

In the popular imageries of state, a dominant image is that of the state as an 'external and distant entity', which may be seen 'either as an oppressive intruder of the affairs of the local community or as a benevolent protector of people against local oppressors' that is determined contextually (Chatterjee 1997: 295–6). This imagery of state as up above the local communities is well articulated by Ferguson and Gupta (2002). They point out that notion of the supremacy of the state over local communities often tends to depict the state and local communities through spatial and scalar hierarchies, finding expression through verticality and encompassment. According to Ferguson and Gupta:

> Verticality refers to the central and pervasive idea of the state as an institution somehow 'above' civil society, community and family. Thus the state planning is inherently 'top down' and state actions are efforts to manipulate and plan 'from above', while 'the grassroots' contrasts with the state precisely in that it is 'below', closer to the ground, more authentic, and more 'rooted'. (2002: 982)

Being 'above' the local community, the main concern of the state is planning for the benevolence of local community and intervening in a top-down manner through its routinized functions of bureaucracy. In contrast to the state, local communities are perceived as 'on ground' (Ferguson and Gupta 2002: 982). Similarly, through the idea of encompassment the state is viewed as superior to, and encompassing the diverse institutions of power situated at the local level. However, the vertical imagery of the state has come under critical scrutiny. Community participation and democratic decentralization have been propagated as tools to counter such a top-down approach of the state.

The interesting paradox in India is that while, the state in principle ostensibly supports the notion and ideology of community participation, it is simultaneously ensuring its bureaucratic presence in village communities through the garb of community participation. In reality the vertical imagery of the state remains intact. For instance, in appointing community-level health workers, such as anganwadi workers (AWW) and accredited social health activists (ASHA), while the village community approval is sought in the guise of ensuring community participation. Once selected, the community-level health workers are easily inserted into the bureaucratic structures of the state. So these community-level health workers by virtue of occupying the space between the state and community are often perceived in terms of their dual roles: as agents of the state, located at the margins of the bureaucratic structure, and as representatives of the local community. This is true of both AWWs and ASHA workers.

These intersecting zones between community and state are of immense significance in the context of implementing state-health interventions because the community-level workers become the key agents in carrying forward the state agenda at the local level. In other words, these community-level health workers serve as village-level bureaucrats in carrying forward state agenda. In a way the villagers experience the state through these village-level bureaucrats routinely, everyday. In fact, the community-level health worker functioning in village space as an 'agent' of the state certainly challenges the dominant notion that the state is an 'external and distant entity'. The following section discusses how the assertion of the state power at the village level is made through the everyday mundane work of its village-level bureaucracies.

GENDER, CLASS, AND REPRODUCTIVE SURVEILLANCE

It has been well acknowledged in feminist scholarship on health that women's reproduction has gained specific attention in the post-colonial development discourse (Chatterjee and Riley 2001; Hollen 2003; Kumar 2006; Ram 1998). Myriad relationships among different sectors such as poverty, education, and health have come to be linked to women's reproductive behaviour. With the nation being drawn to the global ranking system of development, women's reproductive behaviour has come to be linked to indicators of development. Improper management of women's reproduction is conceived to be having the potential of creating an obstacle in India's narrative of development in the world stage. Generating knowledge about women's reproductive behaviour, extensive planning, and surveillance remains a key in designing development interventions. This rationale takes an elaborate form in the everyday pedagogical functions of the state.

In the everyday practices, the increasing intervention of professionals has become a reality (also see Anagnost 1995; Escobar 2010). However, scholars like Ram (2001) and Hollen (2003) also point out that in this discourse not all women are drawn to the statist developmental discourse on an equal footing. Women from marginalized categories such as rural women, urban slum women, tribal women, dalit women, and women from Muslim community are constructed as the problem categories, responsible for the backwardness of the country. Hence, most of the interventions are directed towards these women. Further, scholars like Mohan Rao (2004) observe that the dominance of selective primary health care (SPHC) approach in the Indian development discourse makes it impossible to acknowledge the structural issues involved in generating the health problems. Rather, health problems have come to be individualized and considered as problems which could be sorted out through the technical interventions of the health functionaries.

Based on a field study conducted among the community-level health workers in the Baunsuni Block of Boudh district of Odisha, we attempt here to map how rural women are drawn into the development discourse through the mundane routinized activity of the bureaucratic machinery. In the rural areas a series of developmental institutional agents like AWWs, ASHAs, Auxiliary Nurse Midwives, and Lady Health Visitors, whatever their stated roles, are charged with reforming women's reproductive behaviour in different ways. Village-level health workers, such as, the AWW and ASHA, for instance, are often projected as the symbols of community participation. In 1975, the Government of India had launched the Integrated Child Development Services (ICDS) programme, through which initiatives were made to appoint AWWs in villages. A woman from among the village community was appointed as AWW. Her responsibility was to look after the health and nutritional needs of mothers and children. The Integrated Child Development Services project was launched in the Boudh District of Odisha in 1993. Further, in 2005, another rung of community-level workers, ASHAs were introduced through National Rural Health Mission. Like the Anganwadi worker, the ASHA is also necessarily a woman functionary, selected from the village community that she is required to serve.

Most of the community-level health workers are women. The gendered nature of the state in drawing women from the economically weaker sections to underpaid, low remuneration community welfare work has been highlighted in feminist scholarship (Dressel 1987; Kabeer 1994). However, the introduction of different layers of women bureaucratic agents is of immense significance. On the one hand, in employing primarily women as community-level workers, the state in a way proactively acknowledges women's health needs, and more particularly, women's reproductive health needs as its main concern.

On the other hand, since the community-level health workers (mainly AWWS and ASHAs) are members of the village community, the state is ever present in the village through these bureaucratic agents.

Such insertion of the bureaucratic agents in the village space keeps women in a double bind. Community-level workers are key agents in making available the state health services, in situations of desperate need. From another angle, now women, are not only under biomedical scrutiny when they visit hospitals, but by virtue of the state health agents being located within the village space, ordinary women can no longer easily escape the statist gaze (also see Ram 1998: 114–43). Working close to village women, as they do, these community-level workers can exercise close scrutiny over women's behaviour. This is well reflected in the views of some of the AWWs. According to one of the Anganwadi workers:

> In the village we establish good rapport with most of the Self Help Group (SHG) women, who inform us about the new pregnancy cases in the village. We also get to know about the pregnancy cases through our daily home visits, from neighbors and while talking to women in the village. After getting confirmation about a pregnancy case, we keep track of the person. After completion of three months of pregnancy we dispense the first TT to the expectant mother and provide iron-folic acid tablets, which she is asked to consume regularly. The woman is also given chloroquine tablets and told about the procedures of consumption. The pregnant woman is asked to attend health camp every month, and is also provided with supplementary food by the Anganwadi centre from the month she takes her first TT. In the fifth month of pregnancy another TT injection is given. In every health camp we enquire whether the woman is taking the iron-folic acid tablets and chloroquine tablets properly or not. Through our daily visits also we ensure that the woman takes medicines properly. When women do not agree to take TT and other medicines during pregnancy we persuade them, and if they do not agree the ANM of the locality and the PHC doctor try to persuade them. From seventh month onwards we ask the pregnant woman to take proper food and also ask them to remain prepared for the delivery. They are supposed to inform ASHA as soon as the delivery pain comes and go to the health centre for child birth.
>
> (Extracts from fieldwork)

The above narrative foregrounds the complexities involved in such a close scrutiny of women's behaviour. For instance, what happens when women refuse to conform to the prescribed medical practices that operationalize the medicalized reformatory agenda of the state (as for instance, if a woman were to refuse to take TT or chloroquine or refuses regular medical checkups or to go for hospital delivery)? The moment women refuse to conform to the medicalized discourse propagated through the village-level bureaucrats, they come to be labelled as irresponsible, superstitious, stubborn, backward women, responsible for risking the life of their children as well as themselves. Responsible behaviour gets defined as that which is in agreement with the highly medicalized discourse. Their nonconformity to the statist agenda makes them subjected to persuasion by various state functionaries. This vocabulary of persuasion in actual practice turns out to be a pressure building mechanism.

Through a series of bio-medically rationalized interventions such as hospitalization of childbirth, medicalization of pregnancy and child-rearing practices, execution of sterilization and sanitation programmes, women become the key objects of statist reformist agenda. This idea of reformed, responsible woman is very much structured by their caste and class location. Many illustrations maybe cited of the way in which the lower-caste and lower-class women confront the class-based challenges in their everyday life in meeting this normative standard of responsible motherhood. We elaborate two examples.

Over the last few decades there has been a renewed focus on breastfeeding that has been operationalized at the community level by the state's functionaries. In the villages the main agenda is to prompt women to adopt breastfeeding, promoting it as being a scientifically approved method. Many breastfeeding campaigns have taken place at the PHC sub-centre level over the last few years in the Baunsuni PHC area. Health functionaries counsel women to exclusively breastfeed new born children for at least six months. Not surprisingly it is the lower class labouring women who bear the brunt of such campaigns. An older generation of lower-class women are now being glorified for having 'traditionally' breastfed their children, while new mothers are perceived as challengers who may upset such 'traditional' practices through their 'irresponsibility' (Hollen 2003). In recasting an old and traditional practice as a scientific/ medical practice in whatever the situation, the health workers/agents of the state acquire the moral authority to judge rural women from a lower-class. This is reflected in the narrations of an Anganwadi worker:

> In this locality, many women do not take care of their children properly. After two-three months of their delivery, they join the work in the field by leaving the child under the supervision of some family members.

Mothers need to pay full attention to their children during their infancy. The agricultural ripping period is going to start from next month. From now onwards the mothers will be busy in the agricultural work for coming five to six months. Under my Anganwadi center now all the children are in the 'normal' category. But I know in the coming two months the children's health standard is going to fall. Since most of the mothers will be busy in the agricultural work, they will not take proper care of their children. Therefore, during agricultural season we need to pressurize mothers and remind them more often to take proper care of their children.

(Extracts from fieldwork)

It is evident that this is one of the pathways by which the health worker gets to shift the responsibility of the well-being of the child entirely on the woman rather than the state's health system and social conditions. This also relieves the entire family/community from the responsibilities of child care. A biological function, that of breastfeeding, becomes the linchpin for the statist reordering of social relationships.

There has been constant advocacy by the state to promote hospitalization for childbirth. Different schemes are initiated to lure poor women to use hospital for childbirth. In 2005, the Janani Surakshya Yojana was launched through National Rural Health Mission. This scheme was to bring modifications in the maternity benefit scheme. It further intended to integrate antenatal care during pregnancy, institutional care during delivery, and immediate post-partum period. Through this scheme institutional delivery was promoted, by providing financial assistance to women who go through hospital delivery. While the programme promised cash benefits to women up to two live births, the monetary assistance for the third childbirth was assured to women only if they accepted sterilization after the third delivery. Further, for undergoing family planning operation after delivery, women were assured additional cash incentive (Government of India 2005).

As is evident, hospitalization for childbirth is very closely tied to family planning programme in general and female sterilization, in particular. One of the major duties of ASHAs in the villages is to motivate the pregnant women for hospital delivery and accompany them to hospital for delivery. And since most of these women are from the poorer classes, it is they who are the main targets of the statist propaganda of female sterilization. So the scheme indirectly pressurizes them to seek sterilization. The statist agenda of hospitalization for childbirth may be seen as a ploy to regulate and discipline the reproduction of women from lower economic background.

The vertical/hierarchical imagery of the state gets well defined through the mundane routinized practices of community-level health functionaries. They become the key institutional agents through whom the verticality of the state gets well depicted. For example, one of the main responsibilities of the Anganwadi worker is to maintain records of the weights of children in her Anganwadi area. As part of the job, she is expected to persuade mothers to be very attentive towards maintaining a certain weight level of the children. The Anaganwadi worker while on the one hand exercises surveillance over women's child-rearing practices, on the other hand her own managerial skills are closely scrutinized by her higher authorities, her supervisors. The Anganwadi workers, being in the lowest rung of the hierarchy in the state machinery also remains a vulnerable worker, who is prone to be blamed as being irresponsible and/ or inefficient. Her efficiency is determined by her ability to pressurize the mothers to ensure their children do not fall out of the 'normal' contour, the normal standards. This fact that she performs her job efficiently lends weight to her moral authority to intervene in the reproductive health behaviour of women.

COMMUNITY HEALTH WORKERS' EVERYDAY NEGOTIATIONS WITH GENDER, CASTE, AND PROFESSION

In discussion so far the institutional agents of the state mainly appear to be guided by the statist ideology of class inequality. As agents of the state, they are ideally expected to take up the 'universal roles' and their embodied caste, class, ethnic, and religious identity, is expected not to interfere with their professional responsibility. However, the fieldwork among the community-level health workers in Baunsuni reveals that the caste identities of women play a crucial role in not only determining who can be a suitable community health worker, but also how the community health worker is going to deliver her service.

Scholars like Debabar Banerji (1982) and Mark Nichter (1986) have pointed to the way the democratic process is subjugated by the village power structure to serve the interests of the privileged communities. Such a trend is also well reflected in my field site. The caste of the women remains a major influencing factor in the appointment of the community-level workers such as AWWs and ASHAs. They are seen as symbols of community participation. Hence, the involvement of the village community is sought during their recruitment. The Baunsuni sector of ICDS programme has 21 Anganwadi centres and every centre has one Anganwadi worker. Of these 21 Anganwadi workers five are from Brahmin castes, 13 are from Other Backward caste groups,[2] more particularly belonging to Dumbal, Hatua, Teli, Sudo, Bhulia Meher, and Bania castes, and one is from Keuta[3] caste, a group that is a recent entrant to the Scheduled Caste category. Two of the AWWs are from Scheduled Caste categories, considered to be untouchables[4] (who self-identify themselves as 'harijans'). So although the Brahmins are a minority community in Boudh district, they form a sizeable number of AWWs. Further, the discussions surrounding the appointment of ASHA in the village showed that castes of the women become a major decisive factor in their appointment.

Recent studies on community-level workers especially ASHAs have mainly drawn attention to the functioning of the ASHA in the local village community (see Roalkvam 2014), the mutual trust of relationship between ASHA and villagers (Mishra 2014), performance of ASHAs (Bajpai and Dholakia 2011). Though a study by Farah N. Fathima et al. (2015) in Karnataka has focused on the selection processes of the ASHAs, they have mainly drawn attention to the participants' class backgrounds.

As stated earlier, the involvement of the institutions of the village community, such as, *gram sabha*, the village panchayat, and the village heath and sanitation committee is required in the selection of ASHA (Government of India 2005). ANMs and male multipurpose health workers also play observer roles in the selection process of ASHA, while the AWWs of the village along with the village committee members play an important role. The responses of the AWWs, ANMs, and Multipurpose Health Workers (MPHWs) of the Baunsuni PHC, make it clear that women from the untouchable Dalit communities are least likely to be appointed as ASHA. They point out that on most occasions the members of the gram sabha and the panchayat do not want to appoint an ASHA belonging to untouchable Dalit group. According to one of the ANMs in the Baunsuni PHC:

> No harijan woman is selected in our sub-centre area as ASHA. In one of the villages, one woman belonging to the harijan caste community had applied for the post. Though I was interested to select her, the village committee did not want to select a harijan woman as ASHA. Hence, I could not do anything. In most cases the Anganwadiworker does not want to select an ASHA from harijan caste communities, because she has to work with her on a day-to-day basis. Again the village committee

and the panchayat have to get involved in the selection of ASHA, and they do not want to appoint a woman belonging to the harijan caste group. They want to accommodate a woman who belongs to their touchable caste. Hence, the selection of a harijan woman as ASHA becomes difficult.

(Extracts from fieldwork)

While most of the time though the ANMs, AWWs, and MPHWs in their own way contribute in producing such a hegemonic discourse, the responsibility for such decisions is often shifted to the other members. However, some of the ANMs and MPHWs belonging to the untouchable Dalit community pointed to the fact that as a survival strategy, they often consciously take a decision of not supporting the candidature of applicants belonging to their community. One of the MPHWs of Baunsuni PHC said:

Nine ASHAs have been selected in our sub-centre area. Though one ASHA is from scheduled caste, she is from touchable keuta caste. Because of the caste feeling, women belonging to untouchable communities do not get appointed as ASHA. Though I belong to a *harijan* caste, I have not selected a single ASHA who belongs to my caste. Even though sometimes women belonging to my community apply for the post, I am compelled to support the candidature of an upper caste woman rather than the woman belonging to my caste. To survive in the locality I need to be in good terms with the panchayat and the village leaders. If I support the candidature of a woman belonging to my community as ASHA, the village community is going to stand against me. Hence to avoid such situation, most of the time I advise the interested candidates from my caste community not to apply for the post.

(Extracts from fieldwork)

In most village communities women belonging to the untouchable Dalit groups are, clearly, the least preferred candidates for the ASHA post. It is easy to see that what gets recognized as the 'village community' is, in fact, the dominant section of the village. Hence, their hegemonic public opinion gets construed as *the* 'public opinion' of the village. Though the state's guidelines for the formation of village health committee emphasizes the involvement of members belonging to the Scheduled Caste, the 'touchable' caste like Keuta caste is most often preferred and co-opted as the representative of the Scheduled caste community rather than a person belonging to the untouchable Dalit groups.

The testimony of one of the respondents draws attention to the fact that on one of the occasions only one untouchable Dalit woman had applied for the post and while the village committee had to give its approval for her appointment, the ANM of the locality openly expressed her displeasure over her appointment. According to her, women from the touchable caste groups would have access to the households of the upper caste groups, while a lower caste woman would not be entertained by the upper caste households. In such articulation the interest of the upper caste groups comes to be equated with the interest of the village community as a whole.

On a few occasions, the ANMs and MPHWs perceived that the lower caste women are the most suitable candidates for the ASHA post because, the ASHAs have to deal with women during their childbirth period, which is considered to be polluting. It was argued, as an ASHA is required to escort and accompany women to the health centre during their pregnancy and engage with neonatal care (considered to be a polluting state), women from lower caste groups would be more suitable. As an ANM pointed out:

> In our sub-centre area two ASHAs are from 'untouchable' *ganda* community. People were initially opposing the appointment of these women as ASHAs. Though some upper caste women had applied for the post, none of them were meeting the eligibility criteria. The women belonging to the lower caste communities were meeting the eligibility criteria. Hence I convinced the villagers saying, if an 'untouchable' woman becomes an ASHA, she need not touch you always and go to your home. She is mostly required to help women during their pregnancy and after pregnancy. Anyway, women stay in a pollution state till the fifth day of their pregnancy. Hence, the physical contact of an untouchable ASHA is not going to be a problem during the pollution state of women. And after fifth day, anyway women are going to purify themselves. Since ASHA is going to help women during pollution state, lower caste women are good for such job.
>
> (Extracts from fieldwork, emphasis present in original)

To interpret the above, upper caste women are often invited into the statist discourse in taking up the public role of being the agents of development with an unmarked universalized identity. However, the lower caste women enter into such a discourse of development only as governed bodies and objects of surveillance. Here, it is interesting to note that when lower caste women's inclusion in the public role is sought, their caste marked stigmatized bodily identity itself becomes the idiom through which their entry gets legitimized (see Pinto 2006).

Even though upper caste women enjoy the advantageous position of taking up public role in getting appointed as community-level health workers, they cannot afford to emphatically shun social contacts with the lower caste communities. They are required to exercise a 'statist gaze' over the lower caste community women, as a part of their bureaucratic function. However, this does not mean the disappearance of the practice of caste from the lives of these modern professionals. In the pursuit of professionalism, new boundaries seem to have been drawn. Many frontline health workers in the field articulate this duality of roles. According to an AWW:

> Children from all caste groups come to study in the Anganwadi. We do not practice any kind of caste discrimination. But while serving food to children in the Anganwadi centre, the upper caste children are served food in the Anganwadi and the children from harijan caste groups are sent home with the food. They are not served food in the Anganwadi. This system has been practiced because the upper caste groups do not want their children to sit beside a child belonging to the harijan caste group, while having their food. I need to conform to some of the minimum caste norms as a woman from upper caste group.
>
> (Extracts from fieldwork)

Further she says:

> In this village I have survived as an Anganwadi worker because I have tried to strike a balance between the upper caste groups and the harijans. I do not neglect harijans while providing service. While delivering the service I have to keep in mind the interests of both the upper caste groups and the harijans. For instance, while measuring the weight of children, I cannot skip measuring the weight of harijan children. If I come to the upper caste pada after measuring the weight of harijan children, the upper caste people will not allow me to measure the weight of their children. Hence I try to solve the problem by measuring the weight of upper caste children in the morning and going to the harijanpada in the afternoon to measure the weight of their children, on the health check up days. Being a married woman from a Brahmin caste, I also need to conform to the customs of the family and caste. Hence each time I come in contact with the untouchable communities I take bath before entering into the inner space of house.
>
> (Extracts from fieldwork)

One often encounters situations where the interests of state actors comfortably colludes with the dominant group interest, resulting in keeping the lower caste groups at the margins in accessing state services.

However, such a discriminatory attitude often seeks a refuge through the justification such as 'facing pressure' from 'village community'. The community-level health workers often find an escape route by putting the blame on the 'village community', which seem to be less accountable. Further, the community-level health workers from the dominant communities often try to justify their own caste practices through suggesting dichotomies in their roles and practices in terms of public/private, state/familial responsibility. They often try to justify their attempts of maintaining bodily purity, by taking a bath each time they come in contact with the untouchable castes, as a private practice, which does not come into conflict with their public roles.

Gopal Guru (2009b: 55) suggests this kind of dichotomization of space into public/private and domestic/state provides an opportunity to 'feel sovereign over controlling the domestic space'. Such sovereignty remains unattainable in continuous time and space. Hence, fragmentation of time and space gives the upper caste health functionaries an opportunity to escape from the universal identity and feel sovereign at the domestic space. This fragmentation of time and space allows them to perform two seemingly contradictory roles such as conforming to the dominant gender role of being the bearer of caste purity on the one hand, and taking on the universal role of health worker of the whole village community on the other hand. The attempt of conforming to the gender-based caste norm is expressed in several ways, such as taking care to maintain bodily purity by making minimal visits to untouchable Dalit pada and taking a bath after each visit. Fragmentation of time and space is also achieved through arranging separate time slots for untouchable Dalit women and upper caste women for health checkups and food distribution.

While the upper-caste community health workers can often afford to have the luxury of fragmenting their time and space in performing their professional responsibility, community-level health workers from the untouchable communities enter their public roles with a deep sense of reduction (also see Guru 2009a). The acceptance of servility by the community health workers belonging to untouchable communities, becomes one of the ways through which the cordial relation with the village community is sought. This exercise of self-restraint while performing her public role is evident with the discussion with an AWW belonging to untouchable caste:

> Though the Anaganwadi worker is supposed to measure the weight of children, I cannot measure the weight of upper caste children because

of my caste status. The upper caste people will not like me to touch their children and measure their weight. I also need to maintain cordial relation with all the caste groups. Hence I abide by all the caste rules and do not try to transgress it. The Anganwadi helper, who is from gaud caste (a middle level caste), measures the weight of upper caste children and I only stand at a distance and monitor it and note down the weight of children. Also during cooking food and serving food in the Anganwadi, I keep a distance from the site.

(Extracts from fieldwork)

So far the discussion has focused on how the community health workers' complicity is established with the hegemonic caste interest in the village community. This in turn gives us the impression that these hegemonic tendencies go uncontested. However, voices from the field often reinstate the fact that assertion against such domination is often made, though not in an organized form. Further, in such cases of fragmented assertions one may witness that different power structures, from state machineries to non-state actors, try to come together to suppress such assertion.

An incident involving the shifting of an Anganwadi centre from a space located at the interface of the 'untouchable' Dalit pada and upper caste pada to a 'proper' upper caste pada of the village demonstrates the way the assertions by the untouchable caste groups are suppressed. In that village in the Baunsuni Block, initially the Anganwadi centre was established at a space very closer to untouchable pada, at one end of the upper caste pada. As the general practice in almost all the Anganwadi centres in Baunsuni, here too cooked food was being served only to upper caste children with the untouchable children being sent home with their share (since neither the AWW nor the helper, both upper caste women, wanted to clean up after these children had eaten).

At some point, a member of the untouchable caste group came inside the Anganwadi and demanded that either the children belonging to untouchable castes should also be served food inside the Centre, or no child should be served food inside. This incident was, later deliberately misconstrued as the unreasonable demands of drunken man, projecting it to be an attack on the modesty of the AWW and her helper. Hence, a demand for social justice, that is, assertion of the right of the children from untouchable communities to consume food within Anganwadi centre, got construed as an act outraging the modesty of upper caste women. The village committee, Anganwadi supervisor, as well as

Community Development Project Officer of ICDS (CDPO) held meetings and decided to shift the Anganwadi centre to the upper caste pada. To be sure, the shifting of the Anganwadi in a way was seen as a response to a larger change in the village landscape, where untouchable Dalits were seen to be overstepping the limits of their caste status, which is defined by submissiveness (also see Kannabiran and Kannabiran 2003: 249–59). In such a situation, it was seen to be dangerous for the upper caste women to perform their public role in the space. This incident draws our attention to the complex ways in which gender and caste intersect.

* * *

The chapter began with analysing the dominant imaginary of the state as a supreme agent over the local communities, as discussed in the scholarship. It is also argued that the state justifies its position based on the claim that it works on a rational principle vis-à-vis the supposedly irrationality of the local communities. Planning and intervening in the lives of local communities through its bureaucratic apparatus, for the benevolence of the local communities is projected to be the main concern of the state. However, the study with community-level health workers in the Boudh district of Odisha shows that though the state tries to project itself to be working on a principle of universal rationality, class, caste, and gender bias remain an underneath theme. Women from marginalized categories become the main target of the statist health interventions, who are in many ways pressurized to conform to the biomedical agenda of the state. Further, in analysing the everyday routinized practices of the CHWs in delivering their services across caste groups also challenges the dichotomized understanding of state and local communities. The bureaucratic hierarchy of the state and the hierarchies of the local communities seem to converge on many occasions. What could be derived from the working of the state agents at the local level is that through dispersed communitarian networks the state power is coordinated and consolidated. Hence, the caste and gender hegemonies at the local level could be seen to be playing a crucial role in the statist process of governance. In contrast to Ferguson and Gupta's proposition that hierarchized model of state and local communities gets challenged in contemporary times with new forms of transnational governmentality, the chapter argues that even outside the transnational networks, the way the interaction between state and local communities gets played out on a day-to-day basis, such neatly hierarchized model of state vis-à-vis local communities also gets challenged.

NOTES

1. This chapter draws on an ethnographic study conducted during 2006–07 among the community level health workers in the Baunsuni Block of Boudh District of Odisha. The broader term community level health workers, is used in the study to refer to the grassroot level health workers such as Anganwadi workers (AWWs), Auxiliary Nurse Midwives (ANMs) and Multi-Purpose Health Workers (MPHWs). Though AWWs, ANMs, MPHWs broadly carry out the health services, they belong to different institutional setups. While the ANMs and MPHWs are a part of the state health sector, the Aangnwadi Worker functions as a part of the Integrated Child Development Services (ICDS) programme. In-depth interviews were carried out with all the 21 AWWs of the Baunsuni sector of the Boudh Sadar Block ICDS programme. In addition to this, responses were also collected from 16 ANMs and 12 MPHWs. The years 2006 and 2007 mark a significant period in terms of the study with the community level health workers, because in the year 2005 NRHM was launched, which introduced a new rank of community level health worker ASHA. During 2006 and 2007 the procedures of appointment ASHAs was getting carried out in the Baunsuni PHC area. This particular time becomes significant because enthusiastic discussions about the suitability of diverse categories of women for the post of ASHA was carried out among both community level health functionaries as well as different sections of population within the village community.

2. Boudh district is considered as one of the Backward caste zones, having high concentration of population belonging to backward caste groups. As per 2001 census, the scheduled caste population of the district is as high as 21.90 per cent in comparison to the state average of 16.20 per cent.

3. The Keuta caste community is formally included in the scheduled caste category in Orissa in the year 2002. Since, the community belongs to a touchable caste group, on most occasions the village community members find it most convenient to include Keuta caste group member for fulfilling the requirement of scheduled caste representative, rather than including a person who belongs to untouchable caste group.

4. In the context of inclusion of Keuta and Dhibara caste groups in the Scheduled Caste category, the ex-untouchable communities have started organizing protest against such inclusion. The organized protest has started reclaiming the untouchable identity, by forming an organization named 'Asprusya Dalit Sarankhyana Surakshya Samiti'. Hence, hereafter I would be using the term 'untouchable Dalits' to refer to the Dalit caste groups who have been historically subjected to untouchability.

REFERENCES

Anagnost, Ann. 1995. 'A Surfeit of Bodies: Population and the Rationality of the State in Post-Mao China'. In *Conceiving the New World Order: The Global Politics of Reproduction*, F. Ginsburg and R. Rapp (eds), pp. 22–41. Berkeley: University of California Press.

Bajpai, Nirupam and Ravindra H. Dholakia. 2011. 'Improving the Performance of Accredited Social Health Activists in India', *Working Paper no-1, Working Paper series*. Columbia Global Centres South Asia, Columbia University.

Banerji, Debabar. 1982. *Poverty, Class and Health Culture in India*, Volume 1. New Delhi: Prachi Prakashan.

Chatterjee, Nilanjana and Nancy E. Riley. 2001. 'Planning an Indian Modernity: The Gendered Politics of Fertility Control', *Signs* 26(3): 811–45.

Chatterjee, Partha. 1997, 'Development Planning and the Indian State'. In *State and Politics in India*, Partha Chatterjee (ed.), pp. 271–97. New Delhi: Oxford University Press.

Das, Veena and Deborah Poole (eds). 2004. *Anthropology in the Margins of the State*. Santa Fe: School of American Research Press.

Dressel, Paula. 1987. 'Patriarchy and Social Welfare Work', *Social Problems* 34(3): 294–309.

Escobar, Arturo. 2010. 'Planning'. In *The Development Dictionary: A Guide to Knowledge as Power*, Wolfgang Sachs (ed.), pp. 145–60. London: Zed Books.

Fathima, Farah M., Mohan Raju, Kiruba S. Varadharejan, Aditi Krishnamurthy, S.R. Ananthkumar, Prem K. Mony. 2015. 'Assessment of "Accredited Social Health Activists"—A National Community Health Volunteer Scheme in Karnataka State India', *Journal of Health, Population and Nutrition* 33(1): 137–45.

Ferguson, James and Akhil Gupta. 2002. 'Spatializing States: Toward an Ethnography of Neoliberal Governmentality', *American Ethnologist* 29(4): 981–1002.

Government of India. 2005. *National Rural Health Mission: Framework for Implementation 2005–2012*. New Delhi: Ministry of Health and Family Welfare.

Guru, Gopal. 2009a. 'Rejection of Rejection: Foregrounding Self Respect'. In *Humiliation: Claims and Context*, Gopal Guru (ed.), pp. 209–25. New Delhi: Oxford University Press.

———. 2009b. 'Archaeology of Untouchability', *Economic and Political Weekly* 44(37): 49–56.

Hollen, Cecilia Van. 2003. *Birth on the Threshold: Childbirth and Modernity in South India*. Berkeley: University of California Press.

Kabeer, Naila. 1994. *Reversed Realitites: Gender Hierarchies in Development Thought*. London: Verso.

Kannabiran, Vasanth and Kalpana Kannabiran. 2003. 'Gender and Caste: Understanding Dynamics of Power and Violence'. In *Gender and Caste:*

Issues in Contemporary India, Anupama Rao (ed.), pp. 249–60. New Delhi: Kali for Women.

Kumar, Rachel Simon. 2006. *'Marketing' Reproduction? Ideology and Population Policy in India*. New Delhi: Zubaan.

Mishra, Arima. 2014. 'Trust and Teamwork Matter: "Community Health Workers' Experiences in Integrated Service Delivery in India"', *Global Public Health: An International Journal of Research, Policy and Practice* 9(8): 960–74.

Nichter, Mark A. 1986. 'The Primary Health Centre as a Social System: PHC, Social Status and the Issue of Team-work in South Asia', *Social Science and Medicine* 23(4): 347–55.

Pinto. Sarah. 2006. 'More than a Dai', *Seminar* 558. February, 41–50.

Ram, Kalpana. 1998. 'Maternity and the Story of Enlightenment in the Colonies: Tamil Coastal Women, South India'. In *Maternities and Modernities: Colonial and Post-Colonial Experiences in Asia and Pacific*, Kalpana Ram and Margaret Jolly (eds), pp. 114–43. Cambridge: Cambridge University Press.

———. 2001. 'Rationalizing Fecund Bodies: Family Planning Policy and the Modern Indian Nation-State'. In *Borders of Being: Citizenship, Fertility and Sexuality in Asia and the Pacific*, in Margaret Jolly and Kalpana Ram (eds), pp. 82–117. Ann Arbor: The University of Michigan Press.

Rao, Mohan. 2004. *From Population Control to Reproductive Health: Malthusian Arithmetic*. New Delhi: Sage.

Roalkvam, Sidsel. 2014. 'Health Governance in India: Citizenship as Situated Practice', *Global Public Health: An International Journal for Research, Policy and Practice* 9(8): 910–26.

Sharma, Aradhana and Akhil Gupta (eds). 2006. *The Anthropology of the State: A Reader*. Malden, USA: Blackwell Publishing Ltd.

Scott, James C. 1998. *Seeing Like a State: How Certain Schemes to Improve the Human Condition have Failed*. New Haven, CT: Yale University Press.

12

Legitimizing Violence
A Narrative of Sexual Health

Asima Jena

If caste, class, poverty, religion, and gender are the more familiar axes of discrimination, sexuality is clearly another axis along which women face certain kinds of violence. This chapter delineates violence from sexual axis by treating regulation of sexuality, that is, sexual policing as a form of violence albeit its legitimacy. The governance of sexuality takes place through the production of discourse, which orders the subjective position and persuasive approach. In a Foucauldian sense, it conceives violence both at corporeal level as well as metaphoric level. This chapter explains how the routine monitoring of the sexual activities of the female sex workers (FSWs) are met with resistance. Further, how social inequality, subjugation, and stigma that gets reproduced through the discourses of community-oriented sexually transmitted infection (STI) management programme has been elaborated. It also argues that this community-oriented STI management programme is part and parcel of neo-liberal economic policy, which scripted the withdrawal of state by slashing budget for the social sector including health.

Violence and health are closely interconnected and the struggle to end sexual violence, in discourse and practice, has been central to health analysis and practice. The widespread violence of men against women, whether physical, sexual, or psychological, has its roots in patriarchal power structures, ideas, and practices. In fact, it has been a major collective task to identify how sexual violence is played out at all levels of power structures within both the private and public realms. This presupposes the availability of health care to strategize and respond to violence. However, the most challenging task is—how to articulate or theorize sexual violence in a social milieu where violence has been rationalized and has become a regular occurrence than the exception in the daily lives of the marginalized. Clearly, this concern accelerates with the existence of different kinds of sexual violence and the assignment of unequal values to these multitudes. In other words, the violence of normal times is neither equally condemned nor even equally recognized (Kannabiran 2005). Thus, for instance, in the 16 December 2012 Delhi gang rape case, it is argued that the system or 'state apparatus' needs to be empowered to curb these incidents. However, in the case of rape and sexual violence in conflict zones of India (the North-East states, Jammu and Kashmir, and Naxalite zones), it is a known fact that it is the very system that has used rape as a weapon to control dissent or voice against the state, particularly the armed occupation (Kannabiran 2005; Mittal 2015). In the case of the latter, violence against women is tolerated and repressed by underscoring the security of the nation state. As a result, violence becomes an everyday affair and so ubiquitous in the lives of women from marginalized backgrounds like Dalit women, Muslim women, lesbian women, women in sex work, that it is no longer seen as a serious issue. As Phadke (2010) asks, 'Is it the internalization of these power hierarchies that certain kinds of violence, exercises of power, appear legitimate?'

The legitimacy of violence is not just confined to the sphere of geopolitical security. Rather, this notion of security is extended to the realm of health. Sexual minorities have faced discrimination and criminalization in the past on the pretext of maintaining health security. For instance, the panic around sexual health reinforced the puritanical and moralistic agenda like deportation and repatriation of FSWs, incarceration of intravenous drug users, and tight measures against female migration by conflating trafficking and migration with sex work (Desouza 2004; Gopal 2013; Kotiswaran 2012; Ramasubban 1998; Shah 2006; Seshu 2005). While this approach is a reactionary and conservative stance on the issue of HIV/AIDS, another approach stresses the significance of the prevention of HIV infection, the tackling of workplace discrimination, and the striving for workplace equality and rights. This latter approach is understood to be progressive and community-oriented.

This chapter narrates the experience of violence experienced by a sexual minority community, FSWs, in their participation in community-led STI management programme, which is otherwise termed as anti-discriminatory and equality-based. It suggests that this community-driven health programme is also limited and paradoxical in some important respects and, in particular, is limited by a lack of recognition of issues of sexuality (Adkins 2002). Secondly, while delineating the story of violence in the everyday lives of FSWs, it does not see violence in straightforward manner, that is, physical violence, nor does it deal with violence in a symbolic or metaphoric sense. Rather, it explains violence in a much more complex manner, in its corporeal as well as representational terms. But what makes it further perplexing is when this violence is regarded as 'rational' or 'legitimized' from a public health view by simultaneously categorizing the workers as 'danger' and as 'agents of change'. By drawing from Foucauldian concept of 'governmentality' that Foucault treats as a form of violence (Gordon 1991), this chapter analyses the resistances of FSWs in Rajahmundry against asymptomatic case management, which is a treatment component in STI management programme and a prevention strategy of HIV/AIDS through community participation. Following Tambe (2009), Ghosh (2005), and others, I consider this as ethically sound that FSWs should not be the targets of the many forms of violence to which they are routinely subjected. In this direction, this chapter explains how social inequality, stigma, and marginality get reproduced when state and civil society are consistently engaged in surveillance of sexual minorities. This chapter is structured into four sections. The first section provides the broader social context through which the community-oriented STI management programme was initiated. The next section examines the daily surveillance of FSWs through a persuasive approach. The third section narrates the characteristics of surveillance, its inter-linkages with macro-political process, and FSWs' protest against STI management programme and the final section discusses the legitimization of sexual violence and explains why this violence has to be questioned.

This chapter draws from the experiences of a research project, Project Parivartan, as part of the Avahan programme[1] to study the implementation and impact of a peer-led structural intervention among FSWs in Rajahmundry, Andhra Pradesh, India. Avahan was a global health initiative and funded by Bill and Melinda Gates Foundation to prevent HIV/AIDS among FSWs, drug users, and men who have sex with men (MSMs) in six states of India through a three-prong strategy—collectivization through community mobilization, empowerment in terms of community ownership of the health project, and provision of conducive environment via advocacy against police violence, stigma, and ostracization.[2]

SITUATING COMMUNITY-CENTRIC STI MANAGEMENT PROGRAMME

Before outlining the kind of violence FSWs were subjected to and subversion tactics deployed by FSWs, here is a brief background of the community-centric STI management programme that explains the context (larger as well as specific) through which this programme was operationalized in Rajahmundry. The paranoia and sexual tag associated with HIV/AIDS, influenced the public as well as the state response in early 1990s till 2000. Public health initiatives were reductionists and individualistic in terms of prescribing self-control in order to change individual lifestyle and behaviour such as abstinence, prohibition of premarital and extra-marital sex, condom use, and others—along with greater policing in order to purify social bodies.

The AIDS Prevention Bill (1989) provided policing powers to the health authority to force high-risk groups (essentially implying FSWs) to accept mandatory testing, prosecuting MSM on the grounds of upholding national values or Hindu values. Thus not surprisingly, even as sexual minorities became the object of control they continued to face stigma and discrimination, police atrocities, and so on, which became the main impediments for the HIV prevention programme. These stringent measures received criticism from public health activists, lawyers, feminist scholars as well as international civil society on the grounds of violation of human rights and prompted the evolution of a different approach to tackle HIV/AIDS among the marginalized community (Grover 2005; Kotiswaran 2001: 174). Correspondingly, the successful STI reduction among FSWs of Sonagachi of West Bengal through a community-led health intervention provided an impetus to design an alternative HIV prevention programme (Gopalan 2005). Significantly, it emphasized the 'empowerment and active participation' of FSWs in the health programmes under the rubric of 'community health' rather than an isolated and vertical approach oriented to technological imperatives (Gangoli and Gaitonde 2005; Ghosh 2005; Nag 2002, 2005; Ramasubban and Rishyasringa 2005).

To illustrate, the rising STI and HIV incidence rates reiterated the importance of comprehensive or integrationist health programme where basic needs like education, environmental sanitation facility (sanitary napkins for adolescents and condoms at affordable price), mitigation of poverty through enhancement of capability (like employment-generated schemes or skill-building programmes), and issue of equity[3] and protection of human rights such as demand for decriminalization of sex work and repeal of Section 377 were stressed (Gangoli and Gaitonde 2005; Grover 2005; Nag 2005; Pai and Seshu 2014; Sen 2008; Seshu 2005). Notwithstanding the significant contribution of these programmes, these community-led HIV/AIDS prevention programmes may not be isolated from global politico-economic changes occurring during that phase. In other words, these HIV prevention programmes, which are in fact financed by these transnational organizations are in tune with the new global political economic policy. In fact, these transnational organizations (which are elevated to a position of 'messiah') are part and parcel of neo-liberal economic policy. This approach corresponded well with the structural adjustment programme in terms of transferring the health responsibility from the state to people.

Besides this macro context, there is a specific reason for which the STI management programme was rolled out in Rajahmundry. East Godavari has been identified as a highly vulnerable district on the basis of HIV/AIDS prevalence rates. It was ranked third, as the HIV prevalent rate was 2.75 in 2006 and as seventh in 2007.[4] An international public health initiative (Avahan) initiated an HIV/AIDS project in Rajahmundry (during 2004–09) inspired by Songachi[5] as a model to be emulated in the rest of the country. The management of STIs is an important component of HIV prevention programmes because STIs, especially ulcerative STIs, increase the risk of HIV transmission. In rural and resource-poor settings where laboratory facilities are not available for testing, syndromic case management where reported symptoms are treated with medications and asymptomatic treatment provided where populations at high risk are treated regardless of whether they show symptoms, are regarded as effective strategies for managing STIs. Several surveys showed that there are high levels of STIs and HIV in coastal Andhra Pradesh. Further, 68.2 per cent of FSWs had at least one curable STI and 48.5 per cent were HIV positive (Steen et al. 2006). However, there is great amount of uncertainty in the data as the data which is collected from the sentinel centre does not represent the total population, and the source of collection of the data is from anonymous testing centres. Based on prevailing international standards Indian researchers along with the western colleagues initially only looked at the FSWs for evidence of disease and thus found their theses proven when evidence of the disease was found (Karnik 2001). From the public health perspective, treating and preventing STIs among FSWs was a critical goal of the initiative (Avahan) to protect women's and community health. The provision of treatment to asymptomatic FSWs is especially considered an effective measure from the medical point of view. These approaches are not new, but they are receiving renewed attention as public health practitioners struggle to find appropriate interventions for high prevalence, resource-constrained settings with social problems that fuel STD transmission (for example, substance abuse, homelessness, lack of education, and family dissolution).

Consider the following exchange encapsulating the rationale for switching to asymptomatic treatment:

> Clinic staff stated in May 2006 that the clinic DO (Document Officer) found asymptomatic treatment to be a better option than syndromic management because not every kind of STI is visible. Prophylactic treatment reduces the chance of STI infection, and SCAs are not able to identify most of the STI symptoms correctly, except for white discharge.
>
> (Excerpts from the observation of an Arogya Brindam meeting with SCAs and clinic staff)

PERSUASIVE AND DISCURSIVE APPROACH

Although, asymptomatic treatment is considered useful from the medical perspective, it also involved close surveillance of women's bodies. Surveillance is operationalized through a political discourse where scientific representation treats heterosexual masculinity as an ideal and makes other bodies (FSWs) as pathological. Additionally, it entailed depersonalization and disembodiment during treatment and test where FSWs virtually did not have rights over their body and decide on treatment. Indeed, this not only exemplifies the contradiction and limitations of an empowerment programme but also its continuity with the conservative approach discussed above. In other words, both approaches, reactionary and progressive, relied on 'disciplining of bodies'. For instance, though proponents of community health approach advocate prevention and critique the 'technological fixes' associated with the curative approach, they do not oppose the mundane regulation of FSWs for the protection of public health. Nonetheless, what sets apart this approach from the former is that it does not use 'force' as a method or 'government by others'. It rather calls for a 'persuasive approach' or 'government of oneself' to put in the words of Foucault. In this way, the monitoring component is couched in subtle ways. For example, the governance of FSWs is done through the method of confession and scientific discursivity—collection of detailed information on their intimate relationships, as well as the questioning and governing of those activities. Social Change Agents (SCAs) (from the sex work community) were recruited to motivate FSWs to accept the asymptomatic treatment every three months, STI check-ups, and avail syndromic case management services reported the kinds of sexual activity such as (oral, anal, vaginal, and with condom), the numbers of sexual encounter, and ascertained whether condoms were really used in every sexual encounter. Further, in the context of an empowerment intervention, there are additional layers of surveillance, with the staff monitoring and evaluating the activities of SCAs. This narrative of an SCA is about her work and how the staff evaluates her work.

> The girls come to the hospital and they tell then. They tell that I have come and worked with them. Even if they don't tell they (staff) will know when they don't use condoms and they will know if I don't tell them about STDs and about keeping good health. If she goes to the hospital with a complaint they give her medicines and when she goes the second time to the hospital they will know she is fine and is using condoms. Then if she is sick even the third time they (staff) will have a doubt; whether she is not using condoms or not, if she is using then why is she getting the infections. Maybe the temporary husband is not using condoms as they generally don't. Then they will doubt why are these sex workers from Namavaram coming like this. Is the SCA there not giving them proper instructions? Is she not telling them the use of condoms? So, they too should be brought to the hospitals. (Excerpts from a personal interview with an SCA)

The last form of scrutinization was undertaken through direct medicalization process—examining FSWs every month and treating them on the basis of findings from the screening. Presumptive treatment is given if symptoms are not found; if they are found with symptoms, treatment is provided through syndromic case management. Consider the following case:

> Interviewer: Why do you bring them? SCA: It is better to get them tested. We don't know whether they are using the condoms properly with the customers or not. They might say they are using but in reality they might not be using them. After all who sees those things? So I bring them for tests.

(Excerpts from an in-depth interview with an SCA)

These accounts not only show layers of surveillance but also the way an empowerment programme made icons of FSWs, the very portrayal it aimed to question. The latter part will be clear once we reflect on the subtle processes of persuasion or micro level working of the STI regimen. Highlighting its anti-discriminatory approach, this STI management programme was rolled out with a particular discursive text. It was embarked on the endeavour to challenge the stigmatized notions that then prevailed in Rajahmundry (particularly AIDS Awareness for Sustained And Holistic Action (ASHA) programme undertaken by Andhra Pradesh State AIDS Control Society (APSACS) in July 2006) that FSWs were diseased bodies and vectors of HIV infection. This programme produced a counter discourse that FSWs not only protect their own sexual health but prevent the transmission of HIV among the greater public. In this scenario, STI management programme became the reference point aimed to destabilize these images by showing FSWs (more so the SCAs) as disease free and responsible citizen since they participated in STI management programme and in turn secured the health of the public. On the other hand, asymptomatic regimen of the STI management programme withers from the very portrayal of FSWs as role models by suspecting their participation in safe sex which has been elaborated in the fourth section. In fact, the cost-effective and participatory angle is paraphrased in order to mobilize FSWs for these programmes. So, the disciplining of the body of marginalized communities is imposed through the subtle processes of persuasion by soliciting sentiments of attachment on the part of citizen subject. In this scenario, surveillance mechanisms are fiercely framed as a 'choice' of FSWs with a range of incentives like programme staff lobbying for welfare benefits like pension, the provision of free house, voter-id card from the state, and provision of legal aid during the arrest of FSWs, and disincentives like removing former FSWs from SCA position when they were unable to mobilize FSWs for asymptomatic regimen or speculum examination.

Following internationally recognized STI control guidelines, the STI management programme was implemented as a two-pronged strategy. The first involved the setting up of a clinic and providing STI services that included condom promotion, regular check-ups such as speculum examination every month and HIV test every six months, presumptive treatment, syndromic case management, and counselling. Presumptive treatment requires FSWs to take medicine on a full stomach and FSWs need to be monitored for possible side effects to the drug. For these reasons, the clinic provided lunch to its patients and patients were asked to rest in the waiting room for at least an hour after taking the medicine. The second strategy included the formation of an Arogya Brindam, in order to monitor the programme, ensure quality treatment, provide a platform for FSWs to interact with medical professionals, and give FSWs decision-making authority in clinic management and so on.

Consider the following exchanges:

This is a platform to have dialogue between health care professionals and the community members. Since we found the need of an STI clinic for the community, we opened a clinic and selected some of the community members as SCAs. After that we have started providing training to them. Their role was clearly defined i.e., identifying STI symptoms, identifying STI cases, bringing the STI cases to the clinic. It is not just bringing them to the clinic but explaining to the patient the objectives of the clinic. We have capacitated them to that level. We decided to form an organization for them and it is called N-S. This organization [N-S] has the responsibility of ensuring that FSWs avail STI treatment from the clinic. There are also organizations formed at the local level. There are also some areas which are far away from Rajahmundry and FSWs find it difficult to travel to Rajahmundry from those places, and we have out-reach clinics in those areas. Some of you [referring to the doctors] may know also this. We are doing it because the demand has come from them. We are also giving SCAs a decision-making role.

(Excerpts from the observation of an ArogyaBrindam meeting wherein, the Project Manager introduced the committee to a doctor)

They [SCAs who are member of Health Committee] organize clinics in the ten mandals, sometimes during nights on demand. They observe

whether the doctor is giving proper treatment, whether sterilization is
properly done and how the counselling is done, how they are giving
medicines and about follow up.
    (Excerpts from the observation of a meeting with members of Health
          Committee where a staff member explained the purpose of the
                                                          ArogyaBrindam)

As these instances elucidate, the latter strategy emphasized 'community
ownership' where eventually FSWs would own the programme, run
the clinic, and take decisions especially after the discontinuation of
aid from the international health organization, whereas the former
strategy gravitated towards close surveillance and regulation of FSWs'
bodies. So the surveillance programme is an example of the colonizing
process (Arnold 1993) that is built upon an enormous battery of texts
and discursive practices and channelized through a contradictory
empowerment and anti-stigma strategy. So, these transnational
health organizations have constructed a peculiar kind of citizenship
for FSWs in STI and HIV/AIDS control programme and these are
connected to the broader politico-economic processes. Under the
condition of economic reform, the onus of health security shifts from
state to communities by targeting or reforming factors internal to
the communities rather than structural/external conditions. When the
community takes the responsibility of STI management programme
which is funded by transnational health organizations, the state recognizes
it and provides them incentives and disincentives. For instance,
SCAs and FSWs through the help of programme staff apply for
welfare benefits like ration cards, old age pension, free housing,
and so on, from district collector office upon their participation in
STI management programme and failing to do so, disqualify them
from these entitlements as well as from SCA position. This makes it
a cultural as much as a political and economic process. This is also
linked to wider forms of regulation and modes of social discipline
through which capitalist relations of production and patriarchal
relations of reproduction are organized (Rajan 2003). In simple
terms as indicated earlier, community led STI programme are rolled
out through the finance of Avahan with the objective that after the
discontinuation of the funds from the latter, it is the disenfranchised
(socially and economically) communities like SCA and FSWs who
would finance the clinic and run the STI programme. In 2003, with a
USD 100 million budget, the Gates Foundation formally launched the

Avahan—HIV initiative, which was later increased to USD 200 million in 2004 and this grant was for five years (2003–08) which is referred as Phase I. Phase II (2009–13), started in 2009 in which Avahan transitioned financially to another natural owner. Avahan identified two natural and complementary owners such as communities—FSWs or other sexually marginal communities- and the government's public health system—NACO. This transitioning too occurred in phase manner such as in 2009, 10 per cent of it was transferred to NACO and during the exit—in 2013, 70 per cent of the programme was planned to be transferred to NACO. In other-words, 30 per cent of the programme was expected be owned by the communities like FSWs, MSMs, and drug users (Global Health Delivery 2012). In material terms, it implies SCAs are required to hire doctors, pay rent for the clinic and Drop in Centre (rest room), purchase the mobile van, and so on. Nevertheless, the state agencies especially NACO would also own the programme in terms of supply of drugs, condoms, referral services to ART centre, HIV testing, and others. So this participatory approach is very much in tandem with the broader neo-liberal policy which calls for the public and private partnership. Concurrently, it reinforces patriarchy in terms of treating heterosexual masculinity as the norm and regulates alternative sexual practices by making it pathological.

RESISTING STI MANAGEMENT PROGRAMME

Not surprisingly, this surveillance elicited resistances among SCAs and FSWs. After two years of the STI management programme, the number of FSWs who complied with the routine check-up and asymptomatic treatment did not quite reach Avahan's goal of covering 100 per cent and even adding new FSWs. In this context, the formation of a Health Committee became a turning point and emerged as the space for the SCAs to voice their concerns and communicate FSWs' objections against the STI management programme.

One of the grounds through which the SCAs challenged STI management programme was by questioning the rationale of STI management programme or presenting their own rationale for not complying with it. For instance, the Health Committee was not established with the expectation that FSWs and their representatives would resist STI management programme. Yet resist they did, as revealed in this exchange that we observed between the staff and an SCA during Arogya Brindam meeting:

> Intervention staff: Since the SCAs are role models for FSWs, first of all SCAs should undergo asymptomatic treatment as well as other routine check-ups so that other FSWs could follow them.

> SCA: I have good reasons for avoiding asymptomatic treatment. Since I practice safe sex, I do not want to undergo asymptomatic treatment.

> Intervention staff: The doctor would confirm whether you practiced safe sex or unsafe sex and whether you are safe from diseases.

This exchange shows an empowered FSW, fully aware of the rationale prompting asymptomatic treatment explaining why it does not apply to her. Asymptomatic treatment is an approach used in situations of high-risk behaviour where it is impossible to confirm an STI with lab tests and therefore, it is best to assume that there has been exposure to STIs and to treat it accordingly. Since the FSW is personally not engaging in risk behaviour, she sees no reason to get the treatment. It shows, in turn, how her behaviour is doubly controlled by the programme—an intervention that is premised on her empowerment. First, her authority, based in 'experiential reality', which the empowerment encourages her to express, is rejected in favour of the doctor's authority based in 'scientific or medical reality'. Thus, submission to STI management programme implies depersonalization and disembodiment.

Second, her status as an SCA subjects her behaviour to greater scrutiny in the programme, which lays claim to her body as a role model for other FSWs, essentially telling her that she needs to comply with so that others will follow by example. This is ironic given that she is also supposed to engage in safe sex behaviour, using a condom at every encounter in order to be a role model. To submit to asymptomatic treatment is to imply that she is not practising safe sex behaviour, and to practice safe sex behaviour is to make asymptomatic treatment unnecessary. This illustration also best captures how FSWs' bodies are sites of conflict between the health programme and the empowerment programme. The contradiction is further evident in the fact that the advocacy programme focusing on empowerment of FSWs was ostensibly aimed at developing a 'questioning attitude', whereas here, the FSWs are expected to unquestioningly trust the experts.

The second reason for objecting to the STI management programme was in terms of doubting the effectiveness of the treatment. Technically, the programme encouraged SCAs to use the Health Committee to provide inputs to the STI management programme, which has, at times, rejected their inputs in ways that are quite disempowering. Consider this exchange recorded during observations at Arogya Brindam meeting:

> SCA: After taking this medicine, which is meant to cure STIs, we are experiencing even more STI symptoms. I and the Secretary of N-S have been facing the same problems. We thought we will discuss this issue in the SCA Monthly meeting. Even some of the FSWs told me that they face the same problem.
>
> Intervention staff 2: I explained to you before you take the treatment that there are small side effects i.e., white discharge or vomiting. But these are not STI symptoms.
>
> Intervention staff 3: Do not bring these kinds of issues in the SCA Monthly Meeting. You better discuss these health related problems in the ArogyaBrindam meeting.
>
> Doctor: Why did you not inform me about this when you had come to see me?
>
> SCA: I already informed this problem to the counsellor.
>
> Doctor: But you have another problem. You do not follow as per the instruction of the medicine. It was told to you not to take the tablet before a sexual encounter. SCAs are taking tablets before intercourse. Whenever they are free or the business is over, then only they should take the medicine. But SCAs are first taking the medicine and then going for intercourse. That is why they are experiencing this problem.
>
> Intervention staff 2: Earlier they were talking about vomiting sensation but it is actually related to consuming alcohol. They are taking the medicine and immediately they are consuming alcohol. That is why they have these side effects. They should avoid taking alcohol for 24 hours after consuming the medicine.

According to the mandate of the Arogya Brindam, soliciting inputs of patient satisfaction is important. However, when SCAs voiced the concerns of FSWs, programme staff not only dismissed these charges but also went to the extent of remarking that the problem lay with the FSWs themselves who violated the treatment protocol. This facet revealed the way an empowerment programme reproduced 'whore stigma' while aiming to deconstruct it. A second point of contention was the way medicines were prescribed. When SCAs expressed confusion over the asymptomatic and syndromic protocols in which the same medications are prescribed for a range of symptoms, or no symptoms at all, the medical staff rejected these concerns in terms that seem to accuse them of being ungrateful.

The third ground for the act of subversion was associated with the fear of being scrutinized, which also exposed the intrusive nature of the STI management programme. For instance, SCAs described how the fear of the speculum exam kept many FSWs away from the clinic. Because they were required to bring a certain number of their peers into the clinic each month, they begin to sound like programme staff themselves in trying to convince their peers to tolerate the exam:

Interviewer: Do you think bringing these girls to clinics is difficult?

SCA: It's very difficult.

Interviewer: Why?

SCA: I am saying this because, girls (FSWs) would say, Sister (implying SCA), Do you think I have any disease, what are you saying? I will not come as I don't think I have any disease.

Then I persuaded them that With HIV, one cannot address any disease unless we treat sexually transmitted diseases. Do you know what sexually transmitted diseases are, you complained about stomach pain, day before yesterday, do you know that stomach pain is a symptom of sexually transmitted diseases.

Interviewer: Some people say that bringing them is very easy. Why do you think they could easily bring them?

SCA: For some people, they want their health in good condition. They want to cure their ailments. Those who have awareness regarding health are coming to hospitals. For some others, they are afraid of injection and blood test. They will put the hand inside the vagina, these people would like to sleep with anyone but are afraid of this test. Why because, those clips, iron clips, (speculum) they are called, If they want to put those things, our girls are terrified, this is the main reason, they are terrified about looking at those iron clips. They say they don't want (to be examined). If I say, You readily sleep with a fat fellow, but you are afraid of those clips. They say that it is a different issue and they are habituated. They say that, at hospital they put the hand, which is terrifying.

(Excerpt from personal interview with with an SCA, emphasis in original)

This illustration demonstrated the problem of the 'risk discourse' interactions that are held by the public health specialists. The key point here is that behaviour which is, for public health reasons, considered 'risky' may be viewed as habitual, normal, or mundane by those who engage in them; in addition, they may be seen to carry different meanings of risk. In short, for FSWs STI infection is one of the risks among various other kinds of risks. More than HIV, poverty, stigma related to sex work, police violence, lower caste status, and so on, are the important threats. Concomitantly, FSWs need protection from various health needs than just STI and HIV.

The Sexually Transmitted Infection management strategy also involved considerable scrutiny of sex workers' sexual activities, which is resisted as invasive. This invasive nature was not related with the use of medical instruments per se but rather the questions related to sexual behaviour. The intervention staff asked FSWs as part of the risk assessment component of the STI management programme as follows:

SCA: The problem is if I bring FSWs secretly from my place to this hospital, they subjects us to tests and in the process ask how many men they encounter in a day and how many condoms they use etc. They feel shy to answer. They think it is insulting when they ask such questions pertaining to their secret work and they don't show interest to come here.

Interviewer: Don't they ask in the private hospitals?

SCA: No, they don't. They ask what the problem is and if we say that there is a rash or some infection then they test and say you got some infection and give medicines. But the people here want all details. They feel tired answering these questions about why they are doing sex and with how many they are doing it. If there is no such questioning then I can assure you there will be many patients coming here.

Interviewer: Why are they asking like that, is there any reason?

SCA: The staff at C is always of the opinion that the FSWs alone come here for treatment and so the conversation is always with suscpicion; they don't think regular patients come here. Sometimes they even ask me, how many did I have intercourse with today. I feel why is sir asking that way. Because I am used to these people so I answer them but these new ones get terrified when they ask such questions. The probing questions about sexual encounters make them feel embarrassed. Some women engaging in sex work secretly is not like the road ones. I mean, the road based sex workers don't mind telling they had sex work with five or six a day. But these are afraid. They should be handled differently. They should advise her about the care to be taken. There could be some women who are

not sex workers, but still they get STDs, and then they also should be
treated. When we have a hospital we should be very clever in handling
the patients.

(Excerpt from personal interview with the author,
emphasis in original)

This quote is important as it problematizes the categorization of FSWs
as risk groups in order to subject them for surveillance. It would appear
that there is an absence of shared understanding between the initiative
and FSWs, particularly to arrive at a clear understanding of the high-
risk group for which the STI management programme is designed. For
instance, the initiative defines a high-risk group, that is, the eligible
client for STI service, is based on the number of clients that the FSWs
have. In fact, an excerpt from one of the interviews with the staff
of the initiative favours the placing of FSWs at different risk levels
based on the type of FSW. This kind of classification is said to help
them filter FSWs for inclusion and exclusion in the STI management
programme. For instance, a home-based FSW who transacts sex work
for money twice a day can be disfavoured for inclusion over an FSW
who gets seven clients a day since she has more chance of spreading the
virus (Sengupta and Sinha 2004). But, the criterion for classification
differs from SCAs' understanding that it is the secret FSWs, generally
entertaining limited and regular partners, who do not comply with the
safe sex regimen and use condoms unlike the 'public' FSWs. So, SCAs
recruit those women into clinic that they believe to be transacting sex
for money.

Fourthly, there were several structural barriers, which are linked to the
previous point and pre-empted SCAs and FSWs to meet the requirements
of the STI management programme. Some of these challenges include
losing business hours, constant mobility of the FSWs within and outside
the district, and the fear of being identified. As mentioned earlier, the STI
management programme was implemented through participatory and
empowerment approach that intended to de-stigmatize FSWs by making
their bodies free of STI infections. However, what the intervention does
in this process is place responsibility on the community, which in turn
makes them visible. From the point of view of the FSWs, this visibility
becomes a stake to the very identity of FSWs. In other words, this new
subjectivity clashes with the secret identity of the FSWs and reinforces
the stigma. Here, the 'visibility' (that FSWs are involved in HIV/AIDS
prevention project) is the main factor, which obstructs other FSWs from
associating with the STI management programme. In short, for secret

FSWs, complying with STI management programme implies being identified as FSWs and AIDS cases. This visibility means that they have to dissociate themselves from sex work, just as they had to relinquish working hours from sex work.

Notably, it is not a coincidence that at a crucial juncture when vertical programmes re-emerge instead of a strong public health care setup, factors internal to marginal communities are controlled and handed to the community as their health responsibility. So, this description of submission is the empirical violence of the examination; where FSWs are subjected to tests and procedures and treated as infectious bodies. Their suffering of violence is of a less literal but no less painful kind, which can be described as barbarically inflicting definitions, namely, 'STI case/AIDS case'. In broad theoretical terms, it implies that the empirical violence involved in biomedical practice arises from a prior classificatory violence, the violence of a rational knowledge, which forces its objects to conform to its logic in order that they might be rendered knowable. Waldby (1996) called this surveillance as 'violence of biomedical practice' in the field of AIDS enforced on people who are infected with the virus or groups already required to defend themselves against the toxic intolerance of the dominant order (Waldby 1996: 2, 4). Despite, or perhaps, because, of biomedicine's assertion of its own innocence of historical and political meaning, it constantly absorbs, translates and re-circulates 'non-scientific ideas—ideas about sexuality, social order, culture—in its technical discourses … The preamble relationship between medical and social knowledge implies that biomedical discourse can be treated, at least in part, as a discourse of culture' (Waldby 1996: 23).

After all, for Foucault, the search for freedom in the pleasures of sex is ironically what places a person under the domain of power (Das 1996: 2411). So, these already stigmatized communities are caught in a double bind, hitherto immoral status and new sexual health movements (Jena 2012). More precisely, a society that shuns women who are engaged in selling their sexual services and looks down on them in contempt, now campaigns for decriminalization of sex work as a consequence of HIV and AIDS epidemics. From this angle, the only way the Indian State would accept FSWs is via AIDS awareness and prevention programmes (Gangoli 2004; Merchant 2009: xix; Sathyamala and Priya 2006). That is, FSWs will be considered and recognized by the state if they participate in HIV/AIDS prevention programme. This is why public health activists have advocated decriminalization and de-stigmatization of the profession, defined sex work as work, and supported the liberal feminist position on sex work. In fact, as argued by Kotiswaran (2012), these public health bodies typically call for a rights-based approach to sex work without unequivocally advocating decriminalization. Their utilitarian approach is that they tolerate female sex work to the extent necessary to prevent the spread of HIV to general population and institutionalizes a 'watch care system'. However, this does not contemplate redistributive law reform in favour of FSWs. So, HIV/AIDS is the prism through which FSWs are recognized and bodies of women become cultural signs. In addition, the sexual violence experienced by FSWs is a consequence of the political and economic structure.

* * *

This chapter described violence along the sexual axis by treating the governance of sexuality, that is, sexual policing, as a form of violence through the study of a community-oriented empowerment programme aimed at controlling STI infection among FSWs in Rajahmundry. It showed how surveillance of the lives of FSWs was legitimized for protecting the health of the larger public. Surveillance is operationalized through a political discourse where scientific representation treats heterosexual masculinity as an ideal and makes other bodies (FSWs) as pathological. Secondly, the disciplining of the body is imposed through subtle processes of persuasion by soliciting sentiments of attachment on the part of citizen subject. Hence, this discursive exercise and regulation of FSWs should be contested for multiple reasons.

From the perspective of FSWs, HIV infection is an issue among several other social problems. More than HIV, poverty, stigma related to sex work, police violence, lower caste status, and others are important threats. However, in the STI management programme, the needs of the men and the utilitarian approach are inherent where the protection of the greater public and men from the HIV and STI infection is predicated on the protection of the FSWs from infection. In this manner, asymptomatic treatment is made ubiquitous in the lives of FSWs even though they have to face several challenges, such as, the fear of being identified, dissociation from sex work as a means of intimidation, depersonalization, and a process of subjugation. Secondly, this compulsion is absent in the case of 'savarna' or women from dominant sections. This scenario mirrors the concept of graded inequality (Geetha 2009).

There is a gap between the everyday experiences of the violated women and the relatively comfortable lives of upper caste and class women where 'privacy' is maintained and choice is a matter of right. So, the regulation of FSWs involves a process of exclusion and is concerned with the majoritarian schema of identity marked by a desire to keep the other in the state of otherness and distance, and claims universal validity for itself. So, in a way it has consolidated the existing social hierarchies and built fresh consensus of class, sexuality, and knowledge. Thirdly, the STI management programme, by making asymptomatic case treatment compulsory, reproduces 'whore stigma' while aiming to deconstruct it. It endorses the empowerment of FSWs and recognition of sex work as work. It started out with constructing two opposite images of FSWs, 'sexual marginals are carriers of infection as well as agents of change'. If the second image challenged the negative image associated with sex work, the former reiterated the stigma by justifying the governance of sexuality of only FSWs. The daily surveillance and disciplining of these sexual marginals is deployed systemically or carefully planned where violence is neither recognized nor condemned and instead, is rationalized. The non-recognition of sexual violence has to be understood from the point where force gets transformed as 'consent'. So, Female Sex Workers' sexuality has been so intensely medicalized and so closely associated with the AIDS epidemic that FSWs are effectively treated as if they themselves were the viruses in the public health discourse (Jena 2007). These attributes are sufficient to qualify regulation and surveillance of sexuality as 'violence'.

The risk of STI and HIV infection is a little in determinate because these instances offer fluid and interchanging subjectivities of women. However, the STI and HIV-control programme is cohered around the specific realities or a single trait of sexual marginals who do not experience their life in a compartmentalized manner. So, the chapter not only questions the necessity of compulsory surveillance of FSWs but also exposes the lack of recognition of issues of sexuality.

The violence that occurs through surveillance is material as well as symbolic and difficult to conceptualize because of its many simultaneous meanings and rationalization. The surveillance project points out the simultaneous axes of normativity, each axis invested with the power to discipline anti-norms. It also opens up the space to explain the structural forces and discuss subjectivity in terms of assertions against STI treatment regimen. This violence is inextricably linked to the larger politico-economic processes.

NOTES

1. Avahan is an initiative of Bill and Melinda Gates Foundation launched in 2003 in order to reduce the spread of HIV in India.

2. The insights provided here are based on multi-method research—informal interviews with FSWs (including those who are Social Change Agents (SCAs)) about their experiences of using an STI clinic and STI prevention service, ethnographic observations emanating from various meetings, particularly Arogya Brindam (Health Committee) meetings, informal interviews with the project staff including the doctor and counsellor, observation of satellite clinics in which STI clinic services were provided to FSWs, and review of documents (for example, the manual—*Clinic Operational Guidelines and Standards*). This study was conducted in the year 2006–07, with a follow-up visit was made in March–April, 2010. Initially, while observing STI clinic services and ArogyaBrindam meeting, I was impressed with the clinic services, recognition of sex work as work, and anti-stigma strategy adopted by SCAs with the help of project staff to challenge HIV/AIDS programme organized by APSACS (Andhra Pradesh State AIDS Control Society). I could see the work satisfaction of SCAs and growing sense of self-respect. However, over the course of time I found not only the loss of enthusiasm among FSWs but also the presence of a feeling of subjugation and discontent. This occurred at a juncture when asymptomatic treatment was introduced and acceleration of workload for SCAs, which led them to take retirement from sex work. Complaints of SCAs against staff, clinic work, multiple challenges that FSWs faced in order to meet asymptomatic requirement, I initially overlooked it as a minor issue or an interpersonal one that would be resolved eventually. However, when some of the FSWs equated asymptomatic treatment particularly vaginal test in every three months as a tool of intimidation and power, this provoked me to probe it further. At the same time, project staff, which otherwise tries to address problems of FSWs at the structural level, undermined the issues raised by FSWs and made asymptomatic treatment inevitable. Thus, this sexual surveillance did not remain just as any other monitoring process, rather it generated subversion, reproduced social inequality, and stigma which is a sufficient attribute to qualify it as 'violence'.

3. For instance, Grover's (2005) work highlighted the lobby for the provision of low-cost generic ARV drugs for people living with HIV/AIDS by Indian state.

4. According to Andhra Pradesh State AIDS Control Society (APSACS) the declining rate of HIV/AIDS incident rate is due to the visibility of the international and national NGOs.

5. In fact, the programme kick-started with the exposure visit of staffs and FSWs to Songachi to learn and reflect.

REFERENCES

Adkins, Lisa. 2002. 'Risk, Sexuality and Economy', *British Journal of Sociology* 53(1): 19–40.

Arnold, D. 1993. *Colonizing the Body: State Medicine and Epidemic Disease in nineteenth Century India*. Berkeley: University of California Press.

AVAHAN STI Services-Clinic Operational Guidelines and Standards (COGS). 2005. Family Health International & World Health Organization.

Das, V. 1996. 'Sexual Violence, Discursive Formations and the State', *Economic and Political Weekly* 31 (35/37): 2411–23.

Desouza, S. 2004. 'Razing Baina, Goa: In Whose Interest', *Economic and Political Weekly* 39(30): 3341–3.

Gangoli, G. 2004. 'Women as Vectors: Health and Rights of Sex Workers in India'. In *Unheard Scream: Reproductive Health and Women's Lives in India*, R. Mohan (ed.), pp. 87–108. New Delhi: Zubban.

Gangoli, L.V. and R. Gaitonde. 2005. 'Programmes for Control of Communicable Diseases'. In *Review of Health Care in India*, V.G. Leena, D. Ravi, S. Abhay (eds), pp. 75–100. Mumbai: CEHAT.

Geetha, V. 2009. 'Bereft of Being: The Humiliation of Untouchability'. In *Humiliation: Claims and Context*, G. Guru (ed.), pp. 95–107. New Delhi: Oxford University Press.

Ghosh, S. 2005. 'Surveillance in a Decolonized Space. The Case of Sex Workers in West Bengal,' *Social Text* 23(2): 55–69.

Global Health Delivery. 2012. *The Avahan India AIDS Initiative: Managing Targeted HIV Prevention at Scale*. Harvard: Harvard Medical School.

Gopal, M. 2013. 'Sexuality and Social Reproduction: Reflections from an Indian Feminist Debate', *Indian Journal of Gender Studies* 20 (2): 235–51.

Gopalan, A. 2005. 'Client Advocacy and Service Provision: The NA Foundation's Mission'. In *AIDS and Civil Society: India's Learning Curve*, R. Radhika and R. Bhanwar (ed.), pp. 167–88. Rawat: Jaipur.

Gordon, C. 1991. 'Governmental Rationality: An Introduction'. In *The Foucault Effect Studies in Governmentality*, B. Graham, G. Collin, and M. Peter (eds), pp. 1–52. Chicago: Chicago University Press.

Grover, A. 2005. 'Meeting the Unmet Legal Needs of Positive People: The Lawyers' Collective HIV/AIDS Unit'. In *AIDS and Civil Society: India's Learning Curve*, R. Radhika and R. Bhanwar (eds), pp, 197–224. Jaipur: Rawat.

Jena, A. 2007. 'Struggles for Empowerment: Indian Sex Workers Negotiating, Resisting and Coping with an STI Management Programme', Paper presented at 'Annual Meeting, Society for the Study of Social Problems', New York, August.

———. 2012. 'Body as a Site of Contestation and Reconciliation: Learning from an STI Management Programme in India'. Paper presented at RC–54, 'Body

in Social Sciences: Embodied Action, Embodied Theory, Understanding
Body in Society', Second International Sociological Association Forum,
University of Buenos Aires, Argentina, 1–4 August.

Kannabiran, K. 2005. 'Introduction'. In *The Violence of Normal Times: Essays on Women's Lived Realities*, K. Kannabiran (ed.), pp. 1–45. New Delhi: Women Unlimited.

Karnik, Niranjan S. 2001. 'Locating HIV/AIDS and India: Cautionary Notes on the Globalization of Categories', *Science, Technology, & Human Values* 26(3): 322–48.

Kotiswaran, P. 2001. 'Preparing for Civil Disobedience Indian Sex Workers and the Law', *Boston College Third World Law Journal* 21(161): 160–240.

———. 2012. *Dangerous Sex, Invisible Labour: Sex Work and Law in India*. New Delhi: Oxford University Press.

Merchant, H. 2009. *Forbidden Sex, Forbidden Texts: New India's Gay Poets*. New Delhi: Routledge.

Mittal, D. 2015. 'What about India's Daughters in the Conflict Zones?', www. Countercurrents.Org, 8 March.

Nag, Moni. 2002. 'Empowering Female Sex Workers for HIV/AIDS Prevention and Far Beyond: Sonagachi Shows the Way', *Indian Journal of Social Work* 63(4): 473–501.

———. 2005. 'Sex Workers in Sonagachi: Pioneers in Revolution', *Economic and Political Weekly* 40(49): 5151–6.

Pai, A. and Seshu, M.S. 2014. 'Understanding the De- Criminalisation Demand'. Kafila.org, 7 November 2007. Available at: https://kafila.online/page/180/. Accessed on 2 January 2015.

Phadke, S. 2010. 'If Women Could Risk Pleasure: Reinterpreting Violence in Public Sphere'. In *Nine Degrees of Justice*, D. Bishakha (ed.), pp. 83–113. Delhi: Zubaan.

Ramasubban, R. 1998. 'HIV/AIDS in India: A Gulf between Rhetoric and Realities', *Economic and Political Weekly* 33(45): 2865–72.

Ramasubban, R. and B. Rishyasringa. 2005. 'Introduction'. In *AIDS and Civil Society: India's Learning Curve*, R. Ramasubban and B. Rishyasringa (ed.), pp. 1–39. Rawat: Jaipur.

Rajan, R.S. 2003. *The Scandal of the State: Women, Law and Citizenship in Postcolonial India*. New Delhi: Permanent Black.

Sathyamala, C. and R. Priya. 2006. 'Sex as Work: A Changing Discourse', *Journal of Creative Communications* 1(2): 204–8.

Sen, A. 2008. 'Foreword. Understanding the Challenge of AIDS'. In *AIDS Sutra: Untold Stories from India*, A. Negar (ed.), pp. 1–15. New Delhi: Random House.

Sengupta, J. and J. Sinha. 2004. 'Battling AIDS in India', *The McKinsey Quarterly* 3.

Seshu, M. 2005. 'Organising Women in Prostitution: The Case of SANGRAM'. In *AIDS and Civil Society: India's Learning Curve*, R. Ramasubban, and R. Bhanwar (eds), pp. 137–58. Jaipur: Rawat.

Shah, S. 2006. 'Producing the Spectacle of Kamathipura: The Politics of Red Light Visibility in Mumbai', *Cultural Dynamics* 18(3): 269–92.

Steen, R., V. Mogasale, T. Wi, A.K. Singh, C. Daly, B. George, G. Neilsen, V. Loo, and G. Dallabetta. 2006. 'Pursuing Scale and Quality in STI Interventions with SW Avahan Results', *Sexually Transmitted Diseases* 82(5): 381–5.

Tambe, A. 2009. *Codes of Misconduct: Regulating Prostitution in Late Colonial Bombay.* Minneapolis: University of Minnesota Press.

Waldby, C. 1996. *AIDS and Body Politics.* London: Routledge.

13

Violence against Women as a Health Care Issue

Perceptions and Approaches

Sangeeta Rege and Padma Bhate-Deosthali

Violence is now widely recognized as a global public health concern (Garcia-Moreno et al. 2014a). Evidence shows violence, which may take various forms such as, caste/race violence, homicide, suicide, domestic violence, rape, or that inflicted in war and situations of armed conflict, is common and causes immediate and long-term health and social consequences for survivors/victims and their communities. Violence is a tool used to maintain the existing inequalities and imbalance of power between individuals/groups/communities. The inequalities may be based on gender, class, caste, religion, race/ethnicity, sexual orientation, and disability.

Violence was placed on the international agenda in 1996 when the World Health Assembly adopted Resolution (WHA 49.25: Forty-Ninth World Health Assembly, Geneva 20–25 May 1996), which declared violence 'a leading worldwide public health problem'. This resolution called for a scientific public health approach to prevent violence. It recognized that the health workers are often the first to identify the victims of violence and have the necessary technical capacity to help the victims (WHO 1997). The resolution called upon the WHO to initiate public health activities to: (*i*) document and characterize the burden of violence, (*ii*) assess the effectiveness of programmes, with particular attention to women and children and community-based initiatives, and (*iii*) promote activities to tackle the problem at the international and country level.

Notable advancements in developing a public health approach were made in several developed countries such as the United Kingdom, Australia, and the United States of America. However, in developing countries there are several constraints: Non-recognition of violence against women (VAW) as a public health issue, limited resources, competing public health priorities, lack of clearly enunciated policies and protocols, among others (Bhate-Deosthali and Duggal 2013). Health care professionals play an important role in the treatment of injury, physical and/or psychological trauma, rehabilitation of victims, and prevention of further violence. While the public health system is recognized as one of the most critical sites for addressing the post-violence mechanism, in many countries it currently lacks the capacity and sensitivity to adequately and effectively respond to the needs of victims and survivors of violence. This lack of sensitivity is documented in situations of conflict as well as routine times (Medico Friend Circle [Bombay, India] 2002).

In India, even the medico-legal documentation (where there is a legal binding) of domestic violence, rapes, suicides, homicides, deaths in police custody, and caste or communal violence is neither accurate nor complete as there are no uniform protocols and procedures laid down. Here are some examples of the current health sector response.

> A woman comes for an abortion for an unwanted pregnancy resulting out of rape. She reports that a medico-legal examination was done a month back but she was not provided an emergency contraception (EC) to prevent the pregnancy.
>
> The post mortem reports of women killed in the communal riots in Gujarat 2002 made no mention of the sexual violence inflicted on them— There were injuries related to insertion of rods in vagina (MFC report).
>
> Patient reports to the hospital with a history of consumption of a bottle of insecticide and doctors record it as accidental consumption of poison. (Deosthali and Malik 2009)

These are not isolated examples but reflect common experiences of victims of violence in India.

The women's movement in India brought the issue of VAW into the public domain in the 1980s, campaigned for changes in law, and rallied for the setting up of counselling centres, shelters, and legal aid for survivors (Kumar 1993). The women's movement confronted the health system for its coercive population polices, highlighted the complete lack of gender sensitivity within the system, and the insensitive response to rape, amongst others. However, the role of the health sector in responding to and mitigating violence did not become a rallying point.

Despite the fact that health professionals and health systems have a critical role in caring for survivors of violence, as well as in documenting the violence and collecting relevant evidence, there are several gaps in the provision of care and in the medico-legal response. Legal obligations have been cast upon the health sector for responding to VAW. The Protection of Women from Domestic Violence Act (PWDVA) 2005, recognizes health facilities as service providers and mandates that all women reporting domestic violence must receive free treatment and information about the law and appropriate referral services. The Criminal Amendment to Rape (CLA) 2013 (Government of India 2013), and the Protection of Children from Sexual Offences Act, 2012 (POCSCO 2012) now makes it mandatory for all hospitals, public and private, to provide free treatment to survivors of sexual violence. Despite these amendments, the health sector response to violence, in general, and violence against women and children specifically, remains suboptimal. There is a significant gap between legal provision and its implementation for the benefit of survivors and victims.

Violence against women is not recognized as a public health issue in India. The draft National Health Policy, 2015 does not cover aspects related to health sector response to VAW. At a broader level, the policy makes little contribution to operationalize comprehensive services to women facing violence.

This chapter describes the prevalence of VAW and the health consequences they suffer. It also touches on the perceptions of health professionals regarding violence against women. It then presents different approaches adopted by civil society organizations to engage the health sector to respond to VAW. While doing so it raises concerns about the lack of an institutionalized health care response and draws attention to the policy gaps that keeps the government from committing itself to ending all forms of VAW.

PREVALENCE OF VIOLENCE AGAINST WOMEN

Domestic violence and sexual violence are the most pervasive form of gender-based violence, cutting across caste, class, race, religion, and socio-economic background. But, there is little consistent evidence on the prevalence of these forms of VAW in India.

The National Family Health Survey (NFHS) and National Crime Records Bureau (NCRB 2014), provide some insight into the occurrence and the nature of violence against women. The National Family Health Survey (NFHS 2005–06) (IIPS 2009) included specific questions on domestic violence and its results indicated that the lifetime prevalence of physical or sexual violence among women of 15–49 years was 34 per cent, while about 19 per cent of these women reported being subject to violence in last 12 months preceding the survey. On an average, among married (the category 'ever married') women 36 per cent report cuts, bruises, or aches; 9 per cent report eye injuries, sprains, dislocations, or burns; 7 per cent report deep wounds, broken bones or teeth, or other serious injuries; and 2 per cent report severe burns. Abused women generally seek help from their own families and friends. Very few go to institutions, such as the police (1.5 per cent), medical personnel (0.5 per cent), or social service organizations (0.05 per cent). But this data is 10 years old; no new national household survey has been conducted since then.

The National Crime Records Bureau recorded a total of 124,791 sexual offences against women in 2014. This higher number is probably due to a change in the definition of rape, which now covers all forms of sexual violence beyond the peno-vaginal penetration. Additionally, 8,455 dowry deaths were recorded and 118,866 cases of cruelty by husbands. These data are of those women who mustered the courage of reporting offences to the police stations. A comparison of NFHS and NCRB data shows women's reluctance to seek a redressal mechanism.

These national-level surveys, however, do not record the frequency and impact of domestic violence and sexual violence. Neither do they calculate the impact of violence on women that lead to suicide attempts or repeat incidents of victimization. Emma Williamson (2013) points out that building such measures of impact while collecting data enables a deeper understanding of the prevalence of domestic and sexual violence. She points out that population-based national surveys collected by governments of different countries do not canvas data from independent domestic violence advocates, health professionals, shelter homes, and social workers, and so fail to include the number of women and children seeking support outside the system. This means that the national surveys on prevalence of VAW and children may not be the most reliable sources on this matter.

In the Indian context, community-based studies show a prevalence of VAW ranging from 17 to 80 per cent (Bhate-Deosthali 2016). Amongst the different forms of VAW, the most commonly studied form is domestic violence and a bulk of the research contributes to the evidence on the prevalence of domestic violence against women. Even within domestic violence, the focus is on marital violence. No estimate of violence faced by girls and women from their natal family is available.

The variations related to the prevalence can be attributed to differences in the methodology, the manner in which questions are asked, the extent of rapport established and ways in which data is analysed. Studies conducted by institutions that report high prevalence are due to better tools and processes for enabling women to report violence of various forms. It is important to therefore note that there is no reliable data on VAW in India. Because of the underreporting as above, what is known/available is just the tip of the iceberg.

HEALTH CONSEQUENCES OF VIOLENCE AGAINST WOMEN

Violence against women is associated with a broad array of health consequences. Domestic violence, especially sexual violence has been associated with adverse outcomes to women's physical health including reproductive health, making them more vulnerable to sexually transmitted infections including HIV/AIDS and psychological well being (Garcia-Moreno et al. 2005). A study among 2,199 pregnant women in North India indicated that births among mothers who had faced domestic violence are 2.59 times more likely to lead to peri-natal and neo-natal mortality (Koski and Koenig 2011). Physical and sexual intimate partner violence is associated with miscarriage and reproductive health services should be used to screen for spousal violence and link to assistance (Johri et al. 2011).

Some of the mental health outcomes of routinely suffering domestic violence include symptoms such as crying easily, inability to enjoy life, fatigue and thoughts of suicide; depression, feelings of anger and helplessness, self-blame, anxiety, phobias, panic disorders, eating disorders, low self-esteem, nightmares, hyper vigilance, heightened startle response, memory loss, nervous breakdowns, and it is associated with other risk behaviour associated with adverse health outcomes such drug and alcohol use (Deosthali and Malik 2009; Garcia-Moreno et al. 2005). Further, a study reported that the gamut of these mental health consequences for women facing violence can range from mental stress, anxiety, depression, disturbed sleep, psychosomatic disorders, and suicidal behaviour (Kumar et al. 2005). A study by Chowdhary and

Patel (2008) on effects of spousal violence on women's health in Goa shows that spousal violence is a causal factor for attempted suicide and sexually transmitted infections among women.

HEALTH PROFESSIONALS' PERCEPTIONS OF VIOLENCE AGAINST WOMEN

Despite evidence of the many ways in which violence affects lives of women, health professionals have considered domestic violence against women as a private matter (Deosthali and Malik 2009). They believe that their role is only to treat the disease and the physical manifestations of such violence. Such a biomedical approach does not facilitate the disclosure of domestic violence nor does it elicit appropriate and useful response from health professionals (Garcia-Moreno et al. 2015). Health professionals share sociocultural notions that sanction male dominance over women. These attitudes reinforce violence against women. Blaming women for violence faced by them, considering violence to be a part and parcel of married lives, believing that women must have provoked violence are some of the beliefs reflected amongst health professionals (Deosthali and Malik 2009).

Health professionals believe that their role in dealing with cases of sexual violence is restricted to forensic examination and evidence collection. They are unaware of the therapeutic role that they need to play especially in aspects such as psychological first aid and treatment. Even while carrying out the forensic role, health professionals restrict examination to assessing genitals. A tendency to overemphasize genital and physical injuries has been noted amongst health professionals (Deosthali and Malik 2009). Unscientific practices of examination in the form of finger test, determining hymenal status, and recording height-weight of the survivor to examine the possibility of resistance is the norm in medico-legal examination of sexual violence (Deosthali 2013).

One reason for the suboptimal response from health professionals may be attributed to the gaps in medical and nursing curricula. Analytical reviews of medical and nursing curricula point to the gaps in the curricula which do not equip health professionals to adequately respond to women and children facing violence (Deosthali 2013). This was evident in a study on 250 nursing and medical college students in an industrial city of Maharashtra. The study aimed to understand perceptions of medical and nursing students towards the issue of VAW. Half the respondents were nursing students, the others pursuing medicine. The study found that a larger number of female students than male had more discouraging attitudes towards the issue of VAW. Male respondents were more likely to have victim-blaming attitudes towards those reporting abuse (Agrawal and Banerjee 2015). The differences in the perceptions can be attributed to the social milieu that male and female respondents belong to where gender-based discrimination is a norm. Add to this the fact that medical education in India has not taken cognizance of gender theories and perspectives in treating women and men (Subha Sri 2010). Consequently, the medical profession and system lack a gender sensitive perspective in responding to women facing violence.

Notwithstanding the above, it must be recognized that health professionals and health system can respond to the negative effects of VAW by providing supportive care. Supportive care comprises preventing, as well as mitigating, consequences of violence on women; addressing associated problems like depression, substance abuse, and providing immediate and long-term care.

CURRENT INTERVENTIONS ON VIOLENCE AGAINST WOMEN AS A HEALTH CARE ISSUE

Many developed countries have made steady progress in recognizing the importance of health systems response to VAW. They have integrated the responsibilities of the health sector in their national action plans, earmarked budgets for building capacities of health professionals, developed surveillance and reporting methods, and drafted protocols for documentation and service provision (American Medical Association 1992; Bacchus et al. 2012; Garcia-Moreno et al. 2014b). Developing countries are still struggling to respond to VAW in a systematic manner. Though the important role of the health sector and the need to integrate this concern in policies and programmes has been acknowledged, earmarking financial support for building capacities of health professionals, monitoring, and surveillance has still not been achieved.

The post-2000 era saw the initiation of different forms of engagements with the health sector on VAW (WHO, CEHAT, MoHFW 2016).

Hospital-based Crisis Centre to Respond to VAW

An early initiative in the Indian context was the establishment of a hospital-based crisis centre in a Mumbai suburb called Dilaasa

(Deosthali and Malik 2009). The main objectives of the centre was to equip the health professionals to understand VAW as a health issue and respond to women in a sensitive manner. The second objective was to create psychosocial services within the hospital for women who wanted support in dealing with the violence. Dilaasa represents a redesigned 'one-stop crisis centre' (OSCC), focusing on delivering an integrated response to VAW within the existing roles and responsibilities of health professionals. The model has been found to be more sustainable than a traditional OSCC where a separate cadre of specialists is brought into the hospital setting (Garcia-Moreno 2015).

Women either report violence spontaneously or in response to questions from health care providers prompted by signs and symptoms presented in the outpatient or inpatient consultation. Once identified, they are provided medical treatment, their history of abuse is documented, evidence is collected in case of sexual violence if appropriate, medico-legal support offered and they are told about the Dilaasa crisis intervention centre. The hospital has put up posters and distributed cards, and pamphlets to create awareness about VAW as a public health issue. In instances of sexual violence, health professionals have been trained to use the WHO protocols for medico-legal care in sexual violence. This has enabled health professionals to understand circumstances of sexual violence, reject unscientific aspects such as finger test, hymenal status; conduct a gender sensitive examination along with evidence collection; provide reasoned medical opinion, and explain the absence of injuries and/or absence of forensic evidence which helps survivors in courts (American Medical Association 1992).

Besides equipping health professionals to play a comprehensive role, another core function of the hospital-based centre is that of psychosocial support and crisis intervention services. Such services were conspicuous by their absence in health system. Counselling principles followed by the crisis centre help women to put the onus of abuse on the perpetrator and take away blame from themselves. It also equips women with the necessary tools and strategies to heal from abuse as well as stop it. These principles though drawn from the women's movement in India as well as from literature on feminist counselling in the west, were customized to the context of a public hospital, and a methodology of counselling has also been developed (Bhate-Deosthali, Rege, and Prakash 2013; Rege 2010).

Modelled on the Dilaasa crisis centre is another hospital-based crisis centre set up by the Northeast Network (NEN) (WHO, CEHAT,

MoHFW 2016). Northeast Network, in the course of their work in Meghalaya, found that women faced several health concerns especially related to reproductive health because of the violence faced at the hands of their partners, but were unable to do anything about it despite reaching hospitals for treatment. This prompted them to carry out an assessment at a civil hospital in Shillong to understand the hospital response to VAW. They were alarmed to see that health professionals did not recognize violence as a concern that affected health. In order to ensure that women facing violence receive counselling services, NEN actively worked upon the referral system with the women's hospital in Shillong and after four years of persistence were successful in establishing a crisis centre within the hospital in 2011. Allotting of physical space to the centre and terming it as a crisis centre lent legitimacy to the issues of VAW within the hospital. Efforts are underway to get the crisis centre of the hospital recognized as a department of the hospital.

Another unique effort has been by a feminist organization, *Swati* (WHO, CEHAT, MoHFW 2016), based in rural Gujarat. *Swati* has been actively working on the issue of VAW and has played an important role in equipping rural women to deal with systems such as the police, judiciary, and panchayat and to demand their rights and ensure that they get justice. However they encountered problems with the health system when women accessed health services for violence-related care. This prompted *Swati* to start a dialogue with a community health centre (CHC) in one of the rural areas where they work. The dialogue led to the hospital authorities asking *Swati* to conduct training sessions for nurses and doctors on the issue of VAW. Engagement with the hospital led to a shared understanding that the hospital needs to respond to VAW, but that it did not have social workers and was already understaffed. *Swati* stepped in with a trained cadre of women volunteers from several villages that started providing psychosocial services at the level of the hospital. The relationship with the CHC eventually led to the creation of a dedicated space within the hospital for these services.

Strengthening Linkages with the Health System through Referrals

Since 2001 some organizations have liaised with the health system to facilitate availability of psychosocial services to women and children facing violence. These services are either based in the hospitals or in close proximity to hospitals. *Sneha*, a Mumbai-based organization, founded by health professionals and social workers found that hospitals cater to the physical needs of women facing violence through medical treatment (WHO, CEHAT, MoHFW 2016). But beyond that women had no option but to continue to face abuse. *Sneha* recognized the urgent need to ensure that psychosocial services be provided to women facing any form of violence. This led to linking with the tertiary care hospital, where those women facing abuse could receive services from the *Sneha* counsellors. The allocation of space in the urban health centre of the public hospital and the availability of NGO counsellors made it possible for women to access psychosocial services. *Anweshi*, an organization based in Kozhikode, Kerala, is making similar efforts (WHO, CEHAT, MoHFW 2016). They have been providing counselling services, free legal aid, and shelter services to women facing violence. They have approached the Calicut Medical College to start referral services where women could start accessing different services of the *Anweshi* counselling centre.

Engagement with the Primary Health Care System and Accredited Social Health Activist Workers on Violence against Women

Efforts have also been made at the primary health care system to address VAW. Within the Indian health care setting, the health workers at the community level such as the Accredited Social Health Activist Workers (ASHAs), Auxiliary nurse Midwife (ANM), Integrated Child Developmental Services (ICDS) workers, can be instrumental in increasing awareness on VAW, its health consequences and provide information on available services to respond to violence at the community level. One such initiative called *Soukhya* has been set up at primary health care centres in collaboration with St John Medical College, Bangalore to respond to domestic violence survivors (WHO, CEHAT, MoHFW 2016). The programme involves three cadres of municipal primary health care workers such as doctors, nurses, and community workers. Doctors are tasked with mentoring and supervising nurses and community link workers and assisting in responses to complex cases of VAW. Nurses, who are providing the bulk of primary care services, are responsible for identifying women facing violence, explaining the health impact of violence, and referring them to a social worker. Community-link workers, who are residents of the communities served by the health centre, primarily engage in outreach; for example, they identify pregnant women and mothers of young children and motive them to seek antenatal, postnatal, and immunization services and have integrated an awareness initiative on VAW in their routine work.

Developing a Cadre of Community Health Workers to Respond to Violence against Women

Masum, a community-based women's organization working in Pune for almost three decades found that women faced oppression in their personal lives as well because of their caste and religious affiliations that resulted in violence (WHO, CEHAT, MoHFW 2016) but they were often hesitant to seek health care because the moment a medical diagnosis had been made they would be sent back to their natal families, especially if they suffered tuberculosis or had a mental health concern. Hesitation on the part of women to access health services and lack of specific systems and norms in the formal health system to address violence prompted Masum to develop community-based interventions to address these issues. Masum has a trained a cadre of women health workers from the community equipped with knowledge of women's body and women's health, information about health issues and their management, using local herbs for common ailments. Masum has also engaged the ICDS and Accredited Social Health Activists (ASHA) workers on the issue of VAW and has imparted training programmes to facilitate interlinkages between violence and health and enable these workers to create awareness on such links.

Advocacy Efforts for Health System to Recognize Violence against Women

Advocacy initiatives have been carried out by organizations to improve the health care response to VAW. Sama and Tathapi have engaged both public and private health providers on the issue of VAW. They have carried out research to identify the gaps in responses of the health sector and the need for them to carry out their roles under the law in a systematic manner. Sama has actively worked since 2009 to bring the issue to the Jan Swasthya Abhiyan (JSA) platform.

Vimochana, a Bangalore-based feminist organization, has actively worked with the health system for two decades (WHO, CEHAT, MoHFW 2016). Their work with the health system has been primarily on the issue of burns reported by women and the health care response to it. When they began their work at the hospital, it started as an investigative process of determining whether the burns in women were homicidal, suicidal, or accidental. Vimochana's work has shown that in most instances of burns in women could be homicidal, but women succumb to family pressure, and worry for their children's future prevents them from disclosing the homicide. While Vimochana continues to work with families of women who have suffered burns and ensures access to justice for them, it also engages the health system to treat women with burns in a humane and dignified manner. In the course of Vimochana's work they pressed for infrastructural changes in the burns wards and ensured proper diets for women as both were severely lacking in the hospital. They have steadily advocated for the improvement of recording related to dying declarations by health professionals.

Government Initiated One-Stop Crisis Centres in Hospitals

Taking a cue from the different civil society initiatives along with a legal mandate for the health sector under the prevention of domestic violence act (PWDVA 2005), the Kerala state health department through its NRHM programme set up one stop centres called Bhoomika (WHO, CEHAT, MoHFW 2016). By 2011, these centres had been set up in 14 district hospitals of Kerala and are staffed with a counsellor each. Though the cadre of trained counsellors exists in the 14 districts, they have a heavy caseload. This does not permit them to undertake in-depth counselling and they often have to refer women to other counselling centres. There is little integration of these one-stop centres with the rest of the hospital activities. There is a need for establishing a model that includes participation from different cadres of health professionals in order to create a more integrated approach to the issue of VAW.

There is no single model for addressing VAW in the health sector. The three prominent models namely, ecological model, a multi-sectoral approach, and systems approach have informed the manner in which countries have designed national action plans, policies, and protocols (Columbini, Mayhew, and Watts 2008).

The ecological model has been applied in the primary health care approaches to respond to violence against women as it helps health professionals to identify risk factors and consider them for development of strategies to reduce the risk through broad-based prevention programmes. The model focuses on individual, relationship, community and societal factors, which increases risk of women facing violence. Factors such as early age of marriage, isolation, young age have been identified as individual risk factors. Similarly, a host of factors have been identified at relationship, community, and societal levels. The application of the ecological model is reflected in the work by Masum and Soukhya at the level of primary health care, where health professionals and community health workers are equipped to identify risk factors and develop response with a focus on not just individual health needs but also on creating awareness amongst communities to aim for social change.

The multisectoral approach involves different stakeholders in responding to VAW. Implementing such an approach involves a coordinated response among agencies providing psychosocial support, legal aid, and shelter services and police aid. So a single sector is not responsible for the provision of all services. Such an approach is reflected in the efforts made by Sneha and Anweshi as they include inter-sectoral coordination to ensure comprehensive services for women facing violence as well as monitor referral networks to ensure that women are informed about their services.

The systems approach speaks of direct responsibilities of health service delivery organizations. This approach focuses on building skills and resources across an entire organization and not just individual health professionals. It aims to build an institution where the professional culture of an organization is changed and health professionals are convinced that responding to VAW is a part of their job responsibilities. Key elements of a systems approach would entail improving health professionals knowledge and skills about VAW, improving knowledge on national laws on VAW and role of the health sector, strengthening policies related to privacy and confidentiality of women reporting violence through improvement in clinical and infrastructural policies, drafting protocols for care and support to women facing violence, strengthening medical records and information systems, and ensuring the availability of educational and awareness materials for patient population.

Models such as the Dilaasa focus on the health care delivery approach as whole and integrate the response to VAW in the role of health professionals. Such an integrated approach is closely linked to systems approach where health professionals are equipped to screen women for violence, provide medical care, and basic emotional support followed by a referral in the same health facility to a counselling department.

* * *

This chapter presents various interventions with health system and health professionals for improving response to VAW by different organizations including initiatives by the government. However, few approaches have been properly evaluated and hence it is a challenge to motivate the government to replicate such efforts. Despite legislation on responding to violence against women and the explicit role of the health sector, there are several challenges in implementing these roles on the ground. One of the reasons is the lack of technical and financial resources for implementation of health sector roles.

The preoccupation is with OSCCs and this is true of South Asia. The WHO Guidelines (2013) recommend that the ministries of health must adopt various models for provision of care at different levels of the health system and not focus narrowly on a single model for the entire country. The integration of VAW within clinical care is recommended at all levels from primary to tertiary levels notwithstanding the presence of a full-fledged OSCC. This is an important recommendation as low- and middle-income countries have limited resources across various sectors and OSCCs are highly resource-intensive. However, in India there seems to be fixation on OSCCs. The Ministry of Women and Child Development (MWCD) is currently charged with the setting up of one-stop crisis centres across the states with dedicated budgets (The Ministry of Women and Child Development 2016). Unfortunately, these centres are stand-alone crisis centres and no efforts are being made to foster collaborative partnerships with the health system to support these crisis centres. Nor are these crisis centres located in the hospitals despite global evidence on the utility of health institution based responses to VAW (World Health Organization 2013: 37).

The Ministry of Health and Family Welfare (MoHFW) has recognized VAW as an issue only after the massive campaign post the brutal sexual assault and murder of a young physiotherapist in December 2012. Taking cognizance of the abysmal response to rape by health professionals, the MoHFW has formulated comprehensive medico-legal guidelines for survivors of sexual violence in 2014 (Verma, Seth, and Subramanium 2013). A multisectoral advisory committee was established for the drafting of these guidelines that focus on therapeutic care as well as medico-legal aspects of sexual violence. Despite this progress, the draft NHP 2015 did not include VAW as a health care issue. The guidelines drafted by the advisory committee are an important step and it is now critical that different states in India ensure that these guidelines are adopted and implemented uniformly. However, these cover only sexual violence and not domestic violence.

The World Health Organization clinical guidelines of 2013 have been developed focusing on low- and middle-income countries and the specific recommendations made need to be translated into a clear policy document of a health systems response to VAW by the MoHFW. In the absence of a clear policy the response will remain chequered and not systematic.

The health system in India has been slow in recognizing VAW as a health care issue despite a legal mandate for health professionals to respond to survivors of violence. Several promising interventions are in place that demonstrate what can be done by health workers and how the response can be integrated within the system. There is a need to develop a systems response so that individual doctors and nurses who respond to specific needs of survivors are supported by hospital-based interventions and clear policy guidelines and protocols.

REFERENCES

Agrawal, S., A. Banerjee. 2015. 'Perception of Violence against Women among Future Health Professionals in an Industrial Township', *Industrial Psychiatry Journal* 19(2): 90–93. Available at: http://doi.org/10.4103/0972-6748.90337. Accessed on 7 August 2016.

American Medical Association. 1992. *Diagnostic and Treatment Guidelines on Domestic Violence*. American Medical Association. Available online at: http://www.ncdsv.org/images/AMA_Diag&TreatGuideDV_3-1992.pdf.

Bacchus, L., S. Bewley, C. Fernandez, H. Hellbernd, S. Lo Fo Wong, S. Otasevic, L. Pas, S. Perttu, and T. Savola. 2012. *Health Sector Responses to Domestic Violence in Europe: A Comparison of Promising Intervention Models in Maternity and Primary Care Settings*. London School of Hygiene & Tropical Medicine: London. Available online at: http://diverhse.eu and http://diverhse.org.

Bhate-Deosthali, Padma 2016. *Neither Evidence nor Care: Situational Analysis of Health Sector Response to Sexual Violence*. Geneva: WHO.

Bhate-Deosthali Padma and Ravi Duggal. 2013. 'Rethinking Gender Based Violence and Public Health Policies in India Insights from Dilaasa, Mumbai, India'. In *Gender Based Violence and Public Health-International Perspectives on Budgets and Policies*, Nakray Keerty (ed.), pp. 184–96. London: Routledge.

Bhate-Deosthali, Padma, Sangeeta Rege, and Padma Prakash. 2013. *Feminist Counselling Practices in Domestic Violence*. New Delhi: Routledge.

Chowdhary, N. and V. Patel 2008. 'The Effect of Spousal Violence on Women's Health: Findings from the Stree Arogya Shodh in Goa India', *Journal of Postgrad Medicine* 54(4): 306–12.

Columbini, M., S. Mayhew, and C. Watts. 2008. 'Health Sector Responses to Intimate Partner Violence in Low- and Middle-income Settings: A Review of Current Models, Challenges and Opportunities', *Bulletin of World Health Organisation* 86(8): 635–42.

Deosthali, Padma. 2013. 'Moving from Evidence to Care: Ethical Responsibility of Health Professionals in Responding to Sexual Assault', *Indian Journal of Medical Ethics* 10(1): 2–5.

Deosthali, Padma and Seema Malik. 2009 'Establishing Dilaasa: A Public Hospital Based Crisis Centre'. In *NGOs, Health and the Urban Poor*, Vimla Nadkarni, Roopashri Sinha, and Leonie D'Mello (eds), pp. 140–60. Mumbai: Rawat Publications.

García-Moreno, C.H., C. Jansen Watts, M. Ellsberg, and L. Heise. 2005. *WHO Multi-country Study on Women's Health and Domestic Violence against Women Initial Results on Prevalence, Health Outcomes and Women's Responses*. Geneva: World Health Organization.

García-Moreno Claudia, Cathy Zimmerman, Alison Morris-Gehring, Lori Heise, Avni Amin, Naeemah Abrahams, O. Montoya, P. Bhate-Deosthali, N. Kilonzo, and C. Watts. 2014a. 'Addressing Violence against Women: A Call to Action', *The Lancet* 385(9978): 1685–95.

García-Moreno Claudia, Kelsey Hegarty, Ana d'Oliveira, Flavia Lucas, Jane Koziol-MacLain, Colombini Manuela, and Feder Gene. 2014b. 'The Health-Systems Response to Violence Against Women', *The Lancet* 385(9977): 1567–79.

García-Moreno, C.C. Kelsey Hegarty, Ana Flavia Lucas d'Oliveira, Jane Koziol-McLain, Manuela Colombini, and Gene Feder. 2015. 'The Health-Systems Response to Violence against Women', *The Lancet,* 385(9977): 1567–79.

Government of India. 2005. *The Protection of Women from Domestic Violence Act (PWDVA), 2005*. Available at: http://ncw.nic.in/acts/TheProtectionofWomenfromDomesticViolenceAct2005.pdf. Accessed on 7 August 2016.

———. 2012. *The Protection of Children from Sexual Offences Act 2012*. Available at: http://wcd.nic.in/sites/default/files/childprotection31072012.pdf. Accessed on 7 August 2016.

———. 2013. The Criminal Amendment to Rape 2013. Available at: https://www.iitk.ac.in/wc/data/TheCriminalLaw.pdf. Accessed on 7 August 2016.

International Institute for Population Sciences (IIPS). 2009. *National Family Health Survey (NFHS-3) India 2005–06*. Mumbai: International Institute for Population Sciences.

Johri, M., R. Morales, J. Boivin, B. Samayoa, J. Hoch, C. Grazioso, I. Matta, C. Sommen, E.Diaz, H. Fong, and E. Arathoon. 2011. 'Partner Violence During Pregnancy in Guatemala: A Cross-Sectional Study', *BMC Pregnancy Childbirth* 11(49): 1–12.

Koski, A.R. Stephenson, and M. Koenig. 2011. 'Physical Violence by Partner during Pregnancy and Use of Prenatal Care in Rural India', *Journal of Health Population and Nutrition* 29(3): 245–54.

Kumar, Radha. 1993. *The History of Doing: An Illustrated Account of Movements for Women's Rights and Feminism in India 1800–1990*. New Delhi: Zubaan.

Kumar, S., L. Jeyaseelan, S. Suresh, R. Ahuja, and India Safe Streeing Commitee. 2005. 'Domestic Violence and Its Mental Health Correlates in Indian Women', *The British Journal of Psychiatry* 187(1): 62–7.

Medico Friend Circle (Bombay, India). 2002. *Carnage in Gujarat: A Public Health Crisis.* Pune: Medico Friend Circle.

National Crime Records Bureau. 2014. *Crime in India 2014.* Government of India, New Delhi: Ministry of Home Affairs, National Crime Records Bureau.

Rege, Sangeeta. 2010. *Guidelines for Counselling Women Facing Violence.* Mumbai: CEHAT.

Subha Sri, B. 2010. 'Women's Bodies and the Medical Profession', *Economic & Political Weekly* 14(17, 24 April).

The Ministry of Women and Child Development. 2016. *One stop centre scheme: Implementation Guidelines for State Governments/UT Administrations.* Available at: http://wcd.nic.in/sites/default/files/Final%20Approved%20Guideline%20OSC%20%20%281%29.pdf. Accessed on 7 August 2016.

Verma, Justice J.S., Justice Leila Seth, Gopal Subramanium. 2013. *Report of the Committee on Amendments to Criminal Law.* Available at: http://www.prsindia.org/uploads/media/Justice%20verma%20committee/js%20verma%20committe%20report.pdf. Accessed on 9 August 2016.

WHO, CEHAT, and Ministry of Health and Family Welfare. 2016. *Report on Best Practices in Health Sector for Responding To Violence Against Women.* Bangalore: CEHAT and WHO.

Williamson, Emma. 2013. 'Measuring Gender Based Violence—Issues of Impact and Prevalence'. In *Gender Based Violence and Public Health—International Perspectives on Budgets and Policies,* Nakray Keerty (ed.), pp. 65–78. London: Routledge.

World Health Organization. 1997. *Violence against Women a Priority Health Issue.* Geneva: WHO. Available at: http://www.who.int/violence_injury_prevention/media/en/154.pdf. Accessed on 7 August 2016.

———. 2013. *Responding to Intimate Partner Violence and Sexual Violence against Women: WHO Clinical and Policy Guidelines.* Geneva: World Health Organization.

IV

RIGHT TO HEALTH AND UNIVERSAL HEALTH STRATEGIES

14

Universal Health Coverage
How Viable?

K. Srinath Reddy and Manu Raj Mathur

The concept of Universal Health Coverage (UHC) began to evolve in Europe in the nineteenth century with reforms introduced by Bismarck in Germany (Derickson 1994: 80). The Beveridge Report (1942) ushered in British reforms in the 1940s leading to the introduction of the National Health Service (NHS) by Aneurin Bevan in 1948 (Webster 1998). Since then, universal access to affordable health care has become a widely shared aspiration across the globe. Over the last decade many low- and middle-income countries claim to have advanced along the path, albeit following different models. Mexico announced 100 per cent coverage in 2012 while China and South Africa are now close to it. Many Latin American, several Asian countries, and some African nations are reconfiguring their health systems to achieve UHC soon. *The World Health Report* of 2010 documents and endorses this global movement (WHO 2010).

The terms 'universal health coverage', 'universal health care', 'universal health access', and 'universal health protection' are sometimes used interchangeably, but also often used to distinctively demarcate the nature of services provided as well as the range of health determinants addressed under the rubric of universality. Universal Health Coverage can, when interpreted narrowly, mean only coverage of all or most people in a population by some form of a health insurance scheme. In another sense, it may mean accessibility of health services in a geographical sense, without any assurance of quality or affordability. For that reason, some public health advocates prefer to use the term as encompassing universal access to a wide range of services of assured quality along with affordability assured by a people-friendly health system. Others are concerned that the term health care is limited to preventive and curative health services and excludes the social determinants of health, which play a vital role in influencing the health of populations and individuals. They prefer to use the term Universal Health Protection to include 'health beyond health care'. The term Universal Health Assurance is also used to convey a broad combination of universal health care and health promoting actions on the social determinants of health.

To avoid a narrow interpretation of UHC, as merely some form of health insurance or even extended financial protection through state funding, the High Level Expert Group (HLEG) on UHC, constituted by the Planning Commission of India in 2010, chose a much broader definition. It included the dimension of health care as well as the social determinants of public health relevance:

> Ensuring equitable access for all Indian citizens resident in any part of the country, regardless of income level, social status, gender, caste or religion, to affordable, accountable and appropriate, assured quality health services (promotive, preventive, curative and rehabilitative) as well as public health services addressing wider determinants of health delivered to individuals and populations, with the government being the guarantor and enabler, although not necessarily the only provider, of health and related services.
>
> (Planning Commission 2011, emphasis in original)

Since the World Health Assembly adopted the term 'Universal Health Coverage' in 2005, it has become the most widely used phrase in the global discourse on access and affordability of health services. It also now features among the targets under the overarching health goal of the Sustainable Development Goals (SDGs) which are to be adopted by the United Nations (UN) in 2015 (United Nations 2015). The World Health Organization defines Universal Health Coverage as 'a state of health system performance, when all people receive the quality health services they need without suffering financial hardship' (WHO 2012). It is expected to provide equitable access to affordable, accountable, appropriate health services of assured quality to all people, including promotive, preventive, curative, palliative, and rehabilitative services. This chapter uses the term UHC in conformity with this concept.

While UHC has become prominent in public discourse in recent years, the ethos for promoting equity in all spheres emerged from the anti-colonial and anti-feudal struggles that were part of India's freedom movement. The aspirations of a newly independent India for creating a just and equitable society were enshrined in the Constitution, which committed the Indian state to promote access to health for all citizens. While these aspirations may have been dampened by the manner in which the Indian health system has evolved over the past six decades, it is important to recognize that continued commitment to these values must arise from a wide ranging set of obligations, from the Constitution of India to several international covenants to which India is a signatory.

The Constitution of India places obligations on the government to ensure protection and fulfilment of right to health for all, without any discrimination, as a Fundamental Right under Articles 14, 15, and 21 (rights to life, equality, and non-discrimination), and also urges the State, under the Directive Principles of State Policy, to eliminate inequalities in status, facilities, and opportunities (Article 38); to strive to provide to everyone certain vital public health conditions such as health of workers, men, women, and children (Article 39); right to work, education, and public assistance in certain cases (Article 41); just and humane conditions of work and maternity relief (Article 42); raised level of nutrition and the standard of living and improvement of public health (Article 47); and protect and improve environment (Article 48A). The Union of India has signed various international treaties, agreements, and declarations specifically undertaking to provide right to health including but not limited to: Universal Declaration of Human Rights (UDHR): Article 25 (1); International Covenant on Economic, Social, and Cultural Rights (ICESCR): Article 12; Convention on the Rights of The Child (CRC): Article 24; Convention on the Elimination of All Forms of Discrimination against Women (CEDAW): Article 12; UN Convention on Rights of persons with dis-abilities (UNCRPD): Article 25; Declaration of Alma Ata (1978); Principles for the Protection of Persons with Mental Illness and the Improvement of Mental Health Care (1991); Declaration on the Elimination of Violence against Women (1993), Programme for Action of the International Conference on Population and Development, Cairo (1994); Platform of Action for the Fourth World Women's Conference, Beijing (1995) and the Millennium Development Goals (2000); Declaration of Commitment on HIV/AIDS, 'Global Crisis-Global Action' (2001), World Trade Organization (WTO), Doha Declaration on Trade Related Intellectual

Property Rights (TRIPS) Agreement & Public Health (2001), The Framework Convention on Tobacco Control (2003), International Health Regulations, 58th World Health Assembly (2005); and several other declarations and conventions on health. It is necessary to give effect to these international treaties and declarations under Article 253 of the Constitution of India.

India also commits to the pursuit of SDGs adopted at the UN in 2015. The lone but lofty SDG on health aspires to 'Ensure healthy lives and promote well-being for all at all ages'. Among the nine targets linked to this goal, target 3.8 specifically refers to UHC: 'Achieve universal health coverage, including financial risk protection, access to quality essential health-care services and access to safe, effective, quality and affordable essential medicines and vaccines for all' (United Nations 2015).

Thus the promise of universal access to affordable health services has been implicit in our health policy, even if not explicitly legislated as a Right to Health.

The initial years after Independence saw this commitment to health equity being reflected in the free provision of health services to all persons through public health care facilities. While these were limited in range, the rich as well as poor accessed whatever was available on an equal basis. However, the limited allocation of resources to the health sector fell short of the health system needs, leading to progressive weakening of public sector services. Barriers to access were no longer only geographical. They were also manifest as barriers of cost and quality. The private sector, which had a limited presence in those early years of Independent India, grew by default with initial proliferation of nursing homes and later of corporate hospital chains. Cost of health care escalated, even as public financing of health remained stagnant, and out-of-pocket (OOP) expenditure as well as health care related impoverishment spiralled up. The vision of universal access and health equity faded as an enfeebled and fragmented public health care system and an unregulated private sector, which also benefited from state patronage, engaged in an unequal competition that displayed the worst features of market failure in a sensitive social sector that is expected to embody public good.

In the last decade, new initiatives were launched to increase access to essential health services. The National Rural Health Mission (NRHM) was intended to improve health services in rural areas in states with poor health indicators. However, it focused mainly on maternal and child health and did not cover many other health conditions such as hypertension, diabetes, or mental illness, which are now widely prevalent, and has not yet integrated the many vertical infectious disease control programmes. It, therefore, remained an incomplete programme of primary health care. The Rashtriya Swasthya Bima Yojana (RSBY), the national government subsidized secondary care funding scheme for informal workers, as well as state-level tertiary care funding schemes for the poor, helped to extend access to hospitalized care but did not cover primary health care, outpatient care, or long-term medication. Despite some benefits, these initiatives did not constitute the architecture of universal health coverage. About 63 million persons face the threat of poverty every year due to the high cost of health care, which also continues to be an important barrier cited by people not seeking health care in the first place (MoHFW 2014; Reddy 2015a).

It was in this context that the public discourse on UHC has become more animated over the past five years. This chapter covers the key developments of this period, from the report of the HLEG (Planning Commission 2011) and the 12th Five-Year Plan (2012–17) to the draft of the proposed new National Health Policy and the sequence of union budgets that have deflated expectations that public financing of health would rise to levels where UHC could become a viable concept.

TORTUOUS ROAD TO UNIVERSAL HEALTH COVERAGE: HIGH-LEVEL EXPERT GROUP AND 12TH PLAN

With the aim of incorporating a comprehensive plan for health in India within the 12th Five-Year Plan, the Planning Commission of India, under approval by the Prime Minister, constituted the HLEG on UHC in October 2010. The overall mandate of the committee was to develop a framework for UHC, to be progressively implemented over 2012–22. The findings were presented to the Planning Commission in October 2011 (Planning Commission 2011; Sen 2012). The terms of reference (ToRs) related to: (*i*) human resources for health; (*ii*) physical and financial norms for quality and access; (*iii*) improved management of health; (*iv*) community involvement and public-private partnerships; (*v*) reforms of the pharmaceutical sector; and (*vi*) health financing, insurance and financial protection. In addition to this, the HLEG felt the need to provide additional situational analyses and recommendations pertaining specifically to the (*vii*) social determinants of health as well as (*viii*) gender and universal health coverage.

While financial protection was the principal objective of this initiative, it was recognized that the delivery of UHC also requires the availability of adequate health care infrastructure, skilled health workforce, and access to affordable drugs and technologies to ensure the entitled level and quality of care to every citizen. Further, the design and delivery of health programmes and services, call for efficient management systems as well as active engagement of empowered communities. The original terms of reference directed the HLEG to address all of these needs as part of evolving the framework of UHC. Since the social determinants of health have a profound influence not only on the health of populations but also on the ability of individuals to access health care, the HLEG decided to include a clear reference to them, though such determinants are conventionally regarded as falling in the domain of non-health sectors.

While discussing the principles of adopting and achieving UHC, the HLEG regarded it imperative to consider the right to health as the key underlying theme and recommended that this right be recognized in national law. It stated that UHC should be based on 12 core principles: (*i*) Universality; (*ii*) Equity; (*iii*) Empowerment; (*iv*) Comprehensiveness of Care; (*v*) Non-Exclusion and Non-Discrimination; (*vi*) Financial Protection; (*vii*) Quality and Rationality of Care; (*viii*) Protection of patient's rights, appropriate care, patient choice; (*ix*) Portability and continuity of care; (*x*) Pivotal role of public financing, substantial contribution of tax-based funds, single payer system; (*xi*) Consolidated and strengthened public health provisioning as a key component of UHC; and (*xii*) Accountability, transparency, and participation.

Recognizing the low level of public financing as a key barrier to UHC, HLEG recommended that central and state governments together should increase public expenditures on health from the current level of 1.2 per cent of Gross Domestic Product (GDP) to at least 2.5 per cent by the end of the 12th plan, and to at least 3 per cent of GDP by 2022. Since the expenditure on medicines and outpatient care contributed to 70 per cent of the Out-of-Pocket Spending (OOPS) and its highly impoverishing effect, the HLEG called for the availability of free essential medicines by increasing public spending on drug procurement. It further recommended that all drugs listed in the National List of Essential Medicines (NLEM) must be provided free of cost through a public distribution system which avoids stock outs in public facilities. Quality assured generic drugs were recommended for transparent procurement and assured supply. Appropriate price control of all drugs was also recommended. Protection of domestic capacity for inexpensive generic drug manufacture was also emphasized as a policy priority. To raise the level of public financing and provide financial protection against unaffordable health care expenditure, general taxation was recommended, by the HLEG, as the principal source of health care financing. This was to be complemented by additional mandatory deductions for health care from salaried individuals and tax payers, either as a proportion of taxable income or as a proportion of salary.

The High Level Expert Group was of the view that user fee of any kind militated against the vision of UHC. Based on global experience over the past three decades, it was clear that user fee was administratively inefficient, financially inadequate and highly inequitable, HLEG urged the government not to not to levy fees of any use of the health care services covered under the package of UHC. Even if public financing is increased, the priorities may still be misplaced towards expenditure on tertiary care, to the neglect of primary health services. High Level Expert Group, therefore, recommended that expenditures on primary health care (PHC) (including general health information and promotion, curative services at the primary level, screening for risk factors at the population level, and cost effective treatment, targeted towards specific risk factors) should account for at least 70 per cent of all health care expenditure.

The use of multiple insurance companies as intermediaries in central or state funded 'health insurance' schemes was noted by the HLEG to be inefficient. Global experience too argued in favour of a 'single payer' system. Hence, HLEG cautioned the government against the use of insurance companies or any other independent agents to purchase health care services on behalf of the government. It suggested that purchases of all health care services under the UHC system should be undertaken either directly by the central and state governments through their departments of health or by quasi-governmental autonomous agencies established for the purpose. All government-funded insurance schemes should, over time, be integrated with the UHC system. Universal Health Coverage would need to develop a National Health Package that offers, as part of the entitlement of every citizen, essential health services at different levels of the health care delivery system. Recognizing that, in the mixed health care system of India, the private sector too has to support and supplement the services provided by the public sector, HLEG recommended the drawing up of effective contracting guidelines, with adequate checks and balances, for the provision of health care by the formal private sector under the UHC framework.

The primacy of public sector health services, as a strong vehicle for delivery of UHC, was emphasized by HLEG. The chain of district-level services from the sub-centre to the District Hospital (with primary and community health centres in between), were recommended to be strengthened to enable the public sector to play such a role.

The High Level Expert Group report also pointed to an urgent need to ensure adequate numbers of trained health care providers of different categories. Even here priority was to be given to the provision of trained non-physician frontline health workers for delivering primary health services.

Community empowerment and effective participation of community representatives and civil society organisations were also emphasised by HLEG as essential for the design and delivery of people-friendly UHC. It called for enhancing the role of elected representatives as well as Panchayati Raj institutions (in rural areas) and local bodies (in urban areas). It also suggested that a formal grievance redressal mechanism should be instituted at the block levelat the block level. National Health Assemblies, on the lines of the annual multi-stakeholder conclaves in Thailand, were also advocated.

The High Level Expert Group considered the establishment of new regulatory systems and the strengthening of existing mechanisms to be absolutely necessary to ensure quality of care and good governance. The design and implementation of UHC was to ensure strong linkages and synergies between management and regulatory reforms and ensure accountability to patients and communities.

High Level Expert Group recommendations were drawn from global best practices and lessons provided by Indian experience. The functioning of health systems in states like Tamil Nadu and Kerala, which provided higher levels of efficiency and equity than many other states, were valuable in identifying the essential ingredients of a UHC framework. The experience of RSBY and various state sponsored health insurance schemes also offered lessons on how well-intended schemes for financial protection delivered inadequate results or had an unacceptable opportunity cost in neglected primary health services.

The 12th Five Year Plan (2012–17) incorporated some of these recommendations. Universal Health Coverage was listed as first among the guiding principles of the National Health Mission, which added an urban component to NRHM. However, the promised level of public financing was only 1.87 per cent of the GDP (Planning Commission 2013). Further, there was no clarity on the nature of health financing, with regard to creation of a single payer system from the welter of government-funded social insurance schemes. The role of the private sector was emphasized without caveats on the nature of contracting, accountability, and regulation. While integrated care was mentioned, no pathway was indicated for the continuum of care across primary, secondary, and tertiary services across the maze of India's mixed health system.

The plan encouraged states to design different models of UHC and pilot them for evaluation in a few select districts. The responsibility of guiding this was entrusted to the Ministry of Health and Family Welfare. That implementing ministry was lukewarm about accepting the mandate for UHC, which appeared to subsume NRHM, and was reluctant to proceed with implementation in the absence of committed increase in funding.

The journey towards UHC became difficult due to the absence of a clear roadmap in the 12th Five-Year Plan and the Union Health Ministry's commitment to the restricted mandate of the NRHM within the limited resources. Even more disconcerting was the fact that the states, where the primary responsibility for implementation lies, were not actively engaged in a consultative discussion on the HLEG report, during the development of the 12th Five-Year Plan. These factors, compounded by the absence of new allocations to the health sector in the Union Budgets of 2012, 2013, and 2014 effectively derailed UHC.

DRAFT NATIONAL HEALTH POLICY AND UNION BUDGET 2015

New hope for UHC arose with the advent of the new National Health Policy, which was placed for public comment in early 2015 in a draft format. The policy espouses equity, universality, and affordability among its key principles. Among its listed objectives are:

> achieve a significant reduction in out of pocket expenditure due to health care costs and reduction in proportion of households experiencing catastrophic health expenditures and consequent impoverishment; ...

> ... assure universal availability of free, comprehensive primary health care services, as an entitlement, for all aspects of reproductive, maternal, child and adolescent health and for the most prevalent communicable and non-communicable diseases in the population ...

and

ensure universal access to free essential drugs, diagnostics, emergency ambulance services, and emergency medical and surgical care services in public health facilities, so as to enhance the financial protection role of public facilities for all sections of the population.

(MoHFW 2014)

The National Health Policy draft profiles the state of India's health and the performance of the health system with commendable candour. While listing considerable progress towards the Millennium Development Goals for maternal and child mortality as well as the achievements of the NRHM, the document reports that many of India's health indicators, health service delivery as well as level of public financing for health lag behind many developing countries. While crediting NRHM for several innovations, the draft acknowledges that 'much of the increase in service delivery was related to select reproductive and child health services and to the national disease control programmes, and not to the wider range of health care services that were needed. Action on social determinants of health was even weaker'. Even the increase in service delivery was uneven across the country—more than 80 per cent of the increase in services was contributed by less than 20 per cent of the public health facilities. The draft admits 'hitherto primary care has been very selective, covering less than 20 per cent of primary health care needs' (MoHFW 2014).

While calling for an increase in public financing for health from 1.04 per cent to 2.5 per cent of the GDP, the draft is diffident about achieving this because of anticipated fiscal tightening. While espousing the principles of universality and equity, the policy states that financial protection measures would be directed towards the poor. Since the policy states clearly that over 63 million persons are exposed to the threat of being rendered poor every year by unaffordable health care expenditure, the policy recognizes that financial protection has to be extended to the poor as well as the non-poor vulnerable to such a threat. Hence the need to uphold the principle of universality, which goes beyond, targeted programmes, even while aiming for greater equity. The draft, however, does not reconcile its averred faith in universality with its stated preference for exclusive targeting of the poor.

The bold declaration that the Right to Health would be provided a legal framework through a National Health Rights Act, which will ensure health as a fundamental right, is very welcome. However, the draft also states that that it would be voluntary for the States to adopt this, based on their financial resources and ability to implement. That dilutes the basic premise of UHC, which requires that a citizen should be able to exercise that right to access an assured set of health care services anywhere in the country. A right, which extends only to some parts of the country would create different classes of citizenship.

The policy appropriately places great emphasis on strengthening both rural and urban primary health services. Comprehensive care is stressed as a key characteristic of these services, and their integration with secondary and tertiary care is intended to provide a care continuum. It is appropriate that previously neglected areas like non-communicable diseases are also proposed to be drawn into this integrated framework.

The large unmet need for health service providers, which is a major barrier to delivery of comprehensive primary care, is acknowledged. Engagement of non-physician service providers from different categories of allied health professionals, along with AYUSH professionals, is proposed. However, there is no indication of the timeline or the mechanisms for producing the vast numbers needed. There is no indication of how the vested interests created by flawed regulatory Councils, which presently govern health professional education, will be overcome. A firm commitment is made to provide essential drugs and diagnostics free of cost at public facilities, but specifics on what exactly would be provided are invisible.

As the policy moves to address secondary and tertiary care, the growing dependence on the private sector becomes apparent. Strategic purchasing of services from both public and private providers is proposed as the new mechanism for ensuring access to quality assured services, wherein the central and state governments will pay for a defined set of services. While the draft says this will not be competitive, the nature of purchase may put the progressively weakened public sector at a disadvantage if asked to bid for services against the well-resourced private sector.

Ambiguity regarding the role of the public sector is amplified when the draft says that the mindset must move away from regarding public services as free, but instead to consider them as prepaid care. While this correctly holds the public sector accountable for quality, how will quality improve if resources are not infused to improve infrastructure, recruit more qualified personnel, ensure supply chain efficiency, and grant them greater autonomy? How will these happen if the health budget is not increased and governance of the health system not improved?

The policy calls for all national and state health insurance schemes to be aligned into a single insurance scheme and a single fund pool reducing fragmentation. This is highly desirable and will transform the patchwork quilt of government-funded social insurance schemes into a single payer safety net, if it happens. A beginning can be made when the RSBY moves from the Labour Ministry to the Health Ministry. However the big question is whether the states, who are operating these government financed insurance programmes for gaining popular goodwill from their constituents, will willingly allow their branded schemes to be subsumed by a centrally directed single scheme, from whose implementation they do not draw political mileage?

This question becomes even more pertinent in light of the recent recommendations of the 14th Finance Commission, which have been accepted by the Union Government (Finance Commission 2015). The States would now receive a larger share of the tax revenues and would have far greater autonomy in deciding how they would spend within and across sectors. Would the draft policy's proposed financing and purchasing mechanisms be acceptable to and applied across all states? To what extent does this aspirational draft, which espouses several sound principles of desirable health policy, have a buy-in from the States who have the ultimate responsibility for service delivery? This calls for a countrywide consultation to generate a collective commitment to an effective and equitable health system that delivers UHC.

As a signal, the Union Budget of February 2015 has a clear disconnect with the draft health policy. While there has been a marginal increase in the allocations to the health sector, the actual level of funding incorporates the cut applied towards the end of previous budgetary year. In terms of per cent GDP, public financing from the Centre has actually fallen and, unless the states increase their allocations, would result in a dip in the aggregate level of public financing for health. The increase in tax exemption limits for medical insurance and medical reimbursement may provide some relief to the salaried class, but that too will be limited to what private health insurance and private hospitals will cover for some categories of illness. The poor and informal workers will not benefit, thereby excluding 90 per cent of the population from these limited benefits. Importantly, primary health services will be out of this ambit. Creation of more All India Institutes of Medical Sciences, which provide tertiary care, as enthusiastically proposed in the Union Budgets of 2014 and 2015, will not redress the neglect of primary and secondary care.

The tax concessions provided for higher private health insurance premiums, as well as the door opened for workers in formal employment to opt out of the Employee State Insurance (ESI) scheme, suggest that the Union Government wishes to provide the higher income groups and employees the private insurance route for purchase of health care from private providers. This faith in private insurance is misplaced and can become a dangerous legacy, which will thwart future efforts at implementing UHC through a 'single payer' system. The disadvantages of private health insurance have been clearly pointed out by the Harvard health economist William Hsiao:

> Empirical evidence indicates that a free market for insurance cannot achieve social equity and that serious market failures allow insurers to practice risk selection, leaving the most vulnerable people uninsured. Adverse selection among insurance buyers impairs the functions of the insurance market and deters the pooling of health risks widely. Moreover, the insurance market's high transaction costs yield highly inefficient results.
>
> (Hsiao 2007)

Viability and Affordability of Universal Health Coverage

Even as the debate on UHC continues in India, the following questions need to be addressed to determine the prospects of a UHC framework being adopted and earnestly implemented nationwide.

1. Is there a consensus on the vision for UHC?
2. Is there a political commitment to any agreed framework of UHC?
3. Will the level of public financing go up to levels where UHC becomes viable?
4. What roles will the central and state governments play in financing and implementing UHC?
5. Will comprehensive rural and urban PHC, with its seamless integration with higher levels of care, become the key feature of the UHC design, to ensure a continuum of care?
6. How will UHC optimally utilize India's mixed health system to deliver appropriate and affordable health services?
7. What are the barriers to the strengthening of public sector health services?
8. When the interests of private insurance companies and private health care 'industry' collide with the objectives of UHC, will the political decision makers and health system managers collude with them?
9. How can UHC be governed in the absence of strong and credible regulatory systems?

10. How can UHC be monitored without effective health information systems?

11. Can the civil society create a broad based social movement for a people-centric health system that adopts UHC as a core mandate?

There is considerable confusion about what UHC means to different groups who are engaged in the debate on whether and how it should be implemented in India. Some view it merely as a mandatory health insurance, derived from a combination of privately purchased, government subsidized and employer provided insurance schemes. Others view it as financial protection against high OOP and health care-related impoverishment, to be principally mediated by higher levels of tax based public financing and supplemented by the medley of insurance schemes listed above, blended in to a common pool for operating a 'single payer' purchasing mechanism. Some others view it as an entirely tax-based provision of free health services to all of society. A broader concept of UHC extends it beyond mere financial protection, to include other elements of the health system to ensure that the promised entitlements of assured services can indeed be delivered.

The discourse has become further confounded by senior policymakers in the present central government speaking of National Health Assurance Mission and Universal Health Assurance. Prime Minister Narendra Modi has himself said that he advocates 'health assurance, not insurance'. What is meant by 'health assurance' has not been clarified, giving scope to wide speculation and varied interpretation by different sectoral interests.

For UHC to be viable, it has to be embedded in a broad based framework of health assurance, based on a conceptual model that extends from financial protection, across a well-functioning health system, to the social determinants of health (Figure 14.1). Health assurance and UHC have been frequently mistaken for health insurance. Instead, health assurance should be seen as a combination of three concentric circles. If we draw an inner circle of financial protection, tax has to feature prominently in that, supplemented by social insurance and other insurance schemes. If we draw another circle around that, we can introduce the other elements of a functioning health system: health work force, infrastructure, governance, drug vaccines, and technologies, community engagement, and health management information systems. We do need more robust health information systems with real time data for a ready response. If we add those elements of the health system to

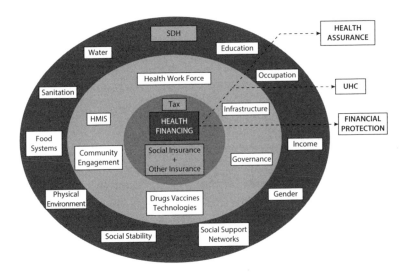

FIGURE 14.1   Vision for Health Assurance

Source: Reddy (2015b).

the financial protection, that is, combine the contents of both circles, we get UHC. But that alone will not suffice. We will also require the social determinants of health, to be addressed to promote and protect health. If we add the social determinants of health in an outer circle to supplement the other two circles of financial protection and broader health system elements, our people will have health assurance. It is that broad vision, of three synergistic circles, that we must develop to deliver appropriate, affordable, and universally accessible health services to all citizens (Reddy 2015b).

Health has not been in the centre of development planning, for any of the leading political parties. References made to universal access and increased public financing for health, in pre-election manifestos, are seldom honoured in subsequent policy priorities. The draft National Health Policy offers an opportunity to catalyse public debate to influence political opinion. All key decision makers in central and state governments must come on board, if UHC is to be implemented in earnest. The private health care sector would like to carve out a large portion of the financial pie by emphasizing the need to step up purchasing of secondary and tertiary care services by the government, exacerbating the fragmentation of health care, and further escalating health care costs. The need for strengthening comprehensive primary health services and providing effective linkages with other levels of care, through a revitalised public sector and responsibly contracted and regulated private sector, has to be advocated as the counterpoint. This should be undertaken by the civil society, which should create a broad-based social movement that will mobilize public opinion and modify policymaker perspectives.

Public financing for health is pivotal for the success of UHC. Both central and state allocations need to increase to a minimum aggregate level of 3 per cent of GDP by 2020. The underutilization of funds by the health ministry is cited by economists advising policymakers as the reason for reducing the allocation or freezing it at a lower level. While this seems logical on the surface, the stark reality is that the public sector in health has been progressively so enfeebled that it has low absorptive capacity. The correct response is to infuse more resources into strengthening infrastructure, expanding the health workforce and providing essential health services, including drugs and diagnostics, with assured access, financial protection, and quality. Only then will the funds be adequately absorbed and appropriately utilized. Otherwise, it would be like starving a sick child and saying it has lost its appetite and energy.

The greater flow of tax revenues to states, as recommended by the 14th Finance Commission, provides a stimulus to states to commit more resources to health and develop viable models for UHC. The increase in tax share from 32 per cent to 42 per cent is also accompanied by greater flexibility in spending the block grants, with less constraints from centrally sponsored schemes. Individual states can now design the framework for UHC as appropriate to their context. This both offers an opportunity and poses a threat. Political will and enlightened policy can galvanize the introduction and implementation of UHC. On the other hand, states may choose to neglect health or wrongly prioritise greater spending on secondary and tertiary care through private sector purchasing via ill-designed insurance schemes. Vigilance of public health advocates and vigour of civil society mobilization are the best defences against such a threat.

Strengthening of primary health services will require urgent action on many fronts. Strengthening of sub-centres and PHCs with technology enabled community health workers, nurses, new cadres of mid-level health workers, other allied health professionals, and AYUSH practitioners will help to deliver these services with greater outreach and effectiveness. Simultaneously, the production of various categories of health professionals must be scaled up. District hospitals must be strengthened and become centres for health professional education. Linkages between primary, secondary, and tertiary services must be established across the mixed health system, in a well regulated manner, so that continuum of care can be assured. Single-payer systems must be established for any payment of services under the UHC and consolidated annual payments for comprehensive health care ('capitation payment') must replace 'fee for service' which provides a perverse incentive for health care providers (especially doctors and hospitals) to order more visits and procedures. Emergency health services too must be made widely available.

Resistance to these reforms will come from a variety of groups: private sector health care providers who favour profit maximization; public sector providers who engage in private practice and have strong conflicts of interest; public health system managers who prefer to abdicate their role to the private sector and escape from the responsibility of ensuring access to assured quality services; private health insurance industry and political decision makers who have a nexus with private medical and nursing colleges or private health care industry. Large sections of our population, which are disenchanted by the performance of public sector in health, may also be unwilling to repose confidence in a UHC framework, which is principally led by government services. It is necessary to restore faith in the public sector by steadily increasing its capacity, infusing more funds, improving the quality, demanding more accountability, and strengthening governance. Only then can the critics of UHC be disarmed and vested interests defeated. This is not an easy task, as UHC is not merely an issue of technical redesign of the health system. It is a political battle that has to be fought with the rallying cry of social solidarity and health justice.

As Martin Luther King said, 'Change does not roll in on the wheels of inevitability. It calls for continuous struggle'.

REFERENCES

Beveridge, W. 1942. *Social Insurance and Allied Services*. H M Station Off London 1942. Available at: http://news.bbc.co.uk/1/shared/bsp/hi/pdfs/19_07_05_beveridge.pdf. Accessed on 12 February 2015.

Derickson, A. 1994. 'Health Security for All? Social Unionism and Universal Health Insurance 1935–1958', *The Journal of American History* 80(4): 1333–56.

Finance Commission. 2015. *Report of the Fourteenth Finance Commission*. New Delhi: Finance Commission India.

Hsiao, W.C. 2007. 'Why is a Systemic View of Health Financing Necessary?', *Health Affairs* 26(4): 950–61.

MoHFW. 2014. *National Health Policy 2015*, Draft. New Delhi, India: Ministry of Health and Family Welfare.

Planning Commission. 2011. *High Level Expert Group Report on Universal Health Coverage for India*. New Delhi. Available at: http://planningcommission.nic.in/reports/genrep/rep_uhc0812.pdf. Accessed on 23 February 2015.

———. 2013. 'Social Sectors', *Twelfth Five Year Plan (2012–2017), Planning Commission of India*. New Delhi.

Reddy, K.S. 2015a. 'India's Aspirations for Universal Health Coverage', *New England Journal of Medicine* 373(1):1–5.

———. 2015b. 'Health assurance: Giving Shape to a Slogan', *Current Medicine Research and Practice* 5(1): 1–9.

Sen, G. 2012. 'Universal Health Coverage in India', *Economic and Political Weekly* 47(8): 45–52.

United Nations. 2015. *Transforming Our World: The 2030 Agenda for Sustainable Development* (Finalised text for adoption). Available at: https://sustainabledevelopment.un.org/content/documents/7891TRANSFORMING%20OUR%20WORLD.pdf. Accessed on 3 August 2015.

Webster, C. 1998. *The National Health Service: A Political History*. London: Oxford University Press.

WHO. 2010. *The World Health Report: Health Systems Financing: The Path to Universal Coverage*. Geneva: World Health Organization.

———. 2012. *What is Universal Health Coverage?* Geneva. World Health Organization. Available at: http://www.who.int/features/qa/universal_health_coverage/en/index.html. Accessed on 24 February 2015.

15

Kerala's Early Experience
Moving towards Universal Health Coverage

Sunil Nandraj and Devaki Nambiar

The concept of Universal Health Coverage (UHC) or Access, widely debated and discussed in India, as in the world (Gwatkin and Ergo 2011; Kutzin 2012; Mishra and Rao 2015; Mukhopadhyay 2013; Sengupta 2013), has long origins. Goals and visions for this are drawn in part from the Alma-Ata Declaration on Primary Health Care (PHC) in 1978 and may be traced even further back, to the post-war and Independence articulations of Beveridge (1942) and Bhore (Government of India 1946) reports. In the current political-economic context, the main motivation for the resurgence of UHC is the grim reality that far from being a free entitlement, health is the cause of impoverishing expenditure globally (Evans, Marten, and Etienne 2012; Sen 2015).

In India, where neo-liberal economic policy since 1991 has meant that even health system strengthening is carried out in 'mission' mode, health reforms have been a matter of public debate for many years. Building on this, UHC was defined by the High Level Expert Group on Universal Health Coverage (HLEG-UHC) in 2011:

> Ensuring equitable access for all Indian citizens resident in any part of the country, regardless of income, social status, gender, caste, or religion, to affordable, accountable, and appropriate, assured quality health services (promotive, preventive, curative, and rehabilitative) as well as public health services addressing wider determinants of health delivered to individuals and populations with the government being the guarantor

and enabler, although not necessarily the only provider, of health and related services.

(Planning Commission 2011)

In order to achieve this vision, the HLEG proposed increase in public financing for healthcare to 2.5 per cent of Gross Domestic Product (GDP) by 2017, with preferential allocation (up to 70 per cent) for primary care. It recommended cashless, primarily tax-funded mechanism that would deliver an essential package of primary, secondary, and tertiary services. The High Level Expert Group proposed the creation of public health and health management cadres, augmentation and skill-based training of health human resources, a substantial allocation for essential drugs, enhancement of community participation, and action on social determinants of health. The expert group was mindful of the agenda of health for all envisioned at the cusp of Independence, recognized the various efforts, experiences, successes and failures of health reform over India's six decades of existence, and attempted to build upon these lessons and the lessons of other nations on the UHC path (Nambiar 2013; Sen 2015). Even as it lacked operational detailing, this report inaugurated a discourse on UHC in India, and served as a frame of reference for debates on health reform (Baru 2012; Mishra and Rao 2015; Sengupta 2013; Srivatsan and Shatrughna 2012) as well as a number of policy moves thereafter, including the 12th Five-Year Plan, the erstwhile National Health Assurance Mission, and the Draft National Health Policy. These policy moves may best be described as ad hoc (Duggal 2016). An implementation framework for UHC is still awaited in the country.

This chapter reflects on early developments for UHC in Kerala, which has been among the early adopters of UHC. The state has evolved a bottom-up model for progressive universalization of health services that places strong emphasis on existing systems, resources, and data. This was the authors' first and enduring impression and lesson in the course of their own engagement in providing technical support to the Department of Health and Family Welfare of the Government of Kerala on UHC from 2014 onwards. Having contributed to and learnt from this process, the main argument presented in this chapter is that UHC is as much about where and how you start as it is about where you want to go. We first lay out the existing scenario in Kerala and the context in which UHC reforms were introduced. Then, we describe the model for UHC propounded in the state and the way in which district pilot assessments were carried out to detail this model. Finally, we indicate what the way forward is with regard to UHC-linked interventions.

THE KERALA STORY

Kerala's story is peculiar and offers many lessons. Ramachandran (1997), writing about the Kerala model, pointed out several factors contributing to Kerala's unique situation: the historical specificities of nineteenth century Kerala, the missionary activity, and the government policy in the erstwhile princely states (particularly Travancore), the pervasive influence of the matrilineal system, anti-caste social reform, mass political movements led by the Communist Party from the 1930s and the Communist governments that came to power in 1957, 1967, 1980, and 1987 (Drèze and Sen 1997). When the state of Kerala was established in 1956, the Communist Party was the only political organization in the state with a programme for socio-economic and political change. They point out, 'Despite its relatively short periods in the leadership of the government of the state…. The left in Kerala has mobilized the people for kinds of social change unprecedented in the rest of the country' (Drèze and Sen 1997). Thus in 1985, Kerala was seen as an exemplar of 'good health at low cost' (The Rockefeller Foundation 1985).

This was, however, short-lived: fiscal pressures constrained such efforts in the later 1980s onwards. Health expenditure as a percentage of the Net State Domestic Product (NSDP) declined from 1.75 per cent in 1990–2001 to 1.12 per cent in 2009–10 (Oommen 2014). Simultaneously there was a massive increase in health expenditure per capita, borne largely by the population, not by the government. The National Sample Survey Organisation (NSSO) data from 2014 shows that both men and women in Kerala are doubly likely to go to a private doctor or hospital than to a public hospital or health centre for their most recent ailment (National Sample Survey Office 2015). Further, only one in 10 people seek care at primary-level facilities, like primary health centres (PHC), dispensaries, and so on. There is a clear preference for hospital-based care, which in turn is driving up 'mediflation' (Oommen 2014). A 2000 study found that while the poor were engaged in catastrophic spending (over 40 per cent of their income on health care), the rich were spending about 2.4 per cent of their income on health care (Kunhikannan and Aravindan 2000).

When a team revisited 'Good Health at Low Cost' in 2013, Kerala could no longer be counted a success story. Rather it was the neighbouring state of Tamil Nadu that was highlighted (Balabanova et al. 2013). The very fact that costs had escalated in Kerala booted it from consideration in this new report. However, it bears mentioning that a sample survey, conducted a year after the report was published, found that hospitalization costs were higher in the state of Tamil Nadu as compared to Kerala, driven up by urban expenses (National Sample Survey Office 2015). Regardless, Kerala now bears the ignominy of poor health at escalating cost.[1] Further, in 2005–06, the weighted incidence of catastrophic expenditure (defined as more than 10 per cent of pre-payment expenses put towards health) was 29.52 per cent in rural areas and 22.32 per cent in urban areas, with substantial concentration of these expenses among the poor.

The equity hallmarks of the Kerala model—of accessible and quality health protection and promotion, publicly provided along with education, and social security, run the risk of becoming artefacts of nostalgia and utopia.

BEGINNING OF UNIVERSAL HEALTH COVERAGE PATH

Seized of this, Kerala was among the first Indian states to act on implementing UHC. In 2013, the Draft National Health Policy of the state committed to developing its own 'template' for UHC. The Public Health Foundation of India, which served as the secretariat of the HLEG, was identified to provide technical assistance for the implementation of the programme at the district level. Thus began a partnership, that included extensive fieldwork in Malappuram and Palakkad districts (from 2014 to 2015) on which, this chapter is based.

Universal Health Coverage in Kerala was not so much the adaptation or incorporation of global concepts and categories as it was a deepening of our understanding of the state's history and current situation. We were keen to understand services, utilization, human resources, health burdens as they existed in the state, and link them to a vision of UHC that made intuitive sense to district and state officials running the system as well as to citizens making use of it. It was decided to conduct an assessment of both pilot districts to help shape the strategies for UHC intervention.

While carrying out this assessment, we were keen that the use of research evidence and knowledge should not stand pari passu with the existing running system, but should be woven in and out, be generated and used as intelligence in the system to drive programme design and action. Thus rather than carry out primary data collection, we relied on existing secondary data sources. So as not to burden the system, at the district and state level, programme coordinators were positioned to compile and standardize data, and be present and understand the needs and constraints of the health system. A government order was issued for the activity, following which there was collaborative creation of assessment formats and determination of key domains for data collection. Coordinators cleaned and compiled data and analyses were repeatedly presented at state- and district-level disseminations.

In the assessment, adapting the UHC cube (Roberts, Hsiao, and Reich 2015), we sought to understand the diverse services and resources being utilized by the different population groups. In addition to the elements of population coverage, service coverage, and financial risk protection, we were also interested in institutional mechanisms. For instance, we wanted to identify the services provided by each departments/sectors (public sector, private sector, health department, other departments) at which levels, and using what resources (that is, human, physical, financial, and knowledge resources). We wanted to gauge the strengths and weakness of the system in delivering care, and identify and prioritizing gaps for the pilot phase of UHC. Based on this logic, over eight months, we collected and analysed over 500 indicators for the year 2013–14 from over 60 sources.

A central question was: What are the top illness/disease conditions affecting populations in the districts? To answer this, our team collected utilization data from four major financial risk protection schemes operational in the districts: Rashtriya Swasthya Bima Yojana—Comprehensive Health Insurance Scheme (RSBY-CHIS), CHIS Plus, and Karunya Benevolent Fund. This allowed us to focus on the illness/diseases conditions/events that are proxies for catastrophic expenditure: that is, the poor using these schemes to pay for conditions that are not subsidized enough for them to otherwise afford. We also compiled routinely reported data from public facilities, that is, reporting of communicable and non-communicable diseases from the District Statistician. The findings are detailed in our report (Nandraj et al. 2016). We summarize below, two of the key findings from this study.

Health Burden Patterns Vary by District and Are out of Step with Health Services and Provisioning

The top mortality burdens in both districts were from non-communicable diseases (cardiac arrest, followed by respiratory distress), while, as can be expected, top morbidity burdens in both districts were from communicable diseases (with acute respiratory disorder topping the list in both districts, followed by hypertension) (see Table 15.1).

The differences among the districts are instructive. In Malappuram, we saw a high burden of deaths from non-communicable diseases

TABLE 15.1 Top 20 Mortality and Morbidity Burdens (2013)

	Malappuram			Palakkad		
*Profile**						
Total Area (square kilometres)	3,032			4,480		
Total Population in Lakhs (2011)	41.13			28.1		
Total Number of Females in Lakhs (2011)	12			11.01		
Mortality†	*Number*	*Proportion (per cent)*		*Number*	*Proportion (per cent)*	
Non-Communicable Diseases	15,304	76.1		10,741	59.4	
Communicable Diseases	254	1.3		500	2.8	
Injuries/Accidents/Suicides	747	3.7		1,188	6.6	
Senility, Ill-defined causes, and non-attributed	3,807	18.9		5,642	31.2	
Total	**20,112**			**18,071**		
Top 20 Morbidity Events/Conditions‡	*Number*	*Proportion of top 20 (per cent)*	*Proportion overall (per cent)*	*Number*	*Proportion of top 20 (per cent)*	*Proportion overall (per cent)*
Communicable Diseases	756,999	63.3	9.4	544,519	65.1	14.0
Non-Communicable Diseases	403,372	33.7	17.5	235,362	28.1	32.4
Injuries/Accidents	32,689	2.7	0.8	54,612	6.5	3.3
Reproductive, maternal and child health events	2,722	0.2	0.1	1,641	0.2	0.1
Others	3,118,022	Not applicable	72.3	842,769	Not applicable	50.2
Total of Top 20	**1,195,782**	**100**	**27.7**	**836,134**	**100**	**49.8**
Total	**4,313,804**			**1,678,903**		

Source: *Kerala State Planning Board. Economic Review 2014. Thiruvananthapuram: State Planning Board.

†SEVANA Local Self Government Civil Registration System 2015.

‡Non-Communicable Disease and Communicable Disease district reporting (including Integrated Disease Surveillance Programme), Rashtriya Swasthya Bima Yojana/Comprehensive Health Insurance Scheme, Comprehensive Health Insurance Scheme Plus, and Karunya Benevolent Fund claims. Top 20 conditions account for 27.7 per cent of all morbidities in Malappuram and 49.8 per cent of all morbidities in Palakkad.

(76.1 per cent), accounting for one in three of the most common events/conditions faced in the state. In this district, non-communicable diseases appear to be highly fatal and likely to be diagnosed at late stages. However, people in Malappuram suffer from a wide range of morbidities, possibly including a spectrum of conditions in the Non-Communicable Disease (NCD) category. In Palakkad, in contrast, we note that causes of death are more diversified (with injuries, accidents, and suicides accounting for 6.6 per cent of deaths). In fact, suicide was the cause of 571 deaths in 2013, more than double the number seen in Malappuram. In Palakkad, moreover, the causes of morbidity are more clustered: The top 20 conditions account for close to half of all morbidity reported in the state (see Table 15.2).

None of these considerations is reflected in the design of services. Three of four allopathic facilities in Malappuram have chest and tuberculosis specialties with one of five posts lying vacant, while only one of three facilities in Palakkad has a chest and tuberculosis specialty. There are no cardiologists in the public sector, even as in Malappuram, there are 31 cardiologists in the private sector. Further, there are almost five times as many chest and tuberculosis doctors in the private sector as there are in the public sector.

At lower levels of care, the average outpatient load is as low as three patients per day at dispensaries in Palakkad to as high as 140 patients averaging per day in 24 × 7 PHCs in Malappuram. Accredited Social Health Activists (ASHA) are largely in place, but in the absence of protocols for non-communicable diseases and conditions like acute respiratory disease, their ability to intervene and support communities for these top conditions is limited.

Further, the highest patient volumes are seen in Taluka Headquarters Hospitals (761 outpatients on average per day in Palakkad and 828 in Malappuram district), suggesting that primary-care facilities are underutilized and may not be performing preventive and promotive functions adequately. This crowding at higher levels puts pressure on the ability of the system to handle its current load, and to plan services using a public health frame/orientation.

Care Is Sought at Secondary Levels, Where the Private Sector Dominates

Private sector facilities far outnumber public sector institutions (see Table 15.3). There were 11 times more private allopathic hospitals

TABLE 15.2 Top 20 Conditions, Procedures, and/or Events in Malappuram and Palakkad (2013)

Rank	Top condition/procedure/events	Malappuram total[#]	Rank	Top conditions/procedures/events	Pallakkad total[#]
1	Acute Respiratory Infection	653,427	1	Acute Respiratory Infection	476,192
2	Hypertension	123,924	2	Hypertension	75788
3	Diabetes Mellitus Type 2	107,547	3	Diabetes Mellitus Type 2	60451
4	Chronic obstructive pulmonary disease	85,030	4	Acute Diarrheal Disease	59489
5	Acute Diarrheal Disease	83,498	5	Accidental Injuries/Road Traffic Accidents	54612
6	Asthma	54,862	6	Chronic obstructive pulmonary disease	44,518
7	Accidental Injuries/RTA	32,689	7	Asthma	30,092
8	Mental Disorders	9,593	8	Cancer	8,928
9	Ischemic Heart diseases	9,120	9	Ischemic Heart diseases	4,935
10	Cancer	8,465	10	Mental Disorders	4,688
11	Dengue Fever	8,321	11	Chronic Kidney Disease	3,556
12	Pneumonia	3,778	12	Dengue Fever	2,458
13	Cerebro Vascular Accident	3,474	13	Cerebro Vascular Accident	2,406
14	Enteric Fever/typhoid	3224	14	Pulmonary TB	2,125
15	Viral Hepatitis A	2,688	15	Snakebite	1,682
16	Delivery (CS & normal)	1,863	16	Enteric Fever/typhoid	1,300
17	Chronic Kidney Disease	1,357	17	Pneumonia	1,273
18	Pulmonary TB	1,249	18	Delivery (Caesarean & normal)	924
19	Urinary tract infection	859	19	Urinary tract infection	717
20	Leptospirosis	814	20	Acute gastroenteritis	474
	Total of Top 20	**11,95,782**		**Total of Top 20**	**836,134**
	Remaining conditions/Procedures/Events	**31,18,022**		**Remaining Conditions/Procedures/Events**	**842,769**

Source: Authors.[2]

[#] Total reflects addition of cases of communicable and non-communicable diseases, RSBY, CHIS Plus, and Karunya Benevolent Scheme claims in 2013.

TABLE 15.3 Public and Private Health Facilities in Malappuram and Palakkad, Kerala (2013–14)

Type of facility/Service	Malappuram			Palakkad		
	Public	Private	Ratio of private to public	Public	Private	Ratio of private to public
	Allopathic System of Medicine (Number of facilities)					
Medical College	1*	1	1	1*	3	3
Hospital	10#	113	11.30	9	79	8.78
Community Health Centre	20	Not Applicable		19	Not Applicable	
Primary Health Centre	88	Not Applicable		78	Not Applicable	
Dispensary	19	Not Applicable		14	Not Applicable	
Sub Centre	589	Not Applicable		504	Not Applicable	
Eye Hospitals	0	11		0	5	
Dental Clinics	0	150		0	65	
	Other Systems of Medicine (Number of facilities)					
AYUSH Hospitals	13	57	4.38	7	35	5.83
AYUSH Dispensaries	156	424	2.72	161	1	0.01

(Cont'd)

TABLE 15.3 (Cont'd)

Type of facility/Service	Malappuram			Palakkad		
	Public	Private	Ratio of private to public	Public	Private	Ratio of private to public
	Diagnostics (Number of each type of equipment)					
Cath Lab	0	7	—	1	4	4.00
X-Ray	8	250	31.25	11	139	12.64
USG scan	5	47	9.4	6	79	13.17
Laboratory	61	244	4	58	155	2.67
	Other services (Number of each type of service)					
Ambulance	30	111	3.7	47	91	1.94
Medical Shops	166	2,028	12.22	134	921	6.87
Dialysis Machines	26	130	5.00	18	37	2.06
	Utilization (Number of beneficiaries)					
Deliveries	16,214	70,244	4.33	9,003	30,042	3.34
Caesarian Deliveries	4,858	19,952	4.11	2,966	8,755	2.95
Full immunization	76,486	1,501	0.02	39,492	4,098	0.10

Source: Authors.

*Newly sanctioned medical colleges.

#Includes General, District Specialty and Taluk Hospitals.

in Malappuram than public; the ratio was close to nine in Palakkad. Even for non-allopathic facilities, there were roughly five times more hospitals and dispensaries in the private sector than in the public. The disparity for diagnostic services is greater—there are almost three times as many private laboratories in Palakkad than public, while there are 31 times more x-ray machines in the private sector in Mallapuram than public. In fact, as many as 150 private dental clinics were found in Malappuram and 65 in Palakkad, which have no public sector equivalent. Private eye hospitals numbered 11 and 5 in Malappuram and Palakkad, respectively.

How are these facilities used? Health system data for patient volumes across sectors was only available for immunization (where the public sector dominates) and childbirth (where the private sector dominates). Data from the National Sample Survey 71st Round for Kerala overall (see Table 15.4) suggest that the state is better off than the national average, but not by much (National Sample Survey Office 2015). Roughly two out of three spells of ailment in the state, as against every three out of four spells of ailment all-India, are treated in the private sector. There are no appreciable differences by gender. It is also evident that in Kerala, both individual doctors and hospitals get similar patient volumes in the private sector (whereas nationally, private doctor load is roughly double that of the hospital load). However, in the public sector, there is about twice the patient volume in hospitals as there is in lower, primary-care facilities. This means that patients are either presenting at later stages of disease (where they must go to secondary and higher-level facilities), or they have a preference for hospital-based care.

TABLE 15.4 Per Thousand Distributions of Spells of Ailment Treated on Medical Advice over Levels of Care for Each Gender

State	Kerala		India	
	Male	Female	Male	Female
HSC/PHC and other	97	118	79	90
Public hospital	216	242	164	174
Private doctor	360	350	513	497
Private hospital	327	291	243	239
All	1,000	1,000	1,000	1,000

Source: National Sample Survey Organisation (2015).
*Others includes ANM/ASHA/AWW/Dispensary/CHC/MMU.

Neither situation is desirable from a UHC perspective, where care should ideally be sought at lower levels and at earlier stages of illness. The implications of the skew of medical shops may have for mediflation are obvious: There are 12 times as many medical shops as are in the private than public in Malappuram and almost seven times in Palakkad. Patients going to the private sector will likely be referred to these private medical shops and be spending out of pocket.

Across both districts, health system data indicate that there is both overcrowding and understaffing at block level facilities (especially Taluka Head Quarters Hospitals, THQH). The magnitude of understaffing was highest for specialists in the public sector, which is likely to be correlated to the high reliance on the private sector. The public sector is thus left with Sophie's Choice: Whether to provide urgent, sought services—secondary care—or focus on important services—primary care. These levels of care in the public sector were found to be in a kind of competition instead of being in a continuum.

THE WAY FORWARD

These findings suggest that nothing short of a substantial re-engineering of the public health system will be needed to advance on the UHC path. For this reason, it has been proposed that comprehensive care pathways be developed for the top 20 conditions at the district level, which entails developing an essential health package using an entitlements framework (looking at specific health issues and developing interventions all the way from the community non-clinical level, through to specialized, tertiary level care). To implement these pathways, Kerala's health system will have to be re-engineered with norms for appropriate services at appropriate levels of care. Linked to the current emphasis on strengthening CPHC, it is proposed that two Taluka hospitals per district be focused upon in a phased manner and made nodal institutions with autonomy to upgrade human resources, streamline drug logistics, diagnostics services, and human resources for provision of wider range of services and infrastructure which provide secondary care for high burden of ailments (the top 20 conditions). Linked to these will be PHCs and Community Health Centres with an effective referral system that are equipped to deliver the top 20 care pathways with role clarity and adequate human resources. This would improve the inpatient services in Taluka hospitals, decongest the higher facilities, and provide comprehensive preventive and promotive focused patient care at primary facilities and community levels. These areas may also be linked to and thus strengthened by larger development planning exercises currently underway as part of the next Kerala Five-Year Plan.

If Kerala has to move towards UHC, the government sector has to emerge as viable in a highly privatized and tertiarized health-seeking context. This may be achieved by placing emphasis on the burdens that citizens face, with a focus on prevention, early detection and promotion of health, as well as quality provision of care for acute management of disease. This should help reduce out of pocket expenditures a priori and in the long term, reduce reliance on financial risk protection schemes. Eventually, risk protection could be built into the system just as UHC could be embedded into a larger human development agenda for the state.

NOTES

1. But clearly, our definition of good health has changed. Low mortality—specifically infant mortality—and long life expectancy were seen as proxies of good health back in 1985. Now, with the spectre of non-communicable diseases, all eyes are on morbidity. For every 'average' Indian reporting an ailment in the past two weeks, Kerala has three. But is that not to be expected of a state further along the epidemiological transition?

2. Based on raw data taken directly from District Statistician (Palakkad), Non-Communicable Diseases. Palakkad: District Medical Office, 2015; District Statistician (Malappuram), Non-Communicable Diseases. Malappuram: District Medical Office, 2015; District Statistician (Palakkad), Communicable Disease. Palakkad: District Medical Office, 2015; District Statistician (Malappuram), Communicable Disease. Malappuram: District Medical Office, 2015; Comprehensive Health Insurance Agency Kerala (CHIAK). RSBY-CHIS Plus data. Trivandrum: CHIAK, 2015; Integrated Disease Surveillance Programme (IDSP) Cell, Palakkad. - IDSP data, Palakkad: IDSP Cell, Palakkad District Medical Office, 2015; Integrated Disease Surveillance Programme (IDSP) Cell, Malappuram. IDSP data, Malappuram: IDSP Cell, Malappuram District Medical Office, 2015; Palakkad District Lottery Office. Karunya Benevolent Fund data. Palakkad: District lottery office, 2015; Palakkad District Lottery Office. Karunya Benevolent Fund data. Palakkad: District lottery office, 2015; Malappuram District Lottery Office. Karunya Benevolent Fund data. Malappuram: District lottery office, 2015.

REFERENCES

Balabanova, D., A. Mills, L. Conteh, B. Akkazieva, H. Banteyerga, U. Dash, L. Gilson, A. Harmer, A. Ibraimova, Z. Islam, A. Kidanu, T.P. Koehlmoos,

S. Limwattananon, V.R. Muraleedharan, G. Murzalieva, B. Palafox, W. Panichkriangkrai, W. Patcharanaramumol, L. Penn-Kekana, T. Powell-Jackson, V. Tangcharoensathien, and M. McKee. 2013. 'Good Health at Low Cost 25 years On: Lessons for the Future of Health Systems Strengthening', *The Lancet* 381(9883): 2118–33. Available at: http://doi.org/10.1016/S0140-6736(12)62000-5. Accessed on 25 November 2017.

Baru, R. 2012. 'A Limiting Perspective on Universal Coverage', *Economic and Political Weekly* 47(8): 64–6.

Beveridge, W. 1942. *Social Insurance and Allied Services*. Cmd. 6404, London: H.M.S.O.

Drèze, J. and A. Sen. 1997. *Indian Development: Selected Regional Perspectives*. Oxford, UK: Oxford University Press.

Duggal, R. 2016. 'Is NITI Aayog Even Thinking about Health?', *Economic and Political Weekly* 51(20): 12–14.

Evans, D.B., R. Marten, and C. Etienne. 2012. 'Universal Health Coverage is a Development Issue', *The Lancet* 380(9845): 864–5. Available at: http://doi.org/10.1016/S0140-6736(12)61483–4. Accessed on 25 November 2017.

Government of India [Bhore Commission]. 1946. *Report of the Health Survey and Development Committee* (4 volumes). New Delhi: Government of India.

Gwatkin, D.R. and A. Ergo. 2011. 'Universal Health Coverage: Friend or Foe of Health Equity?', *The Lancet* 377(9784): 2160–61. Available at: http://doi.org/10.1016/S0140-6736(10)62058-2.

Kunhikannan, T.P. and K.P. Aravindan. 2000. *Changes in the Health Status of Kerala, 1987–1997*. Thiruvananthapuram: KRPLLD, Centre for Development Studies.

Kutzin, J. 2012. 'Anything Goes on the Path to Universal Coverage? No', *Bulletin of the World Health Organization* 90(11): 867–8. Available at: http://doi.org/10.2471/BLT.12.113654. Accessed on 25 November 2017.

Mishra, A. and Seshadri S. Rao. 2015. 'Unpacking the Discourse on Universal Health Coverage in India', *Social Medicine* 9(2): 86–92.

Mukhopadhyay, I. 2013. 'Universal Health Coverage: The New Face of Neoliberalism', *Social Change* 43(2): 177–90. Available at: http://doi.org/10.1177/0049085713492281. Accessed on 25 November 2017.

Nambiar, D. 2013. 'India's "Tryst" with Universal Health Coverage: Reflections on Ethnography in Indian Health Policymaking', *Social Science & Medicine* 99: 135–42. Available at: http://doi.org/10.1016/j.socscimed.2013.08.022. Accessed on 25 November 2017.

Nandraj, S., J. Joseph, K. Mannethodi, Y. Thankachy, D. Nambiar, R. Shastri, and P. Ganesan. 2016. *Moving Towards Universal Health Coverage in Kerala: Piloting in the Districts of Malappuram and Palakkad*. Delhi/Trivandrum: Public Health Foundation of India/State Health Systems Resource Centre/Department of Health Services, Government of Kerala.

National Sample Survey Office. 2015. *Key Indicators of Social Consumption in India NSS 71st Round (January–June 2014)*. New Delhi: Ministry of Statistics and Programme Implementation, Government of India.

Oommen, M.A. 2014. 'Growth, Inequality and Well-being: Revisiting Fifty Years of Kerala's Development Trajectory', *Journal of South Asian Development* 9(2): 173–205.

Planning Commission. 2011. *High Level Expert Group Report On Universal Health Coverage For India*. New Delhi: Government of India (GOI). Available at: http://planningcommission.nic.in/reports/genrep/rep_uhc0812.pdf. Accessed on 25 November 2017.

Ramachandran, V.K. 1997. 'On Kerala's Development Achievements'. In *Indian Development: Selected Regional Perspectives*, J.P. Drèze and A.K. Sen (eds), pp. 205–326. Oxford: Oxford University Press.

Roberts, M.J., W.C. Hsiao, and M.R. Reich. 2015. 'Disaggregating the Universal Coverage Cube: Putting Equity in the Picture', *Health Systems & Reform* 1(1): 22–7. Available at: http://doi.org/10.1080/23288604.2014.99 5981. Accessed on 25 November 2017.

Sen, A. 2015. 'Universal Healthcare: The Affordable Dream', *The Guardian*. Available at: http://www.theguardian.com/society/2015/jan/06/-sp-universal-healthcare-the-affordable-dream-amartya-sen. Accessed on 25 November 2017.

Sengupta, Amit. 2013. 'Universal Health Care in India: Making it Public, Making it a Reality' (Occasional Paper No. 19). Municipal Services Project. Available at: http://www.municipalservicesproject.org/sites/ municipalservicesproject.org/files/publications/Sengupta_Universal_ Health_Care_in_India_Making_it_Public_May2013.pdf. Accessed on 25 November 2017.

Srivatsan, R. and Shatrughna, V. 2012. 'Political Challenges to Universal Access to Healthcare', *Economic and Political Weekly* 47(8): 61–3.

The Rockefeller Foundation. 1985. *Good Health at Low Cost*. The Rockefeller Foundation: New York.

16

A Financing Strategy for Universal Access to Health Care
Maharashtra Model

Ravi Duggal

Underinvestment in public health has been the hallmark of the Indian state from colonial times, notwithstanding the rich analysis, assessment and recommendations of the Bhore Committee Report (Government of India 1946). In colonial times the various provincial governments were spending a mere 0.35 per cent of Gross National Product (GNP) or around 4 per cent of their budgets on health, not very different from what state governments spend today. The Bhore Report defined eight objectives for its plan for a National Health Service: making adequate provision for the preventive and curative medical care; placing services as close to the community as possible; providing widest possible basis of cooperation between health personnel and the people; enabling involvement of medical and auxiliary professions in health policy formulation; making available diverse diagnostic, treatment, laboratory, and institutional facilities ('group' practice); making special provisions for vulnerable population groups; providing access to health care services irrespective of ability to pay for them; and creating healthy homes, workspaces, and recreational facilities. To realize this the government was urged to spend a minimum of 15 per cent of its budget, which at that point in history was a mere 1.33 per cent of India's GNP (Government of India 1946). Had they been implemented, these measures would have been India's first steps on the path to universal access to health care.

Historically, the Indian State has always been an insignificant player in the provision and/or financing of ambulatory health care. In precolonial times household production dominated, but with modern medicine there was a gradual shift towards commodification. Today the health care system is dominated by modern medicine and health care available largely as a commodity. Even the traditional and non-formal providers use modern medicine in their practice and operate within the market context.

In the case of hospital care the transition has been very different. Right up to the mid-1970s, the State and its agencies were the main providers of hospital care. There were also significant non-state players who set up large charitable hospitals. By 1970s medical education made a major transition. Postgraduation, specialization, and super-specialization became sought after and the character of medical practice changed. Specialists on one hand began setting up private nursing homes and the corporate sector on the other hand began to show interests in entering the hospital sector. Also major changes in medical technology, which hastened the process of commodification of health care, and the entry of private insurance in the health sector made for-profit hospitals a lucrative proposition.

In India, public health expenditures had peaked around mid-1980s with support from the Minimum Needs Program initiated during the 6th Five-Year Plan. The 1980s was a critical period in India's health development because during this period not only did the public health infrastructure, especially rural, expand substantially but also major improvements in health outcomes were recorded. By late 1980s the State was already decelerating investments in the hospital sector and this was a clarion call for the private sector to increase its presence. At the turn of the 1990s structural adjustment reforms, the harbinger of globalization, liberalization, and privatization, impacted the health sector drastically. These macroeconomic reforms rapidly transformed the gains of the public health system made under the Minimum Needs Programme of the 6th and 7th Five-Year Plans into a private sector-led growth that gradually destroyed the public health system. On the one hand the government underfinanced the public health system (with public health expenditure falling from 1.5 per cent of Gross Domestic Product in 1987 to 0.7 per cent in 1994) (see Gangoli, Duggal, and Shukla 2005) and stopped making new investments, and on the other hand private health insurance and corporate investments in the health sector, including the expansion of the medical tourism market and the massive growth of private medical education, provided the vital support for private health care to bloom.[1]

By the turn of the millennium not only had the for-profit hospital sector become dominant, but also privatization via user-charges, as well as through contracting out or leasing had become the order of the day within the state sector. Further evidence from various states which underwent health sector reforms under the World Bank (WB) supported Health Sector Developmental Programme (HSDP) shows huge declines in state public health budgets: From around 10 per cent of the state budgets in 1987 (prior to WB interventions) they are now halved at below 5 per cent (RBI 1987–2015). This reduced budgetary support to public health has led to the destruction of the public health system, a loss of its credibility, and ultimately its ability to achieve the desired health outcomes.

As a consequence of the declining state budgetary support for health, the largest source of financing health care in India is out-of-pocket (OOP) or self-financing. Out-of-pocket spending on health care as a mode of financing is both regressive and iniquitous. The latest estimates based on National Sample Survey Office (NSSO) 71st Round indicate that private expenditure on health care in India is now over Rs 3,200 billion and 95 per cent of this is OOP. Public expenditure on health care is about Rs 1,250 billion additionally. Together this adds up to over 4.5 per cent of Gross Domestic Product (GDP) with OOP expenses accounting for 69 per cent of the share in total health expenditures or 3.1 per cent of GDP. This is a substantial burden, especially for the poorer households in the bottom three quintiles, for whom the ratio of their income to financing health expenditures is two to four times more than the average mentioned above. Further, while this burden is largely self-financed by households much of this does not come from current incomes. Data from the 52nd Round NSS of 1995–6 reveals that over 40 per cent households borrow or sell assets to finance hospitalization expenditures, and there are very clear class gradients to this—nearly half the bottom two quintiles get into debt and/or sell assets in contrast to one-third of the top quintile; in fact in the top quintile this difference is supported by employer reimbursements and insurance. When we combine this data with the ratio of 'not seeking care when ill' in case of acute ailments by the bottom three quintiles in contrast to the top quintile—a difference of 2.5 times, and the reason for not seeking such care being mostly the cost factor—it becomes amply evident that OOP spending has drastic limits and in itself is the prime cause of most ill health, especially amongst the large majority for whom such a mode of financing strains their basic survival (NSSO 1998).

The National Rural Health Mission (NRHM) was launched with the 2005–06 budget to make significant architectural corrections in the public health system. However NRHM, like earlier policies and Five-Year Plans, defined its aim 'to provide effective health care to the poor, the vulnerable and to marginalized sections of society throughout the country' (MoHFW 2005). This narrow approach, however conflicts with the principle of universal access, thus undermining the very objective of a national health programme. It is evident from the history of programme implementation in India that targeted programmes fail to make an impact as compared to universalized initiatives. While these groups need special support from the public health system, the goal of the programme should not be selective because in doing so it distorts the design of universal coverage.

The National Rural Health Mission so far has been merely tinkering with the system. It has not made any significant structural inroads to making the architectural changes it proudly boasts about in the mission document. In fact, NRHM promotes public–private partnerships (PPP) aggressively and a number of initiatives in this line have been launched, the most talked about being the Chiranjeevi scheme in Gujarat for deliveries in private hospitals but financed by government, Rogi Kalyan Samitis, handing over of Primary Health Centres (PHCs)/Community Health Centres (CHCs) to private sector/NGOs in Arunachal Pradesh, Gujarat, and Karnataka, contracting out of specific services in hospitals like laundry, diagnostic, security, catering services, and others. Further, the use of the insurance route to finance tertiary and secondary care for below poverty line populations through programmes like the Rashtriya Swasthya Bima Yojana (National Health Insurance Plan) and its state-level clones like Arogyasri in Andhra Pradesh, Yeshaswini in Karnataka, Jeevan Dayi in Maharashtra, and others, are directing huge resources from the Ministries of Health—in 2010–11 Rs 21.98 billion as premiums for 189 million insured persons—towards such care in the private sector (IRDA 2012).[2] So an increasing proportion of public resources are being directed for the benefit of the private health sector in addition to various subsidies, which already exist.[3]

In sharp contrast, in countries where near universal access to health care is available with relative equity, the major mechanism of financing is usually a single-payer system like tax revenues, social or national insurance, or some such combination administered by an autonomous health authority which is mandated by law and provided through a public–private mix organized under a regulated system. Canada, Sweden, United Kingdom, Germany, Costa Rica, South Korea, Australia, and Japan are a few examples. Experiences from these countries indicate that the key factor in establishing equity in access to health care and health outcomes is the proportion of public finance to total health expenditures. Most of these countries have public expenditures averaging 80 per cent of total health expenditure.[4] The greater the proportion of public finances the better the access and health outcomes. Thus India, where public finance accounts for only 20 per cent of total health expenditures, has poor equity in access to health care and health outcomes in comparison to China, Malaysia, South Korea, Sri Lanka, Thailand (and more recently even Bangladesh and Nepal) where public finance accounts for between 30 per cent and 60 per cent of total health expenditure (WHO 2004).

Thus, if India has to improve health outcomes and equity in access then increasing public health expenditures will be critical. It will have to reverse the post-1991 declining trends in public health spending and move towards the United Progressive Alliance (UPA) government's target of 3 per cent of GDP public health expenditure. Simultaneously, the health care system will need to be organized and regulated in the framework of universal access, similar to countries like Canada or Brazil, or more recently our close neighbour Thailand.

The 12th Plan based on the High Level Expert Group (HLEG) report made a reasonable effort at assessment of the current health scenario and suggested a strategy that would entail a substantial increase in public health spending from 1.04 per cent of GDP at end of 11th Plan to 1.87 per cent by end of 12th Plan, expansion of RSBY, expansion of medical education, access to free medicines in public facilities, regulation of the private health sector, contracting in private services where public facilities are deficient, and so on (Planning Commission 2012a). To accomplish this the Plan made an allocation of Rs 3,000 billion for the health sector, more than double the 11th Plan final allocation of Rs 1,400 billion. The tragedy was that the 11th Plan was able to spend only 64 per cent of its final allocation of Rs 1,400 billion (Planning Commission 2012b: Volume 1). On the face of it the 12th Plan allocation of an average Rs 600 billion per year looks promising because it implies that the total average annual public health expenditure would be Rs 2,400 billion (given that plan expenditure is 25 per cent of total public health expenditure), but for 2013–14 the total budget estimate for public health is about Rs 1,250 billion, almost half of what should be expected to be on target (Rajya Sabha Secretariat 2016).[5]

It must be acknowledged that for the first time a Plan document talks of universal health care, albeit in a limited way, but the process has been aborted with the NITI Ayog rejecting the HLEG as well as the diluted 12th Plan health strategy and pushing for a rapid expansion of health insurance and private sector expansion of the health sector. Even the Draft 2015 Health Policy which has been released recently, speaks the HLEG language of universal access, tax-based financing, comprehensive health care, expansion of public health services, rejection of insurance model of financing etc. has been rejected by the NITI Ayog (Duggal 2016). Further the 14th Finance Commission has altered significantly the fiscal architecture of the country in keeping with the closure of the Planning Commission—there is a substantial shift of untied revenues to the states and the role of the Centre in social sector financing has been considerably reduced consequently. The 12th Plan's health sector allocations are now meaningless. Thus to understand health financing one has to shift focus to the states and how they would prioritize their new found resources and where public health stands in this frame.

TOWARDS A NEW FINANCING STRATEGY

Currently India's health financing mechanism as mentioned earlier is largely OOP and one sees a declining trend in public finance. Table 16.1 indicates trends in health expenditures over the last three

TABLE 16.1   Health Expenditure Trends in India

Year	Total public health expenditure (Rs Billions)	Per cent of GDP	Private health expenditure (Rs Billions)	Per cent of GDP	Per cent private to total health expenditure
1975–6	6.78	0.90	24.66	3.26	78.43
1980–1	12.86	0.99	52.84	4.06	80.43
1985–6	29.66	1.19	90.54	3.61	75.32
1986–7	44.55	1.47	100.00	3.41	69.18
1992–3	64.64	0.74	175.57	2.61	73.09

(Cont'd)

TABLE 16.1 (Cont'd)

Year	Total public health expenditure (Rs Billions)	Per cent of GDP	Private health expenditure (Rs Billions)	Per cent of GDP	Per cent private to total health expenditure
1993–4	76.81	0.98	195.43	2.50	71.78
1994–5	85.65	0.93	278.59	3.04	76.48
1995–6	96.01	0.89	329.23	3.07	77.42
1996–7	109.35	0.88	373.41	3.00	77.35
1997–8	127.21	0.92	458.99	3.30	78.30
1998–9	151.13	0.94	653.40	4.04	81.21
1999–2000	172.16	0.96	835.17	4.76	82.91
2000–01	186.13	0.98	981.68	5.18	84.06
2001–02	194.54	0.94	1,100.00	5.32	84.90
2002–03	197.32	0.88	1,250.00	5.60	86.36
2004–05	258	0.85	1,529*	5	86.82
2006–07	365	0.91	1,854*	5.8	85.19
2007–08	431	0.90	2,042*	5.1	84.78
2008–09	519	0.97	2,249*	4.24	81.25
2009–10	606	0.99	2,477*	4.05	80.34
2010–11	716	0.98	2,730*	3.76	79.22
2011–12	929	1.04	3,007*	3.42	76.40
2012–13	997	0.99	3,312*	3.29	76.86
2013–14	1219	1.06	3,600**	3.13	74.70
2014–15	1498RE[†]	1.15	4,000**	3.08	72.75
2015–16	1570BE[‡]	1.05	4,500**	3.00	74.13

Sources: Public: Finance Accounts of Central and State Governments up to 2011–12 and RBI's Finances of State Governments, and Union Budget Expenditure statements for subsequent years; Private: CSO–GOI–Private Final Consumption Expenditures, National Accounts Statistics, 2003 (1993–4 series).
*Since available PFCE data beyond 2003–04 is only available based on 2004–05 series and not comparable, the estimates have been calculated by author for private expenditures based on the ratio difference of PFCE between 1993–4 and 2004–05 series, for example for 2002–03 the 1993–4 series was 1.6 times the 2004–05 series—overall this appears to be an under-estimate for private health expenditure.
**Author projection.
[†]RE = revised estimate.
[‡]BE = budget estimate.

decades. It is quite evident from the data that public finance of health care is weakening and private expenditure is growing. This needs to change if India has to move towards Universal Access to Health Care. That India needs to commit around 3 per cent of GDP for public health care is a foregone conclusion. Apart from raising budgetary commitments, there would need to be critical structural changes in the way resources are allocated, budgets planned, service delivery organized, the way public health institutions are governed, and so on.

A review of global experience in establishing universal access to health care does not throw up a single common story or path. Each country has done it in a unique way and this indicates that contextual specificity is important. Some common elements and trajectories, may however be identified. For example, the NHS in UK under the Beveridge plan emerged as a post-war crises response with the Labour government at the helm (with Aneurin Bevan as Health Minister), which provided the political will despite huge opposition from the seniors in the medical profession. In Europe it emerged gradually beginning with Bismarck's welfare policies under the pressure of the trade union movements that finally led to the consolidation of the welfare state under post-war social democratic regimes. In Canada it was driven by a political champion Tommy Douglas in Saskatchewan province when he became the first social democrat premier and a few years later he supported the minority Liberal government led by Lester Pearson to pass the Medicare Act at the national level. In Brazil the 1988 reforms under a socialist government created the Unified Health System with a strong decentralization initiative leading towards universal health care access. And more recently Thailand in 2002 with strong legislative and executive backing legislated universal access to health care under the National Health Security Act and the National Health Security Fund. Many other countries like Chile, Mexico, Turkey, China, and Venezuela, and others, have moved close to achieving Universal Access to Health Care (UAHC).

Common elements that emerge from various country experiences are a strong political champion and/or a political party that is convinced about the political value of UAHC and demonstrates the political will to neutralize opposition especially from the powerful medical professional lobby, bringing in a law that mandates UAHC, including several other features: mandating minimum level of budgetary resources; reorganizing the health care system within a strong decentralized governance framework so that services are under local oversight and enable citizen participation; pooling of all resources to finance health care through a single-payer mechanism; developing payment systems and levels that are attractive to the medical professionals to join the system; a regulatory framework that lays out the rules and regulations, and an autonomous health authority that manages the entire health care system. The bottom line is that once UAHC is legislated and the requisite Health Authority put in place, minimum budget levels mandated and the health care delivery system reorganized, it would be difficult for any government or political force to undo. Pressures on the UK-NHS and other European health systems to privatize have been resisted strongly even when conservative governments have been in power.

Thus for realizing UAHC the growth of OOP financing of the health care system will have to be quelled and replaced with a combination of public finance and various collective financing options like social insurance, collectives/common interest groups organizing collective funds, and others. At another level the health care system needs to be organized into a regulated system that is ethical and accountable and is governed by a statutory mandate, which pools together the various collective resources and manages autonomously the working of the system towards the goal of providing comprehensive health care to all with equity.

This will happen only if the entire health care system, public and private, is organized under a common umbrella through a single-payer mechanism, which operates in a decentralized way. Health being a state subject, and given the changed fiscal architecture post 14th Finance Commission it is logical to look at this restructuring at the state level. For instance, in Canada's shift to universal access it was the state of Saskatchewan that took the lead to set up a health system strategy that would give universal access to its residents. Alberta followed and the rest is history.

In India a working group on universal access to health care was set up in Maharashtra by SATHI, an NGO working on health issues and the Tata Institute of Social Sciences, Mumbai drawing in experts in health from across the state. Through deliberations over two years it has developed a framework for a universal access health care system. This is a non-governmental initiative and the idea is to use this framework as an advocacy tool and to get the state government to start thinking about UAHC. The framework has been published as a policy brief[6] and the full report is under publication. The policy brief reviews the current scenario, assesses the gaps and suggests the policy, structural, and functional changes needed to move towards a UAHC system—the service delivery structure, reining in of the private sector, financing strategy, governance and accountability mechanisms, participatory monitoring and planning, and the legislative actions needed. The rest of the chapter elaborates the financing strategy for the UAHC in Maharashtra based on the working group framework.

While Maharashtra has low public spending, OOP expenditures are high and increasing very rapidly because of declining state health spending. For instance, in 2011–12 for the state as a whole the out of pocket expenditure as per the 68th NSS round works out to Rs 212.14 billion or Rs 1,861 per capita or 1.76 per cent of State Domestic Product (SDP) and four times that of public spending for the same year. As is well acknowledged, the NSSO figures are known to be under-estimates. Thus the out of pocket burdens are much higher, and especially so for the bottom three quintiles.

The Universal Access to Health Care framework as an immediate step (and more or less within existing resources) suggests that the state government can resort to certain measures that will make the use of current resources more efficient, accountable and equitable. These are as follows:

1. Allocation of existing resources on a per capita basis to each unit of health service providing outpatient care and per bed for inpatient care (global budgeting) through local government bodies. This will create both fiscal autonomy and responsibility for local governments as well as distributional equity in public health spending. This fiscal autonomy may begin at the zillaparishad (rural) and municipal (urban) levels. This would for instance translate to each district receiving on an average, Rs 215 crore for health services. This is apart from what local governments like municipal bodies and panchayats spend. For instance, the Mumbai Municipal Corporation alone spends over Rs 2,500 crore.

2. Introduce compulsory public health service for medical and nursing graduates passing out of both public and private medical and nursing schools for at least two to three years, with certification/license being withheld for non- compliance with the condition and entry to postgraduate studies denied (the public service can be designed to include credits for post-graduate education). This will raise the availability of medical human power in the public health system substantially. Today over 5,900 (2,800 public) allopathic medical graduates are produced annually in the state and this will not only fill

up all vacancies but also help substantially expand the public health system. Similar compulsory public service for graduates/postgraduates of management schools and other professional courses will bring in the non-clinical skills needed to strengthen the functioning of the public health system as well as other public systems.[7]

3. Strengthen and rationalize use of paramedics/health workers to provide first contact care, both in rural and urban areas. This will substantially enhance availability of ambulatory curative care in addition to preventive and promotive care in the public system as also set up the referral chain in accessing higher levels of care.

4. Strengthen primary medical care in PHCs and urban dispensaries so that hospitals are not used for routine illnesses, and consequently introduce a strict referral system for use of higher levels of care. This will rationalize and economize the use of limited resources.

5. Assure availability of free essential (generic) medicines in all public health facilities. This will improve the credibility of public health facilities and reduce substantially OOP burdens—medicines account for nearly 70 per cent of OOP spending.

6. Wind up the insurance-based health schemes and plough back that money into general health services to strengthen the latter.

7. Stop all forms of user charges in public health facilities.

To raise further resources the state government could do the following:

1. Introduce a health tax on lines of profession tax so that those who are in regular employment or business (and not covered by any social insurance) can contribute to the health budget directly and this will also create accountability pressures for effective and efficient services because those paying such a direct tax are more likely to demand appropriate returns for it.

2. The 6.5 per cent of wages, which are charged for ESIS, could be universalized for all salaried/regular wage employees—the wage ceiling for inclusion should be done away with—and the ESIS system should be merged with general health services. This would increase the employees covered in existing registered establishments from 12 lakh to nearly 30 lakh and a consequent increase in contributions adding substantially to the existing resources for the public health sector. At least half of the self-employed like entrepreneurs, traders, vendors, farmers, and others, could also make contributions for health care by structuring them into occupational groups (similar

to Germany or Japan), increasing the ESIS canvas further as well as further additional resources.

3. Health cess could be charged as part of house/shops and establishment taxes from owners, as part of land revenues, from owners of personal vehicles, from owners of cell phone connections, on health degrading products like alcohol, tobacco products, paan masalas, and so on.

4. An additional VAT of 2.5 per cent earmarked for a State Health Fund as is done for example, in Ghana.

The above are just a few possible ways of innovatively raising resources. There are many other ways of garnering resources from people who have capacity to pay. User charges should be done away with as it is an iniquitous way of making payments. Whenever the state is in a position to raise such resources the target of not only 1.7 per cent of SDP but close to 3 per cent of SDP would be possible.

OPERATIONALIZING THE FINANCING STRATEGY

Let us now look at how the structural changes will be operationalized to move towards UAHC in Maharashtra. Financing is a function of the system we create and it has to be contextualized to that. So the suggestions below begin with a brief profile of what a UAHC system should incorporate based on the Maharashtra UAHC framework document and then a costing is worked out to frame the financing strategy.

PRIMARY HEALTH CARE

1. *Family Practice and Epidemiological Services*: This is the base of the health care system. It is a combination of family medical practice and public health which is delivered to a unit of an average 500 families (ranging perhaps from 100 in sparsely populated areas to over 1,000 in dense habitations), assuming that on any given day between 2 to 3 per cent of the population seeks primary care—preventive, promotive, and curative. For this an epidemiological station (an upgraded version of the current PHC) for between 10,000 to 50,000 population would be needed with a core staff of a public health professionals: paramedics; community health workers, and other support staff to manage public health needs of its area; including outreach through sub centres, health workers and an appropriate number of clinicians based on the

population load, on an average one per 500 to 1,000 families. These clinicians would engage in family practice either as salaried employees or contracted in practitioners under a regulated capitation system of payment similar to the UK NHS, barred from practising privately. All families and individuals in this unit's coverage area will be enrolled under the UAHC and will be entitled to all primary care services (allopathic with progressive integration of AYUSH). These would include curative services, immunization, maternal care, contraceptive, reproductive, dental, ophthalmic, mental health, counselling, health education, environmental and public health, disease surveillance and control, rehabilitation and occupational health, pharmaceutical and basic diagnostic services, ambulance and mobile health services, and others. The Family Medical Practitioner (FMP) could be an allopath or an Ayush practitioner, the latter with crash training in allopathic medicine, or the proposed Bachelor in Health Sciences or the Basic Integrated Doctor who would be located in each sub centre of the epidemiological station area. The head of the epidemiological station would be either an allopath or Ayush doctor who also has training in public health.

2. *First Level Referral Care*: Presently we have the model of CHCs as first referral units but most are non-functional due to poor human resource availability, especially of specialists. Since this infrastructure with 30 beds is already mostly in places it should be retained, upgraded to 45–50 beds and dovetailed with a basic hospital of at least 150 beds like the present SDH (depending of course on the population size but approximately one bed per 1,500–2,000 population). This means that the base referral unit would be the block level hospital and the CHCs (about 3 per Block) would be its ancillary units providing integrated referral and basic specialty services. The block level (in cities the Municipal ward with a single 150–200 bedded hospital that is no CHCs) would be the health district, which will have a local health authority (a sub unit of state health authority) that would administer and govern the basic health care system of the area. For each basic specialty there should be at least two specialists employed or contracted in (those contracted to the UAHC would commit function full time, disallowed private consultative practice). Progressively numbers could be enhanced as they become available towards a goal that each CHC has all basic specialists and the block hospital gradually gets upgraded for higher-level referrals.

SECONDARY AND TERTIARY CARE

The district and large city hospitals of 500–2000 beds, including the teaching hospitals, would provide higher levels of care (about 1 bed per 4,000 population). Where there are inadequate numbers of public hospitals, private hospital beds, including the free beds under the Public Trust Act, would be contracted in through a regulated purchase agreement for exclusive service under the UAHC.

The entire system would be regulated and would have a gate-keeping system through a strict referral mechanism. All non-emergency cases would only come as referrals from the primary health care level.

The above is not a complete description but only an outline to give context to the costing of such a UAHC discussed below. However, it needs to be developed on the lines of the UK NHS but modified to suit the structures and needs within the state.

Working Out the Cost

We are not confining this calculation to the 2–3 per cent GDP commitment of the HLEG report but working out the cost based on the basic health care package defined above. This would of course be a staggered development. Further the costing is being worked out on the basis of an average unit as defined above—1,000 families for a FMP unit, 30,000 population and 5–10 beds for an Epidemiological Station or PHC, one bed per 1,000 population for the basic hospital (SDH) and CHCs, and one bed per 3,000 population per district/tertiary hospital (overall one bed per 1,000 population)—but on the ground will depend on the population covered and the density of an area, with unit rates of payments being adjusted for sparse population (higher rate) and dense population (lower rate). The costing is being done at 2012–13 prices and a population base of 11.4 crore and SDP of Rs 1,400,000 crore.

Primary Care Cost

1. Family Medical Practioner, one per 1,000 families at the rate of Rs 1,500 per family per year, including overheads. For 2.3 crore families 23,000 FMPs needed = Rs 3,450 crore.

   Rationale: Average net income of Rs 12 lakh per year and Rs 3 lakh as overheads, maintenance, assistance, special services etc. of the clinic. The clinic would be located at the sub centre and the ANM and MPW of the sub centre (paid by the ES) would support the clinic for preventive, promotive and outreach activities.

2. Epidemiological Station for 30,000 population at the rate of Rs 500 per capita (Rs 1.50 crore per unit, excluding medicines), including PHC, sub-centres, CHWs, ambulance services, basic diagnostics, public health programmes, health education, social determinants of health surveillance and oversight, audit and community oversight, 5–10 beds, and others. 3,800 ES needed = Rs 5,700 crore.

Rationale: Staff composition for each PHC-FMP unit to include seven doctors (two at the ES-PHC and five clinicians located at sub-centres—the FMPs as above and the latter paid independently as mentioned in (1) above), one PHN or Public Health professional (PHO), two nurse midwives, eight ANMs (females), four MPWs (males), two pharmacists, two clerk/stat assistants, one office assistant, two lab technicians, one dental assistant, one ophthalmic assistant, one physio assistant, one counsellor, three drivers(two for ambulance), one cleaner and 30 CHWs (ASHAs), and others. Doctors and nurses may either be salaried or on contract on a capitation basis as in the NHS of UK. The curative care component should work as a family medical practice with families being assigned to each such provider.

Average of 5–10 beds per PHC, one ambulance, pharmacy, basic diagnostics, ophthalmic, dental, physiotherapy and counselling units, five sub-centres, and others.

Average rural unit to cover 20,000 population (range 10,000–30,000 depending on density); average urban unit to cover 50,000 population (range 30,000–70,000 population depending on density).

All consumables, POL, overheads, and others, except drugs included, with salaries accounting for about 80–85 per cent of expenditures of the unit.

3. Pharmaceutical services for primary care (FMP and ES) at the rate of Rs 45 per capita per annum = Rs 513 crore.

Rationale: Based on NSSO data and the debates we have had over the past years and assuming that generics will be used mostly, and bulk and rationalized buying and elimination of retail purchases will reduce substantially the cost of drugs to the state. (Example of Tamil Nadu and Rajasthan experience in structured and regulated rational procurement.)

4. Basic Hospitals at Block (SDH—two per district for rural and one per 3 lakh population for urban) and CHC at the rate of one bed per 1,500 persons = 76,000 beds @ Rs 750,000 per bed per year would amount to Rs 5,700 crore.

Rationale: Based on costing studies/budgets of public and private hospitals (non-teaching and non-multispecialty). This includes all costs like salaries/fees, diagnostics, medicines and other consumables and admin and maintenance costs, ambulance services, and others.

Secondary- and Tertiary-Care Cost

District level and city hospitals at the rate of one bed per 4,000 population at Rs 15 lakh per bed per year, including medical and health education (doctors, nurses and paramedics). Beds needed 28,500 = Rs 4,275 crore.

Rationale: Based on costing studies/budgets of teaching and multi-specialty public and private hospitals. This includes all costs like salaries/ fees, stipends, diagnostics, medicines and other consumable, admin, maintenance, education, training, and so on. The staff composition as per existing teaching and district hospital norms. All district hospitals are planned eventually to become teaching hospitals so as to decentralize production and improve retention within districts. The range of costs will vary according to the mix of services provided and could range from unit costs of Rs 10 lakh to Rs 20 lakh per bed per year for general and super specialty, respectively.

A note of caution about the costing worked out. In working out the hospital costing I have erred on the higher side since market pricing has been factored. Under a public monopoly and use of rational therapeutics, strict audit and accountability these can be substantially negotiated down, closer to Rs 1 million per bed for teaching hospitals, Rs 0.75 million for the larger general hospitals and Rs 0.6 million for the block-level hospitals. Further the new investment capital spending of 15 per cent would be restricted to the initial years and if proposed infrastructure is in place then in later years this would be much lower.

The minimum requirement as worked out above is Rs 27,834 crore. Presently the state government spends Rs 7,800 crore and the municipal and panchayat local bodies spend around Rs 3,200 crore (Rs 2,500 cores BMC alone). Further around another Rs 500 crore is being spent through social insurance schemes. This means a pool of Rs 11,500 crore (0.82 per cent of SDP) is already being spent from the public exchequer. So the deficit is Rs 16,334 crore.

Where can the state government find these resources?

1. The state government collects a value-added tax (VAT) of around Rs 70,000 crore. If like Ghana, Maharashtra government can institute a 2.5 per cent additional VAT on all goods covered under VAT that is earmarked for a state health fund then approximately Rs 12,500 crore could be generated.
2. The state government can impose a health cess similar to the existing education and EGS cess on various transactions like property taxes, land revenues, cell phone users, on purchase of vehicles, on alcohol and tobacco products, and so on.
3. On the state excise duties which is mainly on alcohol an additional health levy could be imposed that would rein in substantial resources. Similarly on stamp duties and registration and electricity duties a health levy could be imposed.
4. The Maharashtra government could also impose a health tax, similar to profession tax, which could cover all employers/workers and businesses that are not covered under ESIS or other public social insurance scheme. This could easily generate about half the additional requirement.
5. It is estimated that better tax administration and discipline would itself generate an additional one-third of all state taxes. The volume of revenues forgone by the state government is not published, but back of envelope calculations suggest that this could be substantial.

To accomplish the above no great structural changes are needed. What is required is for the various departments like the tax revenue, charity commissioner, finance ministry, labour ministry, and others, to do their work efficiently and as mandated. So raising resources is not the big issue in financing the UAHC; the big issue and challenge is restructuring the health care system—re-energizing the public health system with appropriate resources and good governance and accountability, and regulating the private health sector towards its socialization under the umbrella of UAHC.

To do all of these, an exceptional political will is needed. This is the key element as revealed by the recent Thailand, Venezuela, and Brazil examples. To promote political will we need champions in mainstream politics for the cause of health and health care. We may have one off initiatives like the recent free medicines one in Rajasthan and other states, and so on, but these do not address system issues and hence are only populist schemes to help electoral politics.

Assuming that some political will exists and the resources indicated above are made available then how do we strategize the financing to achieve UAHC goals? At the outset I would like to make it clear that the costing we have worked out above and the resources needed is not for progressive realization. These resources are for a core package that must be made available right from the word go. This has to be a comprehensive approach; parts cannot be separated for prioritization. The government must in principle commit to making these resources available immediately, strategize and design the structural changes needed to make this work. All the resources from taxes, social insurances, cesses, and others should be pooled and transferred to the state health authorities as the case may be and they would transfer these resources to the district/block/municipal health authority as per their requirement based on the units of provision in that region.

As per our working, the resources should be provided to the block-/municipal-level health authority for the areas under its oversight. This block-level health authority would function as the key planning and budgeting unit with participation of providers, managers, elected representatives, and civil society representatives of the region. This authority will also maintain the list of all families/households in the block and enlist them under the UAHC for which appropriate documentation (Health Entitlement card, for example as suggested by HLEG) would be made. To facilitate its functioning this authority will also have a research and information management unit which will maintain all patient records, conduct local health related research, and others. Further, for monitoring and social audits the Community Based Monitoring and Planning system being experimented under NRHM must be appropriately upgraded to work with the UAHC. For accreditation and standards there should be an independent authority with its local branches (and perhaps this should be an authority that covers all social sector and development programmes).

Payment Mechanism and Fund Flow System

The block-health authorities, which will get quarterly allocations from the national and state authorities will purchase health care services from each provider unit as per the cost schedules (detailed cost schedules for each allocation will have to be worked out). The provider units will have to provide detailed budgets of their units (this being done as part of the participatory planning and budgeting exercise) to secure funding. The funds to provider units would be released as monthly advances and at end of each month a utilization statement along with all supporting documents (bills and vouchers) would be sent to secure the release of the next instalment from the treasury, using processes that would improve money management systems. The funds from the central government and states own funds will be pooled in the state health authority, including the other special funds from social insurance, cesses, and others, and allocated as per budget demands from block/municipal health authorities with due diligence.

The plan would have to take account of several issues that have to do with the state of the present system, such as ensuring corrections to the infrastructure right in the beginning; structuring appropriate contracting systems; map functional units required and consistently engage the private health sector and negotiate their terms of engagement with the UAHC. Similarly under the Health Authorities a technical research unit would have to be set up which would work out the detailed costing, pricing mechanisms, and payment systems, audit and reporting systems etc. All this may appear to need a longer-term perspective; however, I do believe that if this cannot be initiated in Plan period and generate the pressure and political will for that it will not happen even in the next 25 years.

To conclude, the financing strategy for UAHC in Maharashtra will have to be evolved keeping in mind the overall restructuring of the health care system, including the involvement of private health provision, and its governance modalities. For effective strategizing a district-level experiment would need to develop the UAHC model but the immediate steps suggested above requires a simple act of political will.

It is important to reemphasize that health care is a public or social good and cannot be left to the vagaries of the market. To realize its social or public value it has to be organized and regulated using both public and private resources for social benefit. Further, health care cannot be planned at the central or state level but has to be decentralized at an appropriate community level as discussed earlier in the chapter. The role of the centre and state is thus to strategize such actions, mobilize and disburse resources and monitor its outcomes. The planning and provision functions (who, how, where) are best left to local governance under community vigilance. Such is the global experience where health care is universally accessible with equity. Why should it be different in India?

As immediate next steps the much talked about architectural corrections under NRHM can be pursued. These would be radical reforms requiring restructuring and organization of the entire health sector, including the private health sector. Such restructuring will be possible only if: health care system, both public and private, is organized under a common umbrella/framework which provides access to all without any barriers; health care is pooled and coordinated by a single-payer system; policy-making and planning of health services is decentralized within a local governance framework; health care system is subject to continuous community monitoring and social audit under a regulated mechanism which leads to accountability across all stakeholders involved.

In order to accomplish the restructuring that we are talking about the following modalities need to be in place: An appropriate legislation mandating the UAHC framework; all resources, financial and human, should be transferred to the district panchayats and municipalities; the district/municipality will work out a detailed district plan which is based on local needs and aspirations and is evidence based within the framework already worked out under NRHM with appropriate modifications; and the private sector of the district will have to be brought on board through appropriate contracting in and payment mechanisms as they will form an integral part of restructuring of the health care system. An appropriate regulatory and accreditation mechanism that will facilitate the inclusion of the private health sector under the universal access health care mechanism will have to be worked out.

NOTES

1. Utilization data from the two NSS Rounds 42nd (pre-1991) and 52nd (post-1991) Round, a decade apart, provide ample evidence of this change. Further the 60th Round in 2004 and 71st Round on 2014, the last such survey, also shows the continuing trend of decline in public facility utilization, especially for hospital care which is now only 39 per cent, perhaps aided by the RSBY type of schemes, in contrast to 60 per cent in 1986. See NSSO (2015,

2006); interestingly OPD utilization in public facilities in the 71st Round has
seen an increase indicating some success of the NRHM, especially in rural areas.

2.   The latest IRDA *Annual Report,* 2015 shows, interestingly, a decline
in government-sponsored health insurance coverage in 2013–14 to 155 million
insured persons and premiums down to Rs 20.82 billion mainly due to some
state governments withdrawing schemes from insurance providers because of
frauds and other adversities encountered.

3.   Some of the prominent subsidies to private health sector include
medical education, with 80 per cent of graduates from public medical schools
joining the private sector; tax waivers to Trust/Society managed hospitals which
do not reciprocate the legal responsibilities of treating 10–20 per cent poor
patients free of cost; supply of patients paid by the public sector to corporate
hospitals like Apollo, Escorts, and others; tax rebates for import of medical
equipment and supplies.

4.   Available at: http://www.oecd.org/document/39/0,2340,en_2649_
201185_2789735_1_1_1_1,00.html. Accessed on 2 August 2005.

5.   The 93rd Parliamentary Standing Committee Report on the 2016–17
Budget released on 27 April 2016 has revealed that the final allocation of the
12th Plan would amount to only 46 per cent of the original allocation. Rajya
Sabha Secretariat 2016–17.

6.   See http://sathicehat.org/images/uhc-policy-brief-english.pdf.

7.   Such a service condition will of course only work if medical education
is adequately revamped to include a more realistic primary-care approach.

REFERENCES

CAG. (various years upto 2011–12). Finance Accounts of Central and State
       Governments, Comptroller and Auditor General. New Delhi: Government
       of India.
CSO. 2013 (1993–4 series). 'Private Final Consumption Expenditures',
       National Accounts Statistics, Central Statistics Organization. New Delhi:
       Government of India.
Duggal, Ravi. 2016. 'Is the NITI Aayog Even Thinking about Health?',
       Economic and Political Weekly 51(20): 12–14.
Gangoli, Leena, Ravi Duggal, and Abhay Shukla (eds). 2005. *Review of Health
       Care in India.* Mumbai: CEHAT.
Government of India. 1946. *Report of the Health Survey and Development
       Committee* (Bhore Committee). Delhi: Government of India.
Insurance Regulatory Development Authority (IRDA). 2012. *Annual Report
       2010–11.* New Delhi: Insurance Regulatory Development Authority,
       Government of India.
Ministry of Finance. 2015. Union Budget Expenditure Statement, Ministry of
       Finance. New Delhi: Government of India.

Ministry of Health and Family Welfare (MoHFW). 2005. *NRHM Mission Document*. New Delhi: Ministry of Health and Family Welfare, Government of India.

National Sample Survey Office. 1998. *NSS 52nd Round–1996*. New Delhi: NSSO, Government of India.

———. 2006. *NSS 60th Round–2004*. New Delhi: Government of India.

———. 2015. *NSS 71st Round–2014*. New Delhi: Government of India.

Planning Commission. 2012a. 'Social Sectors', *12th Five Year Plan 2012–2017* (3). New Delhi: Government of India.

Planning Commission. 2012b. *12th Five Year Plan Volume 1–Faster, More Inclusive and Sustainable Growth*. New Delhi: Government of India.

Reserve Bank of India. (1987–2015). *Finances of State Governments*. Mumbai: Reserve Bank of India.

———. 2016. Finances of State Governments. Mumbai: RBI.

Rajya Sabha Secretariat. 2016. *93rd Report of the Parliamentary Standing Committee on Health and Family Welfare Budget 2016–17*. Available at: http://164.100.47.5/newcommittee/reports/EnglishCommittees/Committee per cent20on percent20Health per cent20and per cent20Family per cent20Welfare/93.pdf. Accessed on 1 May 2016.

World Health Organization (WHO). 2004. *World Health Report 2004*. Geneva: WHO.

17

The Right to Health

A Winding Road to Actualization

Kajal Bhardwaj, Veena Johari, and Vivek Divan

The Right to Health finds no mention in the Indian Constitution, although Part III of that foundational law explicitly provides for the fundamental rights of people, as envisaged in a democratic polity. These include several protections, such as the freedoms of speech and expression, assembly, and religion and the rights to equality, life, and liberty (Constitution of India 1950: Part III). As Constituent Assembly debates make clear, this was a very seriously deliberated part of the Constitution that formed its bedrock (Parliament of India website).[1] Yet, in the panoply of rights that it explicitly mentions, health does not feature. It is only mentioned in the unenforceable yet guiding Directive Principles of State Policy in Part IV of the Constitution: 'The State shall regard the raising of ... the improvement of public health as among its primary duties' (Constitution of India 1950: Part IV, Article 47).

Given its function of judicial review, where the Indian Supreme Court is often required to interpret the Constitution, the court has read the Right to Health into the Fundamental Rights chapter. Particularly, and in order to make available accessible and affordable health care to Indian inhabitants, the court has interpreted the Right to Life under Article 21 by including within its ambit the Right to Health.

The complexity of giving robust meaning to the Right to Health in all its dimensions is underscored by the architecture of health law and policy in India. As the highest law of the land, the Constitution provides the framework within which both central and state governments laws are to be framed and implemented. While 'health' falls within the jurisdiction of states to legislate on, various aspects impacting health care fall under the central or concurrent lists of the Indian Constitution (Constitution of India, Seventh Schedule) resulting in health being legislated at both the central and state levels.

India's health care system is also impacted by international treaties and non-binding commitments undertaken as part of various United Nations (UN) processes. The Right to Health is well recognized and established in international law with its clearest and most important articulation in Article 12 of the International Covenant on Economic, Social, and Cultural Rights (ICESCR 1966). In 2000, the Committee on Economic, Social, and Cultural Rights issued *General Comment 14* on the right to the highest attainable standard of health (*General Comment 14*),[2] '... with a view to assisting States parties' implementation of the Covenant and the fulfilment of their reporting obligations'.[3] The comment focuses on the normative content of Article 12, states parties' obligations to respect, protect, and fulfil the right to health, violations, and implementation at the national level, and also addresses the obligations of actors other than state parties. As India follows the dualist system, treaties and international agreements entered into by the government are not directly enforceable unless Parliament passes a law bringing such treaties and international agreements into effect (Constitution of India). In the absence of domestic laws to the contrary, courts do refer to treaties and international agreements while interpreting the contents of domestic law.

Over the past decade, international trade treaties have also substantially impacted India's health care system. In 1995 India became a founding member of the World Trade Organization (WTO) and signatory to the Agreement on Trade Related Aspects of Intellectual Property Rights (TRIPS). Pursuant to this, in 2005 India amended its decades old patent law to comply with TRIPS and started granting product patents on medicines. India's obligations to the WTO have fundamentally impacted the ability of India to manufacture and supply affordable generic medicines.

India has also been signatory to resolutions at the UN relating to international commitments on health such as the General Assembly Declaration of Commitment on HIV/AIDS 2001 (UNAIDS 2001) and the Sustainable Development Goals adopted in September 2015 (UNDP 2015). These international processes impact health care in India in multiple ways and can be the basis for undertaking legislative efforts (such as the HIV Bill 2014) (Government of India 2014), changes in policies, or in the reasoning of court decisions (*Naz Foundation v. Govt. of NCT, Delhi*). They also impact the flow of international technical assistance and funds to national health efforts.

India also has a widespread and deep-rooted network of policy and planning. The Indian Planning Commission set up in the early 1950s and dismantled in 2014, has drafted and issued detailed five-year policy plans covering several sectors including health, social welfare, and education. These plans were complemented by several sector-specific policies. The first National Health Policy was issued in 1983 (NHP 1983), the second in 2002 (NHP 2002), and a new draft National Health Policy (NHP 2015—Draft) was circulated for comments by the government in January 2015 (Government of India 2015). Specific national policies have also been issued on mental health, access to plasma-derived medicinal products from human plasma, containment of antimicrobial resistance, health research, vaccines, blood, HIV/AIDS, and maternal and child health (NHP).[4] Multiple state-level policies add to the complex framework that governs the provision of and access to health services in India. The legal and policy framework is implemented through a multitude of central- and state-level programmes and institutions, including omnibus initiatives like the National Rural Health and Urban Health Missions (NRUHM) as well as specific programmes such as the Janani Suraksha Yojna, Rashtriya Kishor Swasthya Karayakram, Mobile Medical Units, Drugs and Technology, Health Financing and Risk Pooling, and others (Patel et al. 2015).

The plethora of legislations, policy, and programmes begs the question of why more than 70 per cent of outpatients and more than 60 per cent of inpatient care (Patel et al. 2015) take place within the private sector as opposed to the public sector. Government spending in health has reduced over the years and policy prescriptions are increasingly leaning towards public–private partnerships (PPP) or outright reliance on the private sector for the delivery of health care services with little or no application of the rights framework to the private sector. The private sector has found a place in all NHPs after the 1983 NHP, which proposed to expand health care facilities through the private sector (Thomas and Krishnan 2010). Diminishing political will to upgrade and revive public sector health care facilities has meant a vicious cycle of gross violations at public facilities, which instead of spurring an improvement in services has become the basis for dismantling the public sector, thereby leading to further violations without remedy.

In this scenario, this chapter seeks to examine the scope and limitations of the right to health in India. The chapter comprises six sections including the introduction. The first section traverses key judgments of the Supreme Court that have established the right to health but have also placed limitations on the right. With the plethora of laws, policies, and issues related to health care the following sections examine key aspects of the 'respect, fulfil, and protect' obligations of the State towards the right to health as articulated in *General Comment 14* through selected issues. The next section examines the obligation to 'protect' in the context of the private sector; the following section examines the obligation to 'fulfil' in the context of access to free health services. The chapter further examines the obligation to 'respect' in terms of equal access to health care services and the centrality of people's participation through the example of the HIV programme in the next section. The chapter concludes with reflections on the gaps and lacunae in the right to health framework in India.

THE SUPREME COURT AND RIGHT TO HEALTH

Constitutional silence on the right to health leaves its recognition at the mercy of the legislature—to articulate explicit rights and duties, equal access to health services, and standards of care—and to the courts to interpret existing rights to include the right to health within their ambit. In its constant endeavour to give robust meaning to the right to life guaranteed under Article 21 of the Constitution, the Indian Supreme Court has imbued that right with much substance including health. Yet, the right to health has been circumscribed by the court in a critical way—its exercise extends only to the state, and not to the private sector, except in some circumstances.

In its earlier decisions when the Indian State practised its brand of socialism in name and substance, the court focused on the state ensuring adequate levels of nutrition and standard of living. It also upheld legislative measures that regulated or prohibited consumption of liquor and narcotics as valid public health measures (*State of Bombay & another v. F.N. Balsara 1951*). Later, however, the Supreme Court read the Directive Principles of State Policy, which direct the state to protect health in its various dimensions,[5] into the fundamental right of life and personal liberty, recognizing the right to health as a fundamental right.

For instance, while discussing the rights of workmen to healthy working environments and to be insured, the court, relying on the Universal Declaration of Human Rights and the International Covenant on Economic, Social and Cultural Rights (ICESCR) held that the right to health of a worker fell within Article 21, and that the right did not mean the mere absence of sickness but complete physical, mental, and social well-being (*CESC Limited and others v. Subhash Chandra Bose and others 1992*). In keeping with the idea that the right to health included a safe and healthy working environment, the Supreme Court has directed the state to ensure the installation of safety measures in response to the death of workers at a young age in the slate pencil manufacturing industries due to accumulation of soot in their lungs (*Workmen of Slate Pencil Manufacturing Industries v. State of Madhya Pradesh 1980*).

Over the years the Supreme Court has further articulated the components of the right to health and the obligations of the state in providing health care to the populace by focusing on the health system—the health centre, the hospital, medicines, the rights of patients, and the obligations of providers. While discussing the right of persons to emergency health care (*PB Khet Mazdoor Samiti v. State of West Bengal 1996*) the court held that providing adequate medical facilities is an essential part of the obligations undertaken by the government in a welfare state, and this is discharged by running hospitals and health centres. The failure of a government hospital to provide timely medical intervention to a person in need of treatment results in the violation of their fundamental right to life.

The standards to be followed in government-run hospitals have also been laid down in several cases. In a case involving the administration of a hospital for persons living with mental illness, the Supreme Court observed that the government is required to 'perform its duties by running the hospital in a perfect standard and serving the patients in an appropriate way' and issued detailed directions for changes in the manner the hospital was being administered (*Rakesh Chandra Narayan v. State of Bihar 1989* and other cases). While allowing medical reimbursement for government employees being treated in private hospitals, the Supreme Court outlined the obligations of government-provided health care facilities thus (*State of Punjab and others v. Ram Lubhaya Bagga 1998*),

> No doubt Government is rendering this obligation by opening Government hospitals and health centres but in order to make it meaningful it has to be within the reach of its people, as far as possible, to reduce the queue of waiting lists, and it has to provide all facilities for which an employee

looks for at another hospital. Its upkeep, maintenance, and cleanliness have to be beyond aspersion. To employ the best of talents and tone up its administration to give effective contribution. Also bring in awareness in welfare of hospital staff for their dedicated service, give them periodical medico-ethical and service oriented training, not only at the entry point but also during the whole tenure of their service. Since it is one of the most sacrosanct and valuable rights of a citizen and equally sacrosanct obligation of the state, every citizen of this welfare state looks towards the state for it to perform this obligation with top priority including by way of allocation of sufficient funds. These in turn will not only secure the right of its citizen to the best of their satisfaction but in turn will benefit the state in achieving its social, political and economical goal.[6]

The Supreme Court has also recognized the rights of citizens to safe medicines. Although, at the time, it declined to determine the drug control policy of the state (*Vincent Panikulangara v. Union of India and others 1987*)[7] the court stated that as part of the state's primary obligation to ensure the well-being and health of its citizens, it must formulate and implement an effective and vigilant policy ensuring the safety and affordability of medicines. It also stated that the state's obligation to enforce the production of quality drugs and the elimination of injurious ones from the market must take within its sweep an obligation to make useful drugs available at a reasonable price so as to be within the common person's reach (For a detailed discussion of the later cases relating to drug policy, see Chapter 6, 'Globalization, Intellectual Property Rights, and Pharmaceuticals'). A significant step in this direction was reiterated through the Novartis case in 2013 (*Novartis v. Union of India and others 2013*), where the Supreme Court emphasized the importance of the amendments in the Patents Act, 2005 that would prevent ever-greening of patents for pharmaceutical products, thereby preventing abusive patenting practices in medicines and allowing the grant of patents for true inventions. This, in turn, would prevent monopolies and keep prices of medicines at competitive rates. The Supreme Court upheld the strict application of the patent law amendments referring to Parliamentary debates that had highlighted key concerns related to pricing and availability with the advent of product patents in India.

The Supreme Court has also directed the State to formulate appropriate guidelines and implementation mechanisms that ensure safe and quality blood transfusion.[8] Beyond directives to improve health systems, it has intervened to hold government health schemes accountable through the payment of compensation for gross violations. Where several persons suffered irreversible damage to their eyes after operations conducted at a government eye camp, the Supreme Court directed the State to pay Rs 12,500 to each person apart from interim relief (*A.S. Mittal and others v. State of UP 1989*). Where an excess of fluoride in water obtained from hand pumps sunk by the state government resulted in deformities, the court directed the government to provide free medical treatment, surgery, and artificial appliances at its own expense along with compensation (*Hamid Khan v. State* 1997). The court also steps in to give directions in cases where data before it presents large-scale public health challenges— as it did for the production of iodized salt in a petition filed on the basis of a UN report finding that lack of iodine in the diet had resulted in 60 million people in India suffering from goitre and 300 million being potential patients (*Residents of Well Defined Goitre Endemic Area v. State of Jammu and Kashmir 1982*). The Supreme Court also intervened to halt clinical trials in the country after being made aware of widespread human rights violations of participants; the court is now monitoring a revamp of the regulatory structure to ensure that a system is put in place that protects the right to health of participants in clinical trials (*Swasthya Adhikar Manch and another v. Ministry of Health and Family Welfare & others 2013*).

Although the activism of the Supreme Court in the application of the right to health has been necessary and far-reaching, the power and effectiveness of the court in ensuring the actual implementation of its directions has often been diluted by the indifference of the executive; most of the cases discussed above have taken decades to be enforced with repeated directions and interventions necessitated by the court. Lack of enforcement was evident in the Bhopal Gas Victims cases, where many survivors never received compensation despite multiple court orders. Many reasons have been presented: disputed numbers of the dead and injured,[9] the arbitrary exclusion of almost 90 per cent of those injured by the government (Sarangi 2012) and the filing of fresh claims given that the gas leak was affecting succeeding generations. In recognition of these enforcement challenges, the Supreme Court has sometimes kept cases 'open', even after issuing directions. In a public interest litigation filed to ensure access to first and second line treatment for HIV, the Supreme Court kept the matter open for over a decade during which multiple orders and directions were given to the government. The case was finally closed in 2013 with a clear understanding that the petitioners could re-approach the court for failures in implementing the government HIV treatment programme (*Sahara House v. Union of India 1999*).

Over the years there has been considerable debate over whether the right to health should take the form of a statute. In 2010, Assam led the way in legislating the right to health through the Assam Public Health Act (see Laws of India, Assam),[10] which guarantees the right to health in Section 5 and contains clear provisions on informed consent, confidentiality of health information, and access to affordable and quality health services and commodities for all (Assam Public Health Act, Ss.5–9).[11] This law also envisages a robust health information system that monitors health data, quality of health care, health indicators, and others, with community participation in these processes (Assam Public Health Act, Ss.17–18).[12] Yet, reports from Assam suggest that the enforcement and implementation of this Act appear to be weak.[13] The draft NHP 2015, recommends that the central government enact 'a National Health Rights Act, which will make ensuring health as a fundamental right, whose denial will be justiciable'. A draft of such a law was developed in 2009 (National Health Bill 2009).[14] Comprehensive legislation on mental health has recently been passed and draft legislation on assisted reproductive technologies is being discussed.

Of note is also a draft legislation on HIV/AIDS that was developed through a process of robust consultation which envisioned innovative and cost-effective ways in which rights and obligations could be actualized by affected parties at the local, state, and national levels using existing bureaucratic, quasi-judicial, and judicial systems (Lawyers Collective 2007).[15] The Bill addressed issues of informed consent, confidentiality, and disclosure of health status, non-discrimination, and access to health services, commodities, and medicines (Divan and Bhardwaj 2007). Several of these provisions have been diluted as the Bill has moved through government—the obligation to provide universal access to anti-retroviral treatment, for instance, has been diluted to an ambiguous and legally untenable standard of 'as far as possible' (*Hindustan Times* 2009). Yet, the HIV bill provides a robust template to ensure not only the right to health and other intersecting rights, but also state obligations to ensure delivery of the right through proper implementation mechanisms, with advocacy and participation of civil society in its evolution and enforcement.

However the statutory enactment of various aspects of the right to health may not be the panacea it is often held out to be. Attempts towards the Constitutional recognition of the Right to Education and its subsequent statutory enactment present a cautionary tale. In 2002, the Constitution was amended to include Article 21A—the Right to

Education. It is noteworthy that the Supreme Court had already read the Right to Free and Compulsory Education till the age of 14 into the Right to Life (*Unni Krishnan v. State of AP 1993*). The amendment, however, limited this right to children between the ages of 6 and 14 and included duties for parents thus diluting the more far-reaching interpretation of the Supreme Court. The statutory enactment in the form of the Right of Children to Free and Compulsory Education Act in 2009 (Government of India 2009) resulted in further dilution of the State's responsibility and has been critiqued for, among other things, abdicating the State's obligation by promoting PPPs and compensating private schools for enrolling poor children as well. Legislation on the Right to Food and the Right to Employment have attracted similar critiques of the government using this legislation to limit rather than expand the obligations of the State towards the fulfilment of these rights.

The versions of various Bills aimed to fulfil the fundamental rights and obligations of the State finally introduced in or enacted by Parliament do address substantive aspects of the various rights involved and specify the obligation on the government but they also highlight the importance of public interest groups not only advocating for these laws to expand rather than limit the obligations of the State and to also play a critical role in their proper implementation.

PROTECTING THE RIGHT TO HEALTH: PRIVATE SECTOR

Supreme Court rulings on the right to health have had limited direct application to the private sector. Specifically, the court has held that the right to health is a fundamental right of workmen, and that this right is not only available against the State and its instrumentalities, but also against private industry (*Kirloskar Brothers v. Employees State Insurance Corporation 1996* and other cases). In case of emergency situations, the Supreme Court has held that it is the professional obligation of every physician, whether government or private, to extend medical aid to the injured immediately, to preserve life without waiting for formalities to be complied with under the Code of Criminal Procedure (CrPC) (*Parman and Katara v. Union of India 1989*). More recently, the Supreme Court issued detailed directives to private hospitals to provide treatment to acid attack victims (*Laxmi v. Union of India and others 2015*).[16] The court has also reinforced the provisions of Section 357C of the CrPC, which require all private hospitals to provide first aid or medical treatment free of cost to victims of sexual violence (In re: 'Indian Woman says Gang-raped on Orders of Village Court', published in *Business and Financial News*, 23 January 2014).

Apart from these exigent circumstances, the question of access to health care services in the private sector has seen little consideration. Protection of the Right to Health in private sector contexts thus remains essentially unlegislated even though as stated in *General Comment 14*,

> Obligations to protect include, inter alia, the duties of States to adopt legislation or to take other measures ensuring equal access to health care and health-related services provided by third parties; to ensure that privatization of the health sector does not constitute a threat to the availability, accessibility, acceptability and quality of health facilities, goods and services; to control the marketing of medical equipment and medicines by third parties; and to ensure that medical practitioners and other health professionals meet appropriate standards of education, skill and ethical codes of conduct.
>
> (CESCR 2000: *General Comment 14*)

The ambivalence of the judiciary, executive, and legislature in the application of the right to health can be seen in several instances related to the private sector, the most prominent (and controversial) being in the case of the medical profession itself.

The Indian Medical Council (Professional Conduct, Etiquette, and Ethics) Regulations 2002 (MCI Regulations) govern the practice of medicine, and are closely linked to the right to health since they articulate the manner in which health is to be delivered to patients, and the rights and duties incumbent on medical practitioners. Unfortunately, they betray the low priority given to this most crucial aspect of the health system. For instance, the clause on consent only provides for such to be required in cases of obstetric cases, operations, publication in medical journals, in vitro fertilization, and clinical research (Indian Medical Council Regulations 2002) although the Supreme Court has held clearly that the patient has an inviolable right with regard to her/his body and a right to decide whether or not to undergo a particular treatment or surgery. It has laid down protocols for consent and held that doctors are authorized to do only those procedures for which express consent has been granted (*Samira Kohli v. Dr Prabha Manchanda and another 2008*). The ground reality is, however, quite different. Though consent and confidentiality have to be adhered to, very often patients are unaware of the treatment or medication given to them. Where large numbers of clinical trials take place on vulnerable sections of society, adherence to high ethical standards is of the essence. Despite regulations and guidelines on ethical practices in research, violations do occur, that affect large number of participants in trials. The Supreme Court has intervened in such cases and directed the government to issue rules and regulations to ensure high ethical standards in the conduct of clinical trials are maintained (*Kalpana Mehta & ors. v. Union of India 2012*; *Swasthya Adhikar Manch and another v. Ministry of Health and Family Welfare and others 2013*; *Sama and ors. v. Union of India 2013*).

Similarly, there is utter laxity in laying down stringent standards of confidentiality—with often vague and inappropriate legal terminology. Thus, a medical practitioner is not permitted to 'disclose the secrets of a patient' that have been obtained in the course of the practice except under certain, stipulated circumstances (Indian Medical Council Regulations 2002). Medical negligence is also covered under these regulations in the clumsiest of language, where a practitioner should 'not wilfully commit an act of negligence that may deprive his patient or patients from necessary medical care' (Indian Medical Council Regulations 2002). The enforcement of these regulations by the MCI has attracted criticism and health groups have recently protested efforts by the MCI to dilute the most recent amendments to the regulations that cover the relationship between doctors and the pharmaceutical industry.[17] With the inherent challenge in asking the medical profession to police itself, the ball has been kicked to consumer forums to address private sector health care services. Medical services were brought under the ambit of the Consumer Protection Act by the Supreme Court (*Indian Medical Council v. V.P. Shantha 1996*). Although the Supreme Court has found physicians liable for medical negligence, it has refrained from extending criminal liability against them (Johari 2014). Courts have, however, awarded large amounts of compensation to aggrieved parties, foisting liability on private physicians and hospitals to pay for proven negligence or deficiency in services (*Dr Balram Prasad v. Dr Kunal Shah and others 2013*).

Legislative attempts to regulate specific areas of medical conduct have similarly, been of questionable effect. Ruing the Achilles heel of Indian laws being their non-enforcement, the Supreme Court in relation to the prevention of female foeticide through the pre-conception and pre-natal diagnostic techniques (Prohibition of Sex Selection) Act and the Medical Termination of Pregnancy Act recently noted,

The decline in the female child ratio all over the country leads to an irresistible conclusion that the practice of eliminating female foetus by the use of pre-natal diagnostic techniques is widely prevalent in this country. Complaints are many, where at least few of the medical professionals do perform Sex Selective Abortion having full knowledge that the sole reason for abortion is because it is a female foetus. The provisions of the Medical Termination of Pregnancy Act, 1971 are also being consciously violated and misused.

(Voluntary Health Association of Punjab v.
Union of India and others 2013)

Legislative attempts to prevent hospitals, clinics, and medical professionals from participating in or encouraging the trade in human organs took the form of the Transplantation of Human Organs and Tissues Act 2010 (National Organ and Tissue Transplant Organisation 2010),[18] which was passed in 1994 as a comprehensive legislation to regulate the removal of organs from living and deceased persons as well as transplantation of organs.[19] Transplantation of Human Organs and Tissues Act provides an extensive governance mechanism through an appropriate authority to deal with matters relating to removal, storage, or transplantation of human organs and for tissue banks engaged in recovery, screening, testing, processing, storage, and distribution of tissues (THOTA, S.13[3]).[20] It also makes unauthorized removal of organs or tissues and commercial dealings in them punishable offences (THOTA, Ss.18, 19, 19A).[21]

Under THOTA, the name of the registered medical practitioner who is convicted is to be reported to the State Medical Council to take necessary action including removal of his name from the council's register (THOTA, S.18 [2]).[22] Criminal cases have been filed under THOTA where organs have been taken by donors being misrepresented as near relatives in forged documents, unverified by hospital authorities (*Mrs N. Ratankumari v. State of Odisha 2014*). Some state governments, like in Maharashtra have along with non-governmental organizations (NGOs) started Zonal Transplant Coordination Centres that maintains a list of all patients requiring organs along with the priority, so that there is an equitable distribution of cadaver organs as and when available (see donate life).[23] Yet, despite the legislation and these attempts at enforcement, violations and illegal trade in human organs, particularly kidneys, which often involves the exploitation of the poor and violation of human rights still proliferates. There are reports of trafficking involving clinicians, managers of clinical centres, middlemen, and others (Parliament of India, NHRC letter 2004).[24]

It is of note that associations of medical professionals are themselves at the forefront of resisting legislative attempts to lay down minimum standards of health care facilities and services such as the Clinical Establishments (Registration and Regulation) Act.[25] Unfortunately, instead of this 2010 law being used as an opportunity to ensure non-discrimination in private health care establishments, it only reiterates the Supreme Court's requirement that such establishments are not permitted to deny care in emergency situations (see Law Commissions draft).[26] However, it also provides that such care is to be provided 'within the staff and facilities available' (Clinical Establishments Act 2010), suggesting that even the provision of emergency treatment may be denied on grounds of lack of capacity of the institution. The law appears thereby to have further limited the duty of the private sector to provide emergency health care services. This provides an opening for establishments to deny services, and reports of incidents such as children dying of dengue due to refusals by private hospitals to treat them show the grave repercussions of such a gap in the law.[27] Cases pending in the Bombay High Court have highlighted the plight of patients who have not been given a discharge or dead bodies have not been released to the relatives of the patient due to non-payment of hospital bills (*Arun Chhabria v. State of Maharashtra and others 2013*). Some medical practitioners including those represented by the Indian Medical Association have also demanded that small- and medium-level hospitals be exempt from the ambit of the Clinical Establishments (Registration and Regulation) Act (Rana 2015).

The courts have taken conflicting approaches in relation to access to private hospitals for poor patients. In 2004, a directive by the Bombay High Court to all charitable hospitals required that they provide free or subsidized testing and treatment to the indigent and weaker sections of society by earmarking 10 per cent of total operational beds in the hospital (*Sanjiv Punalekar v. the State of Maharashtra and another 2004*). In 2011, the Supreme Court ordered private hospitals built on subsidized land to ensure that for those from economically weaker sections '25 per cent OPD and 10 per cent IPD patients have to be given treatment free of cost. The said patients should not be charged anything'. However, media reports in 2015 stated that the Jharkhand Human Rights Conference withdrew its petition from the Supreme Court asking for similar orders for hospitals in Jharkhand when the judges are reported to have commented that the court could not give such directions as private hospitals were not obliged to provide such services to the poor.[28]

Reports of violations of the right to health emanate both from the public and the private sectors. The primary difference between the two is that with the former, affected parties can resort to the Constitutional mandate to seek government accountability by filing petitions in the High Court or Supreme Court. For those interacting with the private sector, the road to accountability is greatly limited—patients who pay for medical services may resort to the Consumer Protection Act. An interesting development in recent years has been the use of the Right to Information Act (RTI Act) by patients struggling to prove violations of their right to health. The denial of access to medical records has been used by private hospitals to obfuscate their role and responsibilities to patients. In 2014, the Central Information Commission held that the RTI Act applies to medical records of patients even if they are held in private hospitals.[29] As much as these cases draw praise as progressive legal developments, they are also indicative of the dismal state of affairs governing private hospitals, against whom legal recourse is required even to access one's own medical records.

FULFILLING THE RIGHT TO HEALTH: BY ANY MEANS NECESSARY?

In the cases discussed above, the Supreme Court has clearly held that the State has a constitutional obligation to provide and maintain health facilities. How governments fulfil the right to health has been an area of considerable debate central to which is the question of how health care is financed and delivered. Internationally, the debate around health care financing coalesced around the World Bank-led policy push for user fees in developing countries and its recent dismantling with increasing evidence that user fees have created barriers in access to health care services. This was recognized clearly in 2012[30] in the UN resolution urging countries to adopt universal health coverage, which called on governments

> to ensure that health financing systems evolve so as to avoid significant direct payments at the point of delivery, and include a method for prepayment of financial contributions for health care and services as well as a mechanism to pool risks among the population in order to avoid catastrophic health-care expenditure and impoverishment of individuals as a result of seeking the care needed.

The United Nations resolution moves the emphasis from user fees to what is essentially a call for universal health insurance. The question of whether such mechanisms are provided by public or private actors remains an open and contentious one. *General Comment 14*, for instance, does not favour one system over another as long as it is affordable and thus states that the obligation to 'fulfil' the right to health, includes the provision of 'public, private or mixed health insurance system which is affordable for all'.

The Indian State from the 1990s onwards appears to be favouring just such a mixed health insurance system. Both the Central and State governments run significant public insurance programmes. The Employees State Insurance Corporation (ESIC) scheme covers employees earning up to Rs 15,000 while the Central Government Health Scheme (CGHS) covers workmen and government employees, with medical facilities provided through wellness centres, CGHS dispensaries or ESIC hospitals (National Health Insurance Schemes). The question of whether State insurance schemes should be free of cost arose in the case of *Confederation of Ex-Servicemen Association and others v. Union of India* (2006) where the Supreme Court held that though the right to medical aid is a fundamental right of all citizens including servicemen, framing a scheme for ex-servicemen and asking them to pay 'one time contribution' neither violates fundamental rights nor is it inconsistent with the Directive Principles. It was held that getting free and full medical facilities was not a part of the fundamental right of ex-servicemen and asking them to become members of the Ex-servicemen Contributory Health Scheme by contributing a one-time amount, was according to the Supreme Court in consonance with the law laid down by the court.

With India's adoption of economic reforms in the early 1990s and its commitments at the WTO, private sector insurance companies have an increasingly strong presence in India (IRDAI, Indian Insurance Market).[31] In 1999, the Insurance Regulatory and Development Authority of India (IRDAI) Act was passed to set up a regulator for the insurance sector. In 2015, the Insurance Laws (Amendment) Act sought to amend and consolidate different statutes regulating the insurance sector while allowing for an increase in foreign direct investment in Indian insurance companies up to 49 per cent. Indian citizens covered by private health insurance policies have to rely on contract law, consumer protection law, and the IRDAI to address their grievances.

The experience has been mixed at best. While an increasing number of Indians are now covered by health insurance, the process of getting claims honoured has resulted in a significant increase in litigation. With insurance claims pending or rejected or requiring further resources to pursue in litigation, the positive impact of health insurance on reducing health care spending burden on households is questionable. Investing in affordable insurance rather than investing in affordable health care in the public sector is unlikely to fulfil the State's obligation on the right to health.

The marked difference between the standards applicable to private and public insurance companies was outlined by the Supreme Court, and one may argue that unfortunately the court has practically endorsed the idea that only public sector insurance companies must be held to a higher standard, holding that 'a private player, as the law stands now, may not be bound to comply with the constitutional requirements of the equality clause, the appellants are'. Thus, the Supreme Court held (*United India Insurance Co. Ltd. v. Manubhai Dharmasinh bhai Gajera 2008*) that public sector insurance companies, as part of the State machinery, have a different role to play than their private sector counterparts and, that even though government insurance companies are required to compete with private players, 'fairness or reasonableness' must appear in all their dealings. Quoting the Universal Declaration of Human Rights, the court noted that IRDAI's directions had to keep human rights in mind particularly as the government does to provide social security in the form of compulsory insurance. Noting that it was attempting to strike a balance between human rights and the rights of the State and others that perform public utility functions like insurance companies, the Supreme Court held that:

> Whereas on the one hand we cannot forget the new market economy and the Foreign Direct Investment, we also cannot shut our eyes to the ground realities. There is a huge gap between the high sounded wants of the Government and the realities on the ground. It is essential that while on the one hand, the insurance companies are not put to undue burden keeping in view the changes in the statute as also the policy decisions of the Central Government, they cannot also be permitted to act wholly arbitrarily and unreasonably. They cannot be permitted to create a social condition, which would negate all human rights.
>
> (*United India Insurance Co. Ltd v. Manubhai Dharmasinhbhai Gajera [2008]*)

There is now an increasing trend of state governments providing health coverage and services through private players. Rajasthan has entered into a Memorandum of Understanding with New India Assurance Company to start a health insurance scheme that would cover general sickness to critical illness, on the pretext that it would benefit the poor and needy people to access quality medical and health care facilities in the private sector.[32] Rajasthan is among the few states after Maharashtra, Andhra Pradesh, Gujarat, Kerala, Madhya Pradesh, and Tamil Nadu to start the Swasthya BimaYojna. However, the state does not fulfil its Constitutional obligation of improving and maintaining health care facilities, as the object of encouraging health insurance schemes appears to be to push people towards private sector facilities. Rajasthan has also introduced a scheme outsourcing the running of public health infrastructure to private players. This scheme has been challenged by public health groups arguing that 'the private players are interested in minimum investment and maximum gain. Why the private players will go and serve in those rural areas where government has failed to retain its employees?' (Pandey 2015) According to these groups, the move towards privatization by the state government is really to downsize the free medicines scheme and bring in insurance models (Pandey 2015).

Rajasthan exemplifies the contradictions in the government's approach to health care. Alongside the initiatives towar̶ ̶ :vate health insurance and outsourcing of PHCs, Rajasthan also fe̶ ̶ ̶es an extremely successful free drugs and diagnostics scheme. The success of free drug schemes not just in Rajasthan but in Tamil Nadu, Kerala, and West Bengal spurred the announcement of a similar scheme by the Central Government. The 12th Five-Year Plan estimated the cost of free drugs scheme to be about Rs 6,000 crore a year which was to provide drugs in the National Essential Medicines list consisting of about 348 drugs free of cost. More recently, however, this list was pared down to only 50 drugs free of cost (see Free drugs plan)[33] while the state-run schemes offer hundreds of drugs. The central government has eventually dropped this scheme leaving it to the states. Although Odisha has launched 'Nirmaya', a free drug distribution scheme to provide about 570 medicines and free drugs, it is unclear if other states will follow suit.[34]

Although the Supreme Court held that the right to health does not necessarily include the right to free medical care in the case of the ex-servicemen discussed above, it has issued directions for the provision of free treatment by the Government in the case of HIV (*Sahara House v. Union of India 1999*). How and when the state is obligated to provide free treatment appears to be determined on case-by-case basis. A decision of the Delhi High Court in ordering the government to provide free of cost treatment of an extremely expensive medicine is worth some examination here. The case related to a child born with a rare disease (Gaucher) whose treatment cost Rs 6 lakh per month (*Mohd. Ahmed (Minor) v. Union of*

India 2014). The argument of the government that the treatment cost was too high was rejected by the court, which ordered the government to provide the treatment. The court however, did not examine underlying reasons for the high cost of treatment. In this case, the treatment was patented by a multinational company that had donated only one month of treatment for the child. The Court did not examine or direct the state to examine whether price controls could be imposed, the technology for making the medication could be transferred to public manufacturers or generic companies or if generic versions of the medication could be produced. These avenues, of course, remain open to the government to explore to ensure the affordability of medicines for patients.

RESPECTING THE RIGHT TO HEALTH: HIV IN INDIA

While the previous section has examined the different and contradictory approaches the Indian State appears to be adopting to fulfil the right to health, this section highlights some unique aspects of the evolution of the right to health in India in the context of one of the HIV programme. Respecting the right to health entails among other things that the State refrain 'from denying or limiting equal access for all persons' (*General Comment 14*). The Indian State's HIV response dates back to the mid-1980s and from the beginning, the response has found itself challenged by people living with HIV and NGOs in the various high courts and the Supreme Court. In Lucy D'souza's case (1990), an HIV-positive activist Dominic D'Souza was incarcerated under the Goa Public Health Act, 1985 after he was tested for HIV without his knowledge or consent. Although a challenge to this law failed, subsequent cases established that discrimination against people living with HIV was unconstitutional (*MX v. ZY 1997*).

Since then the government's HIV programme and response has expanded and evolved considerably. In 1992, the National AIDS Control Organisation (NACO) was established within the Ministry of Health and Family Welfare and at the state level, State AIDS Control Societies were established. It took till 2002 for official government policy to recognize the need for a public health response predicated on human rights in the National AIDS Prevention and Control Policy (NAPCP). The National AIDS Prevention and Control Policy recognized the commitment of the government 'to create an enabling socio-economic environment for prevention of HIV/AIDS, to provide care and support to people living with HIV/AIDS and to ensure protection/promotion of their human rights including right to access health care system, right to education, employment and privacy' (NACO 2015). The National AIDS Prevention and Control Policy further committed to providing adequate and equitable provision of health care to people living with HIV/AIDS.

The HIV epidemic in India, is considered to be a concentrated epidemic, with high prevalence among marginalized populations such as sex workers, people who inject drugs, men who have sex with men and the transgender community. These communities remain, in some form or other criminalized under the law and the evolution of the HIV programme in India witnessed the provision of health care services, particular prevention services (formally known as targeted interventions) to these communities despite this criminality. In some cases, the position of the Ministry of Health on continuing criminalization differed considerably from that of the Ministry of Home Affairs. This division arose most sharply in the Delhi High Court during a Constitutional challenge to India's anti-sodomy law Section 377 of the Indian Penal Code, 1860. While the Home Ministry argued for the continuation of the provision, the Ministry of Health submitted an affidavit highlighting how criminalisation was creating barriers in reaching men who have sex with men with HIV prevention and treatment services. While the Delhi High Court struck down Section 377 taking note of among other things the adverse impact of the provision on the right to health (Economic, Social, and Cultural Rights [ESCR]), regrettably in 2012, a division bench of the Supreme Court reinstated the law. In 2016, a three-judge bench of the Supreme Court agreed to consider appeals from this decision.[35]

The National AIDS Control Organization similarly expressed concerns over proposals in 2008 to amend the Immoral Trafficking Prevention Act (ITPA) to expand the scope of criminalization of activities surrounding sex work and punish clients of sex workers stating that such measures were, 'likely to obstruct the efforts made towards controlling the HIV epidemic in India' (NACO newsletter).[36] The provision of clean needles and oral drug substitution to people who inject drugs to minimize their risk of contracting or transmitting HIV similarly has taken place under the HIV programme even though there has been ambiguity over the status of these programmes in terms of the Narcotics Drugs and Psychotropic Substances Act (NDPS Act). It was only in 2014, that Parliament amended the NDPS Act to specifically allow for the 'management' of drug dependence thus legitimizing the provision of such services to drug users (NDPS amendment).

The importance of equal access to health care services was also recognized by the Supreme Court of India in 2013 recognising the rights of transgender persons, directing the government to 'take proper measures to provide medical care to transgender persons in the hospitals and also provide them separate public toilets and other facilities' (*National Legal Services Authority v. Union of India and ors. 2014*). In many respects the HIV programme was far more progressive in fulfilling the right to health than the law on the books.

Another aspect of the obligation to respect the right to health identified in *General Comment 14* is that States should refrain from 'preventing people's participation in health-related matters'. An interesting feature of the government HIV programme has been the extent to which people living with HIV as well as representatives of sex workers, drug users, men who have sex with men, and transgender persons have been involved in the planning of this extensive programme and in service delivery including providing pre- and post-test counselling, ensuring that newly tested people living with HIV register at Anti-Retroviral Therapy (ART) centres, follow up and adherence of those on ART, treatment counselling related to Sexually Transmitted Infections (STIs), Tuberculosis (TB), and hepatitis C. Of the 325 Care and Support Centres aimed at improving survival and quality of life of People Living with HIV/AIDS (PLHIV), 60 per cent are implemented through people living with HIV networks (NACO 2015). In areas where injecting drug use is the driving force of the HIV epidemic, people living with HIV networks are critical in helping drug users adhere to their treatment.

People living with HIV networks and marginalized populations also perform a critical watchdog function regarding the government treatment programme. In the late 1990s Sahara House and Sankalp Rehabilitation Trust, filed public interest litigations in Constitutional challenges to barriers to health care access for people living with HIV. In 2004, the government of India commenced providing HIV treatment and these cases along with other cases in the Supreme Court were tagged together and over the next decade acted as an accountability mechanism for the government treatment programme. During the course of the case, as the HIV treatment programme evolved, commitments from NACO to the top court included the scale up of the ART rollout, phase out of older, harmful drugs like stavudine and the provision and scale-up of second line treatment.[37]

However, more than the use of public interest litigation, people living with HIV have also developed more direct strategies to ensure the provision of uninterrupted treatment by the government programme by keeping a real-time watch on stock-outs of ARVs and diagnostic kits. Supply interruptions are publicized and brought to the notice of NACO for immediate action.[38] In one instance, people living with HIV networks pooled their meagre funds for an emergency purchase of paediatric Anti Retrovirals (ARVs) and donated these to the government programme as emergency procurement was not within the government guidelines.[39]

People living with HIV are also engaging with the legal system in another unique way towards the fulfilment of the right to health. With the government programme overwhelmingly reliant on generic medicines purchased from Indian companies, people living with HIV have since 2005 been filing patent oppositions challenging patent applications and patents on key HIV medicines. Arguably ensuring access to affordable medicines is the remit of the state under the right to health but an extraordinary decade long legal battle in the Indian patent office has been taking place by community groups to ensure generic production and availability of the medicines procured by the government. Using critical public health safeguards introduced by the Indian Parliament in 2005, the majority of these patent oppositions have been successful as can be seen in the Table 17.1 (adapted from UNITAID 2014).[40]

TABLE 17.1   Patent Oppositions in Indian Courts

Medicine	Patent applicant	Opponent (public interest groups that have opposed the patent application)	Status of the patent application
Abacavirsulfate ARV	GSK	Indian Network for People Living with HIV/AIDS (INP+)	Patent application withdrawn
Amprenavir ARV	GSK	Uttar Pradesh Network of Positive People and INP+	Patent application abandoned
Atazanavir ARV	Novartis	Karnataka Network for People Living with HIV and AIDS and INP+	Patent application abandoned

imatinibmesylate *Cancer medicine*	Novartis	Cancer Patients Aid Association	Patent application rejected
lamivudine/ zidovudine *ARV*	GSK	Manipur Network of People Living with HIV/AIDS and INP+	Patent application withdrawn
Lopinavir *ARV*	Abbott Laboratories	Delhi Network of Positive People (DNP+, Network of Maharashtra by People Living with HIV and AIDS and INP+	Patent application rejected
lopinavir/ritonavir (soft gel) *ARV*	Abbott Laboratories	DNP+ and INP+	Patent application abandoned
lopinavir/ritonavir (tablet) *ARV*	Abbott Laboratories	Initiative for Medicines, Access & Knowledge	Patent application rejected
Ritonavir *ARV*	Abbott Laboratories	DNP+ and INP+	Patent application abandoned
Tenofovir disoproxil (TD) *ARV*	Gilead Sciences	DNP+, INP+; Brazilian Interdisciplinary AIDS Association (ABIA) and Sahara (Centre for Residential Care and Rehabilitation)	Patent application rejected
Tenofovir Disoproxil Fumarate *ARV*	Gilead Sciences	DNP+ and INP+	Patent application rejected

Source: UNITAID (2014).

There are several critiques of the HIV programme that point out its vertical nature (Rao et al. 2013) and its over reliance on international funding.[41] With the drying up of international funding, NACO being merged into the Health Ministry, and significant cuts in the domestic health budget, there are serious concerns that this largely successful public sector programme is unravelling.[42] People living with HIV involved in service delivery did not receive payments for months and some programmes even advertised monthly salaries lower than the minimum wage.[43] Questions over proper representation and consultation of community-based groups have also been increasingly raised. Although the programme is attempting integration with broader health programmes this process has been slow and questions over whether such a move would endanger the confidentiality of people living with HIV or increase discrimination against marginalized groups have arisen.[44]

India's HIV programme marked a huge intervention and investment by the public sector in health care at a time when nationally and globally the state was retreating from this sector. Not only was infrastructure for the delivery of HIV prevention and treatment services created, the programme was also based on high, if not entirely ideal, standards of medical ethics in the provision of government services in terms of consent, confidentiality, and counselling for testing and treatment. With the nature of the epidemic, the public health care system was forced to deal with issues of stigma and discrimination while recognizing that only proper treatment through this system could ensure adherence and prevent or limit drug resistance. A crucial and unique aspect of this response was the establishment and evolution of networks of people living with HIV who started out as support groups when care and treatment was not available to becoming a powerful constituency of patient advocates influencing the way in which health care was delivered, health policy was devised and the state was made accountable for the same. Unfortunately, these many remarkable aspects of the HIV response in advancing and shaping the right to health are likely to be lost as international funding dwindles and there is no political will to match it with monies from national budgets.

* * *

Every child has the right to be ensured a fair chance of living a normal, healthy life and of contributing eventually as an adult man or woman, its full share to the general advancement of the community ... The child during every stage of its journey towards adult life needs suitable care and attention. Its proper nutrition, its health care and health education, its physical development are matters of concern to the State, which must see that where parental efforts are inadequate, the child does not suffer. When the necessity arises for medical attention for the individual, there should be an adequate health service to turn to, from which no question of lack of means should cut him off.

(Bhore Committee Report 1946)[45]

In 1946, the Bhore Committee Report articulated one of the earliest expressions of the right to health in an Indian policy and planning document. The fulfilment of this right according to the committee lay in the setting up of a comprehensive national health service. This 'long-term plan' was to be achieved in 'thirty-forty years'. Seventy years after the report, those recommendations remain a distant dream.

Although the right to health as articulated by the Bhore Committee did not find reflection in the Constitution except through the duty of the State towards public health, the Supreme Court has articulated a Constitutional Right to Health. It would be fair to broadly state two aspects of the articulation of the right to health by the Supreme Court that are crucial—that its articulation and establishment has been vital in filling a gap in India's economic and social landscape, and yet, that gap has been only partially filled since the right to health has been made available only in relation to the public sector save some narrow exceptions such as emergency circumstances.

In twenty first century India, where privatization of the health sector has been proposed (NITI Aayog as cited in *The Wire* 2015) as a solution to alleviate its health challenges, and in a country where numbers bear out the fact that most people access the private health system (Patel et al. 2015), this is a huge lacuna. Indeed every aspect of health care that is affected by or delivered through the private sector including medical professionals, health care facilities, health insurance companies, and pharmaceutical companies must be understood within the right to health framework. The approach of the Supreme Court with regard to the obligations of the private sector as they relate to health care should be re-examined. It is increasingly understood that human rights obligations apply to non-state actors like the private sector and it is critical that the jurisprudence in India on the right to health evolves to reflect a deeper understanding of the manner in which violations of the right to health take place, and to provide effective remedies for patients left increasingly at the mercy of the market.

The demand for the application of right to health principles to the private sector is not to make the argument that regulation is sufficient to ensure universal health care to all who need it. As pointed out as far back as 1946, only a comprehensive national health service can achieve this goal. Despite many attempts to shrink the public sector in the area of health care, it has repeatedly demonstrated the ability to deliver high quality care, be it through free medicines schemes or the HIV programme. On matters related to discrimination and criminalization, the public sector has demonstrated its ability to be progressive even when courts are not.

An analysis of the laws, policies, and litigation relating to the right to health also reveals a crucial, positive feature. And that is the central role of peoples' movements and public health groups in the progressive realisation of the right to health. While nearly every aspect of health care and State policy is now being litigated before the courts, the primary actors repeatedly holding the State accountable for the provision of care or the regulation of the private sector are these groups of intrepid people living with HIV, hepatitis C, or cancer who challenge patent monopolies and intervene in cases aimed at diluting the public health safeguards in India's patent law; women's groups who challenge the regulation and oversight of clinical trials, and public health groups who intervene in challenges by pharmaceutical companies to drug price control laws. An increasingly compromised State either sits as arbiter between the private sector and the public interest groups or brings about laws and policies that violate the right to health, that are inevitably challenged on the Constitutional cornerstone of the Right to Life and Health. It is also evident that despite a penchant for drafting bills, enacting laws and issuing policies in attempts to attain legal clarity, the Right to Health in India is a deeply contested space and the Supreme Court and judiciary will remain arenas in which this right is ultimately advanced or stifled.

NOTES

1. Available at: http://parliamentofindia.nic.in/. Accessed on 3 December 2017.

2. Committee on Economic, Social, and Cultural Rights, *General Comment 14*: The right to the highest attainable standard of health (Twenty-second session, 2000), U.N. Doc. E/C.12/2000/4 (2000). Available at: http://www.unhchr.ch/tbs/doc.nsf/(symbol)/E.C.12.2000.4.En (*General Comment 14*).

3. Committee on Economic, Social and Cultural Rights, *General Comment 14*: The right to the highest attainable standard of health (Twenty-second session, 2000), U.N. Doc. E/C.12/2000/4 (2000). Available at: http://www.unhchr.ch/tbs/doc.nsf/(symbol)/E.C.12.2000.4.En (para 6, *General Comment 14*).

4. See National Health Portal. Available at: http://www.nhp.gov.in/state-health-insurance-programmes_pg. Accessed on 29 December 2015.

5. Article 39(e) of the Constitution provides that the State shall, in particular, direct its policy towards securing, 'that the health and strength of workers, men and women, and the tender age of children are not abused and that citizens are not forced by economic necessity to enter avocations unsuited to their age or strength'. Article 41 provides that, 'the State shall, within the limits of its economic capacity and development make effective provision for securing the right to work, to education and to public assistance in cases of unemployment, old age, sickness and disablement, and in other cases of undeserved want'. Article 42 provides that the, 'State shall make provision for securing just and humane conditions of work and for maternity relief'. Article 47 provides that the, 'State shall regard the raising of the level of nutrition and the standard of living of its people and the improvement of public health as among its primary duties and, in particular, the State shall endeavour to bring about prohibition of the consumption except for medicinal purposes of intoxicating drinks and of drugs which are injurious to health'.

6. The Court also stated that the demand on the State cannot be unlimited and would be influenced by its financial condition: 'Investment needs resources and finances. So even to protect this sacrosanct right, finances are an inherent requirement. Harnessing such resources is top priority ... No state or country can have unlimited resources to spend on any of its projects. That is why it only approves its projects to the extent feasible. The same holds good for providing medical facilities to its citizens. Provision of facilities cannot be unlimited. It has to be to the extent finances permit'.

7. The issue of unsafe drugs was also addressed by the court in *All India Democratic Women Association v. Union of India* AIR 1998 SC 1371 which challenged the use of the drug 'Quinacrine' as a method of female sterilization. The Supreme Court disposed of the petition based on the undertaking by the central government that it had already initiated steps for banning this drug. A few months later, the government did indeed ban the import, manufacture, sale, and distribution of Quinacrine as a contraceptive.

8. The Supreme Court gave detailed directions in this regard including the establishment of a National Council for blood transfusion as well as State Councils, licensing of blood banks, elimination of the system of professional donors within 2 years, strengthening of machinery for enforcement of the provisions of the *Drugs and Cosmetics Act* and *Rules*, periodic checking by Inspectors, separate legislation for regulating collection, processing, storage,

distribution, and transportation of blood and operation of blood banks, and submission of report by the Director of Health Services of the Government of India in this regard. See *Common Cause v Union of India* AIR 1996 SC 929.

9. 'Why are Bhopal survivors still fighting for compensation'. See http://www.bbc.com/news/world-asia-india-30205140.

10. Available at: http://www.lawsofindia.org/state/29/Assam.html. Accessed on 4 December 2017.

11. Available at: http://www.nrhmassam.in/pdf/the_assam_public_health_act_2010_041111.pdf. Accessed on 4 December 2017.

12. Available at: http://www.nrhmassam.in/pdf/the_assam_public_health_act_2010_041111.pdf. Accessed on 4 December 2017.

13. See http://www.telegraphindia.com/1130925/jsp/northeast/story_17388214.jsp#.VpMwp_l97IU).

14. Available at: http://www.prsindia.org/uploads/media/Draft_National_Bill.pdf. Accessed on 4 December 2017.

15. Available at: http://www.lawyerscollective.org/files/Final%20HIV%20Bill%202007.pdf. Accessed on 4 December 2017.

16. Available at: https://indiankanoon.org/doc/90443079/. Accessed on 4 December 2017.

17. http://timesofindia.indiatimes.com/india/Activists-seek-health-ministry-intervention-to-stop-MCI-diluting-code-of-ethics/articleshow/31791673.cms.

18. Title amended in 2011.

19. Though the Centre does not have power to make laws for the States with respect to health matters, under Article 252 (1) of the Constitution of India, resolutions were passed by the State legislatures of Goa, Himachal Pradesh and Maharashtra for Parliament to regulate this matter by law. The Act applies to many States now, and to all Union Territories.

20. Available at: http://lawmin.nic.in/ld/P-ACT/1994/The%20Transplantation%20of%20Human%20Organs%20and%20Tissues%20Act,%201994.pdf. Accessed on 4 December 2017.

21. Available at: http://lawmin.nic.in/ld/P-ACT/1994/The%20Transplantation%20of%20Human%20Organs%20and%20Tissues%20Act,%201994.pdf. Accessed on 4 December 2017.

22. Available at: http://lawmin.nic.in/ld/P-ACT/1994/The%20Transplantation%20of%20Human%20Organs%20and%20Tissues%20Act,%201994.pdf. Accessed on 4 December 2017.

23. Available at: http://donatelifeindia.org/the-network/. Accessed on 4 December 2017.

24. Parliament of India. 2004. National Human Rights Commission, letter dated 29.1.2004 to the Prime Minister of India.

25. See http://clinicalestablishments.nic.in/cms/Home.aspx. Accessed on 4 December 2017.

26. Available at: http://indiankanoon.org/doc/100042716/. Accessed on 4 December 2017.

27. See reports in the Indian Express and other media: http://indianexpress. com/article/india/india-others/7-year-old-dead-of-dengue-his-parents-kill-themselves/; http://www.hindustantimes.com/delhi/delhi-boy-dies-of-dengue-father-alleges-hospital-negligence/story-orrOSjUais8Yptxc1MKXwL.html).

28. http://www.livemint.com/Politics/x1LCxLpWxoqOctYcwINHTO/ SC-refuses-to-direct-private-hospitals-to-provide-free-treat.html.

29. RTI order at http://www.rti.india.gov.in/cic_decisions/CIC_AD_A_2013_001681-SA_M_136162.pdf and http://jksic.nic.in/E per cent20-library/ Prabat per cent20KUmar per cent20- per cent20Fortis.pdf.

30. See from http://www.un.org/en/ga/search/view_doc.asp?symbol=A/RES/67/81. Accessed on 27 December 2017.

31. IRDAI, Indian Insurance Market, available at: http://www. policyholder.gov.in/indian_insurance_market.aspx.

32. http://resurgent.rajasthan.gov.in/news/mou-signed-with-new-india-assurance-company-for-bhamashah-health-insurance-scheme-. Accessed on 29 December 2015.

33. Free Drugs Plan available at: http://timesofindia.indiatimes.com/ india/Free-drugs-plan-gets-a-quiet-burial/articleshow/46809394.cms. Accessed on 30 December 2015.

34. See http://www.thehindu.com/news/national/other-states/free-drug-distribution-scheme-launched/article7163048.ece. Accessed on 30 December 2015; http://timesofindia.indiatimes.com/india/Free-drugs-plan-gets-a-quiet-burial/articleshow/46809394.cms. Accessed on 30 December 2015.

35. http://www.thehindu.com/news/national/supreme-court-refers-plea-against-section-377-to-5judge-bench/article8183860.ece.

36. NACO News, Vol. IV Issue 2, April–Jun 2008. Available at: http:// naco.gov.in/sites/default/files/april%20-june08n%20final.pdf. Accessed on 4 December 2017.

37. For more information see, Lawyers Collective HIV/AIDS Unit, Current Cases—Sankalp Rehabilitation Trust v. Union of India—Supreme Court of India. Available at: http://www.lawyerscollective.org/hiv-and-law/current-cases.html. Accessed 8 September 2015.

38. 'Pressure from AIDS Activists Resumes ARV Supply in UP', *Citizens News Service*, May 2011. Available at: www.citizen-news.org/2011/05/pressure-from-aids-activists-ensure-arv.html. Accessed on 8 September 2015.

39. http://www.livemint.com/Politics/n2svOmWwLqMsZu ViMKwHmJ/Is-Indias-AIDS-programme-disintegrating.html.

40. Available at: http://www.unitaid.eu/images/marketdynamics/publications/ TPPA-Report_Final.pdf.

41. http://forbesindia.com/article/cross-border/how-bill-gates-blew-$258-million-in-indias-hiv-corridor/852/0?id=852&pg=0.

42. http://www.ndtv.com/india-news/hiv-aids-success-becomes-the-enemy-656385.

43. http://www.thehindu.com/news/cities/bangalore/hiv-prevention-project-workers-not-paid-regularly/article7356014.ece.

44. http://www.business-standard.com/article/news-ians/naco-nrhm-integration-will-increase-hiv-infections-114090101214_1.html.

45. *Report of the Health Survey and Development Committee*, Survey, 1946. Available at: https://www.nhp.gov.in/bhore-committee-1946_pg. Accessed on 4 December 2017.

REFERENCES

CESCR. 2000. *General Comment 14: The Right to the Highest Attainable Standard of Health (Art. 12)*. Adopted at the Twenty-Second Session of the Committee on Economic, Social and Cultural Rights, on 11 August 2000 (contained in Document E/C.12/2000/4). Available at: http://www.refworld.org/pdfid/4538838d0.pdf. Accessed on 4 December 2017.

Citizen's News. 2011. 'Pressure from AIDS Activists Resumes ARV supply in UP', *Citizens News Service*. Available at: www.citizen-news.org/2011/05/pressure-from-aids-activists-ensure-arv.html. Accessed on 8 September 2015.

Divan, V and K. Bhardwaj. 2007. 'HIV/AIDS Legislation: An Opportunity for Health Care Reform', *Indian Journal of Medical Ethics* 4(2): 66–7.

Government of India. 2009. The Rights of Children to Free and Compulsory Education Act, available at: http://eoc.du.ac.in/RTE%20-%20notified.pdf.

Government of India. 2014. The Human Immunodeficiency & Acquired Immune Deficiency Syndrome (Prevention and Control) Bill, 2014. New Delhi: Ministry of Health and Family Welfare. Available at: http://www.prsindia.org/uploads/media/HIV/HIV-AIDS%20Bill,%202014.pdf.

———. 2015. National Health Policy-Draft. (All versions). New Delhi: Ministry of Health and Family Welfare.

Hindustan Times. 2009. 'Patients protest HIV/AIDS draft bill', *IANS*, 21 October. New Delhi. Available at: http://www.hindustantimes.com/delhi-news/patients-protest-hiv-aids-draft-bill/story-85NvK1Bsq7ZD518pd1wkhM.html. Accessed on 4 December 2017.

ICESCR. 1966. *International Covenant on Economic, Social and Cultural Rights*. Geneva: Office of the United Nations High Commissioner for Human Rights (OHCHR).

IRDAI. (undated). *Indian Insurance Market*. Available at: http://www.policyholder.gov.in/indian_insurance_market.aspx.

Johari, V. 2014. 'Professional Misconduct or Criminal Negligence: When Does the Balance Tilt?', *Indian Journal of Medical Ethics* 11(2): 117–20.

Lawyers Collective. 2007. *HIV/AIDS Bill, 2007*. Available at: http://www. lawyerscollective.org/hiv-and-law/draft-law.html. Accessed on 8 September 2015.

Indian Medical Council Regulations. 2002. Codes of Medical Ethics. Available at: http://www.mciindia.org/RulesandRegulations/CodeofMedicalEthics Regulations2002.aspx.

NACO. 2015. 'NACP IV Component 3', National AIDS Control Organization. New Delhi: Ministry of Health and Family Welfare. Available at: http:// naco.gov.in/nacp-iv-components. Accessed on 2 February 2018.

NAPCP. 2015. *National AIDS Prevention and Control Policy 2002*, Ministry of Health and Family Welfare. New Delhi: Government of India. Available at: http://naco.gov.in/documents/policy-guidelines. Accessed on 8 September.

National Organ and Tissue Transplant Organisation. 2010. Transplantation of Human Organs and Tissues Act 2010. Available at: http://notto.nic.in/act-end-rules-of-thoa.htm. Accessed 8 September 2015.

Pandey, K. 2015. 'Rajasthan Moves to "Privatise" Basic Health Facilities', *Down to Earth*, 20 June. Available at: http://www.downtoearth.org.in/news/rajasthan-moves-to-privatise-basic-health-facilities-50259. Accessed on 2 February 2016.

Patel, Vikram, Rachana Parikh, Sunil Nandraj, Priya Balasubramaniam, Kavita Narayan, Vinod K. Paul, A.K. Shiva Kumar, Mirai Chatterjee, K. Srinath Reddy. 2015. 'Assuring Health Coverage for All in India', *The Lancet* 386(10011): 2422–35.

Rana, Swati. 2015. 'IMA Demands Amendments to Clinical Establishments Act for Survival of Small and Medium Hospitals', Pharmabiz.com, 14 November. Available at: http://www.pharmabiz.com/NewsDetails. aspx?aid=91683&sid=1. Accessed on 28 December 2015.

Rao, Krishna D., S. Ramani, I. Hazarika, S. George. 2013. 'When do Vertical Programmes Strengthen Health Systems? A Comparative Assessment of Disease-Specific Interventions in India', *Health Policy Plan* 29 (4): 495–505. Available at: http://heapol.oxfordjournals.org/content/29/4/495.full. Accessed on 8 September 2015.

Sarangi, S. 2012. 'Compensation to Bhopal Gas victims, Will Justice Ever be Done?', *Indian Journal of Medical Ethics* 9(2) April–June. Available at: http://ijme.in/index.php/ijme/article/view/114/183. Accessed on 27 December 2017.

The Wire. 2015. 'NITI Aayog against Free Healthcare, Bats for More Private Sector Role'. Available at: http://thewire.in/2015/08/25/niti-aayog-against-free-health care-bats-for-more-private-sector-role-9181/.

Thomas and Krishnan. 2010. 'Effective Public Private Partnership in Health Care: Apollo as a Cautionary Tale', *Indian Journal of Medical Ethics* 7(1): 2–4.

UNAIDS. 2001. General Assembly Declaration of Commitment on HIV/ AIDS. Available at: http://www.unaids.org/en/aboutunaids/unitednationsd eclarationsandgoals/2001declarationofcommitmentonhivaids.

UNDP. 2015. *Transforming our World: the 2030 Agenda for Sustainable Development*, Sustainable Development Goals, September. New York. United Nations Development Programme. Available at: https:// sustainabledevelopment.un.org/?menu=1300.

COURT CASES

Arun Chhabria v. State of Maharashtra, Writ Petition No. 352 of 2013 (medical records not given); *Trevor Nerves Britto v. State of Maharashtra*, Criminal PIL No. 41 of 2014 (earlier Writ Petition No. 2359 of 2014); *Sanjay Prajapati v. State of Maharashtra*, Criminal PIL No. 42 of 2014 (earlier Writ Petition No. 2136 of 2014); and *N. Mohanlal and Co. v. Maharashtra Medical Council*, Writ Petition No. 832 of 2014—have all been tagged together.

AS Mittal and others v. State of UP and others. AIR 1989 SC 1570.

CESC Limited and others v. Subhash Chandra Bose and others (1992) 1 SCC 441. See also *State of Punjab v. Mohinder Singh Chawla and others* (1997) 2 SCC 83.

Workmen of Slate Pencil Manufacturing Industries v. State of Madhya Pradesh, Civil *WPB KhetMazdoorSamity v. State of West Bengal* AIR 1996 SC 2426writ Petition No. 5143 of 1980.

Confederation of Ex-Servicemen Association and ors. v. Union of India &ors. AIR 2006 SC 2945.

Dr. Balram Prasad v. Dr. Kunal Shah & ors., Supreme Court, Civil Appeal No. 2867 of 2012, judgement dated 24.10.2013.

Hamid Khan v. State. AIR 1993 MP 191.

Indian Medical Council v. V.P. Shantha. (1996) CPR 1.

In re: 'Indian Woman says Gang-raped on orders of Village court' published in *Business and Financial News* dated 23 January 2014: SuoMotu Petition (Criminal) No.24 of 2014.

Mrs. N. Ratankumari v. State of Odisha. 2014 Cr.LJ 443.

Kalpana Mehta &ors. v. Union of India. W.P. 558/2012 and *Sama & ors. vs Union of India*, In the Supreme Court of India W.P. 921/2013.

Kirloskar Brothers Ltd. v. Employees State Insurance Corp. 1996 (2) SCC 682. See Also *Consumer Education & Research Centre v. Union of India*. AIR 1995 SC 922.

Lucy D'Souza v. State of Goa. AIR 1990 Bom 355.

United India Insurance Co. Ltd v. Manubhai Dharmasin hbhai Gajera. (2008) 10 SCC 404.

Unni Krishnan J P v. State of Andhra Pradesh. (1993)1 SCC 645.

Mohd. Ahmed (Minor) v. Union of India. W.P. No. (C) 7279/2013, order passed by Delhi High Court on 17 April 2014.

MX v. ZY. AIR 1997 Bom 406.

National Legal Services Authority v. Union of India and ors. AIR 2014 SC 1863.

Naz Foundation v. Govt. of NCT of Delhi 160 Delhi Law Times 277.

NDPS amendment. Available at: http://www.lawyerscollective.org/updates/parliament-passes-ndps-amendment-bill-2014-gains-losses.html. Accessed on 4 December 2017.

Novartis AG v. Union of India and ors. AIR 2013 SC 1311.

ParmanandKatara v. Union of India. AIR 1989 SC 2039.

PB Khet Mazdoor Samity v. State of West Bengal AIR 1996 SC 2426.

Rakesh Chandra Narayan v. State of Bihar. AIR 1989 SC 348. See also *RC Baruah v. State of Bihar.* 1986 (Supp) SCC 576, *Chandan Kumar Banik v. State of West Bengal.* 1995 Supp (4) SCC 505, *SheelaBarse v. Union of India.* (1993) 4 SCC 204, *Supreme Court Legal Aid Committee v. State of Madhya Pradesh.* (1994) 5 SCC 27, *UpendraBaxi v. State of UP* (1983) 2 SCC 308, *Peoples Union of Civil Liberties v. Union of India.* 1992 Supp (2) SCC 647 and *BR Kapoor v. Union of India.* (1989) 3 SCC 387.

Residents of Well Defined Goitre Endemic Area v. State of Jammu and Kashmir, Civil Writ Petition No. 5047 of 1982.

Sahara House v. Union of India, In the Supreme Court of India, Writ Petition No. 535 of 1998 along with *Sankalp Rehabilitation Trust & another v. Union of India,* Writ Petition No. 512 of 1999.

Samira Kohli v. Dr. PrabhaManchanda& another. AIR 2008 SC 1385.

Sanjiv Punalekar v. The State of Maharashtra and another in W.P. (PIL) No. 3132 of 2004, order dated 17 August 2006.

State of Bombay & anr. v. F.N. Balsara. AIR 1951 SC 318.

State of Punjab and others v. Ram LubhayaBagga and others. (1998) 4 SCC 117.

Swasthya Adhikar Manch & another v. Ministry of Health and Family Welfare & others in W.P. 779/2012, order dated 21.10.2013 pursuant to which DCGI has brought changes in the law. HPV vaccine cases, Kalpana Mehta & ors. *v.* Union of India, W.P. 558/2012 and Sama & ors. *v.* Union of India, W.P. 921/2013.

Voluntary Health Association of Punjab v. Union of India and others. AIR 2013 SC 1571.

Vincent Panikurlangara v. Union of India and others. (1987) 2 SCC 165.

Index

Editors and Contributors

RENU ADDLAKHA is Deputy Director and Professor at Centre for Women's Development Studies, New Delhi. She did her doctoral research on the psychiatric profession in India with a particular reference to the treatment of women. Her areas of specialization include the sociology of medicine, mental illness and the psychiatric profession, anthropology of infectious diseases, bioethics, and disability studies. Currently she is engaged in research on gender and disability at the CWDS. Email: addlakhar@gmail.com

MALINI AISOLA is a public health advocate working on pharmaceutical policies impacting affordability and access to medicines. She has previously worked with Knowledge Ecology International (based in Washington DC), the Public Health Foundation of India, Lawyers Collective and Oxfam India. She is affiliated with the All India Drug Action Network (AIDAN) and Medico Friend Circle. Email: malini.aisola@gmail.com

RAMA V. BARU is Professor at the Centre of Social Medicine and Community Health, Jawaharlal Nehru University, New Delhi. Her major areas of research interests include commercialization of health services, infectious diseases, comparative health systems, and health inequalities. She has been awarded the Shastri Indo-Canadian Faculty Enrichment Award and also has the Balzan Fellowship, University of London. Email: rama.v.baru@gmail.com

KAJAL BHARDWAJ is a Delhi-based lawyer working on health and human rights. Her areas of interest and work focus on legal and policy issues related to HIV and the impact of trade and intellectual property on health and access to medicines.

MADHUMITA BISWAL is Assistant Professor at the Centre for Studies in Society and Development, School of Social Sciences, Central University of Gujarat, India. She teaches Sociology of Gender, Gender and Sexuality, Rural Society, Research Methodology, Theories of Society, Social Development: Theories and Practices. Email: madumita25@gmail.com

PADMA BHATE-DEOSTHALI worked as Director CEHAT from 2006 to 2016. Her research interests include standards of care in private health sector and its unregulated growth, integrating gender in medical education, women's work and health, and violence against women. She was member of the Steering Group of the GDG-WHO for developing policy and clinical practice guidelines for responding to violence against women. She was a member of the National Committee under the Ministry of Health and Family Welfare, India for drafting the 'Guidelines and Protocols for medico-legal care for victims/survivors of sexual violence', 2014. She is currently pursuing her PhD at the Tata Institute of Social Sciences, Mumbai. Email: padma@cehat.org

VIVEK DIVAN is a lawyer and works on the intersections of law, health, and sexuality. From 2012–14 he was a policy specialist at UNDP's HIV, Health, and Development Group in New York, USA, where he provided advisory and technical support on law, access to justice, and human rights in the context of key populations affected by HIV. He served on the Secretariat for the Global Commission on HIV and the Law and as a member of its Technical Advisory Group from 2009–12, and as senior HIV advisor at the Royal Tropical Institute, Amsterdam (2008–09), where he taught the master's programme in Public Health (ICHD). He was the coordinator of Lawyers Collective HIV/AIDS Unit in India from 2000 to 2007. During that time he was a part of the team that drafted the legislation on HIV/AIDS for India, and was centrally involved in the public interest litigation related to Section 377 of the Indian Penal Code. Email: vivekdivan@gmail.com

RAVI DUGGAL trained as a sociologist, and has worked for over three decades on public health issues. He has worked with FRCH, CEHAT, SWISSAID, Action Aid International, and Ministry of Health, Government of India, and presently works with the International Budget Partnership. His areas of interest include budgets and governance, universal access to health, health financing strategies, and ESCR rights. Email: rduggal57@gmail.com

ROGER JEFFERY is Professor of Sociology of South Asia at the University of Edinburgh, UK, where he has taught since 1972. His research has largely been carried out in the north of the Indian subcontinent, focusing on issues of public health and health policy, maternal and reproductive health, access to medicines, and the transformations of public health and medical services in the context of socioeconomic development and social change. Email: R.Jeffery@ed.ac.uk

ASIMA JENA is Assistant Professor at the Centre for Studies in Society and Development, School of Social Sciences, Central University of Gujarat, India. She teaches medicine, health and society and globalization, and state and social justice. Her research interests include sociology of health, body politics, and development. Email: ashimajena@gmail.com

AMAR JESANI is an independent consultant, researcher, and teacher in bioethics and public health. He is one of the founders of the Forum for Medical Ethics Society and its journal *Indian Journal of Medical Ethics* (IJME) and is presently its editor. He is one of the founding trustees of the Anusandhan Trust, which manages the health research institute, Centre for Enquiry into Health and Allied Themes (CEHAT) in Mumbai, and the health action institute, SATHI (www.sathicehat.org) in Pune. He is also a visiting professor for bioethics at the Ethics Centre, Yenepoya University, Mangalore, India (since 2011) and the Centre for Biomedical Ethics and Culture, Sindh Institute of Urology and Transplantation, Karachi, Pakistan (since 2010). Email: amar.jesani@gmail.com

VEENA JOHARI is a Mumbai-based lawyer and proprietor of Courtyard Attorneys, a legal consultancy firm that works on issues related to human rights and public health. Her main area of work is access to medicines, women, children, HIV, clinical trials, and patent oppositions of pharmaceutical drugs. She serves on the Institutional Ethics Committee for research of the KEM Hospital, Mumbai. She is on the editorial board of the *Indian Journal of Medical Ethics*. Email: courtyardattorneys@gmail.com

NEHA MADHIWALLA is an independent health researcher and activist. She was formerly, Coordinator of the Centre for Studies in Ethics and Rights, Mumbai, and a member of the editorial board of the *Indian Journal of Medical Ethics*. Email: nmadhiwala@gmail.com

VRINDA MARWAH is a doctoral candidate in the Department of Sociology, The University of Texas, Austin. Her primary research interests are in reproductive health and women's labour in contemporary India. Vrinda has worked at the research, capacity building, and policy advocacy levels with Sama—Resource Group for Women and Health, and CREA, Delhi. Email: vrinda.marwah@gmail.com

MANU RAJ MATHUR is a dental surgeon with a PhD in epidemiology and population health from University College London and a masters in public health with specialization in advanced epidemiology from the University of Glasgow, UK. He is currently working as research scientist and adjunct assistant professor at Public Health Foundation of India (PHFI). He is also the Technical Advisor to the President of India. Email: manu.mathur@phfi.org

SAROJINI NADIMPALLY is a health researcher and activist, and Founder of Sama, a resource group working on health and gender issues. She is closely associated with other organizations and networks such as Medico Friend's Circle and People's Health Movement. As Sama's director, she has coordinated national research studies concerning the potential impact on women of reproductive and medical technologies, clinical trials and access to medicines, and the implications of the two-child norm for marginalized communities. Email: sarojinipr@gmail.com

DEVAKI NAMBIAR is Program Head—Health Systems and Equity, The George Institute for Global Health, Delhi, India. Her research focuses on pathways of social exclusion and processes of equity-oriented health systems reform in India as well as other low- and middle-income countries. She was member of the core technical secretariat for India's High Level Expert Group (HLEG) on Universal Health Coverage (UHC). Devaki is a Wellcome Trust/DBT India Alliance Intermediate Investigator working on UHC-linked health equity monitoring in India and supports WHO's capacity-building on this topic globally. Email: devaki.nambiar@gmail.com

SUNIL NANDRAJ is a social scientist by education, health activist by passion, and a full-time researcher in the health sector. He is an advisor to the central government for the implementation of the Clinical Establishment Act, Department of Health and Family Welfare, Government of Delhi for the Aam Admi Mohalla Clinics, Regulation of Health Sector, and Health Insurance, among other reforms being undertaken. He is the co-founder of a website called *medileaks* on the lines of *wikileaks* for documenting irrational practices and irregularities in the health sector in India. Email: sunil.nandraj@gmail.com

PURENDRA PRASAD is Professor at the Department of Sociology and has been working at University of Hyderabad, India, since 2000. His research interests include three broad areas: political economy of health—on questions of health inequalities, role of state and market in access to health care, commoditization of body; agrarian studies—on questions of caste–class inequalities, regional histories, agrarian social structure, and movements; development and its discontents in the context of globalization, urban development, and its processes. Email: purendra.prasad@gmail.com

RITU PRIYA a medical graduate with a doctorate in Community Health, is currently professor at the Centre of Social Medicine and Community Health, JNU, New Delhi. Her work links epidemiology, popular culture, political economy, and health systems analysis for developing an understanding of 'health culture'. She has been an advisor (Public Health Planning) with the National Health Systems Resource Centre under the National Rural Health Mission and has also been actively involved with the people's health movement in the country for over three decades. Email: ritu_priya_jnu@yahoo.com

GERARD PORTER is a Lecturer in medical law and ethics at the School of Law, University of Edinburgh, UK. His research interests include medical law, patent law, and the regulation of the life sciences. He has been a visiting fellow with the Program on Science, Technology and Society at the John F. Kennedy School of Government, Harvard University and at the Centre for Studies in Ethics and Rights, Mumbai, India. Email: gerard.porter@ed.ac.uk

DEAPICA RAVINDRAN is currently a researcher with the Rural Technology and Business Incubator, IIT Madras, India. She has a master's degree in biotechnology and is interested in the ethical and social implications of biotechnology. She has been involved in maintaining a database on the clinical trials registered in the Indian registry CTR-I and the publication of Clinical Trials Watch in the *Indian Journal of Medical Ethics*. Email: deapica@gmail.com

K. SRINATH REDDY is currently President of Public Health Foundation of India (PHFI) and former head, Department of Cardiology, All India Institute of Medical Sciences (AIIMS). In 2009 was appointed as the first Bernard Lown Visiting Professor of cardiovascular health at the Harvard School of Public Health, Harvard University, USA. He is also an adjunct professor of the Rollins School of Public Health, Emory University, and honorary professor of medicine at the University of Sydney. He edited the *National Medical Journal of India* for 10 years and is on the editorial board of several international and national journals. Email: ksrinath.reddy@phfi.org

SANGEETA REGE is currently the Coordinator of CEHAT, Mumbai. Her research interests include health system response to violence against women, gender sensitive health care to survivors of sexual assault, and integrating gender in medical education. Email: sangeeta@cehat.org

SALLA SARIOLA is Senior Lecturer in Sociology at University of Turku, Finland. She holds a fellowship at University of Oxford, Ethox Centre, Nuffield Department of Population Health in the UK. She has conducted ethnographic fieldwork in India, Sri Lanka, and Kenya with research focusing on social studies of biomedicine and bioethics as well as gender and sexuality. She is the author of *Gender and Sexuality in India: Selling Sex in Chennai* (2009). Salla is the coordinating editor of the journal *Science and Technology Studies*. Email: salla.sariola@ethox.ox.ac.uk

AMIT SENGUPTA is a medical graduate and works on issues related to public health, pharmaceuticals policy, and other S&T policy issues like Intellectual Property Rights. He has been associated with the Delhi Science Forum, a public interest organization working on S&T policy issues for the past twenty years. Email: amit37064@yahoo.com

S. SRINIVASAN (CHINU) is an Ashoka fellow (2002) and a Co-founder and managing trustee of Low Cost Standard Therapeutics (LOCOST), a public non-profit charitable trust that allows poor Indians to access drugs at affordable prices, founded in 1983. He is also associated with All-India Drug Action Network (AIDAN) and Medico Friend Circle (MFC). Email: chinusrinivasan.x@gmail.com

ANAND ZACHARIAH is Professor at the Department of Medicine Infectious Diseases, Christian Medical College, Vellore, India. His areas of interests include, infectious diseases and HIV/AIDS, clinical toxocology with a focus on organophosphate poisoning and plant poisoning, and medical education (undergraduate and distance education). Email: zachariah@cmcvellore.ac.in